Arthroscopy

Edited by Carlos Suarez-Ahedo

Published in London, United Kingdom

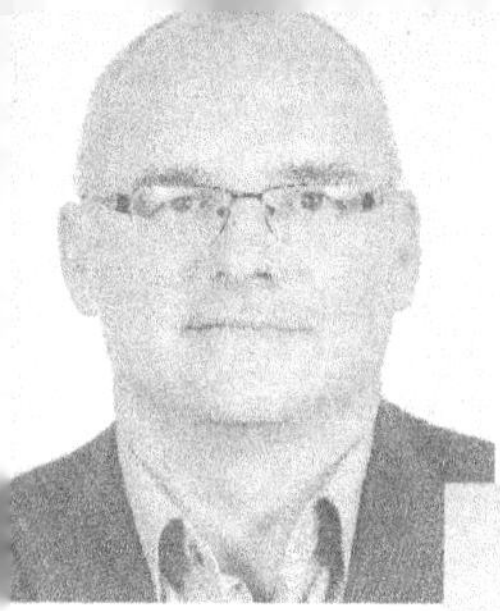
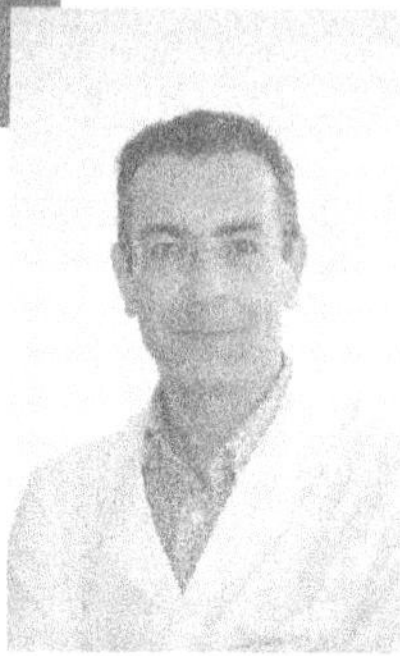
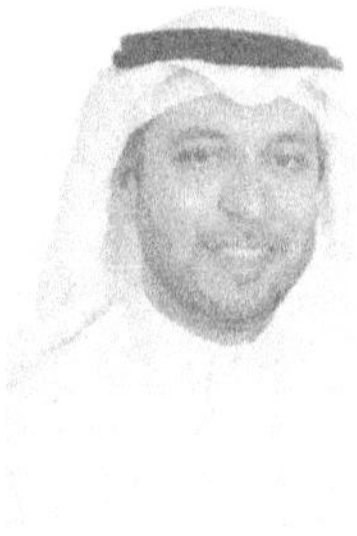
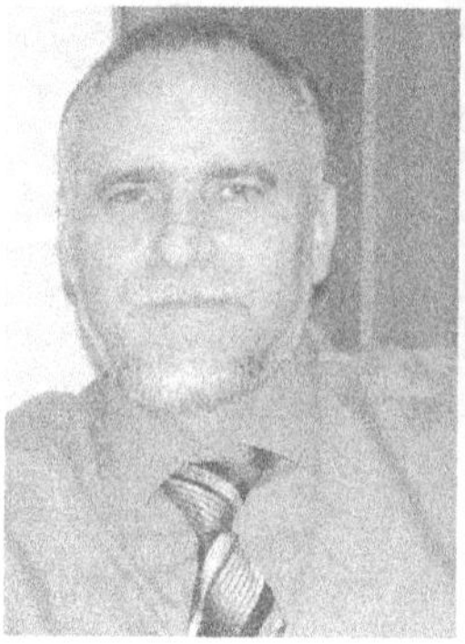
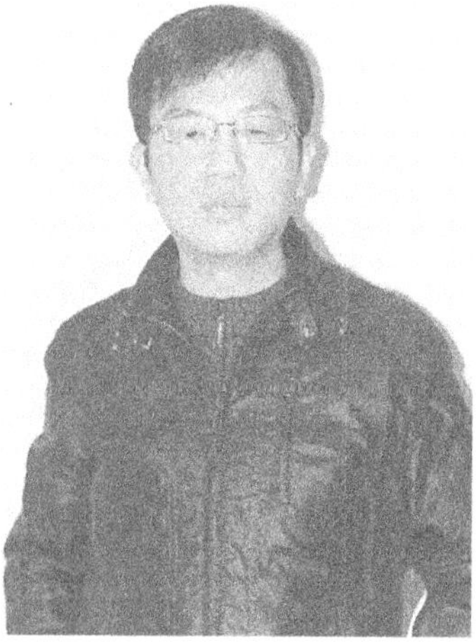
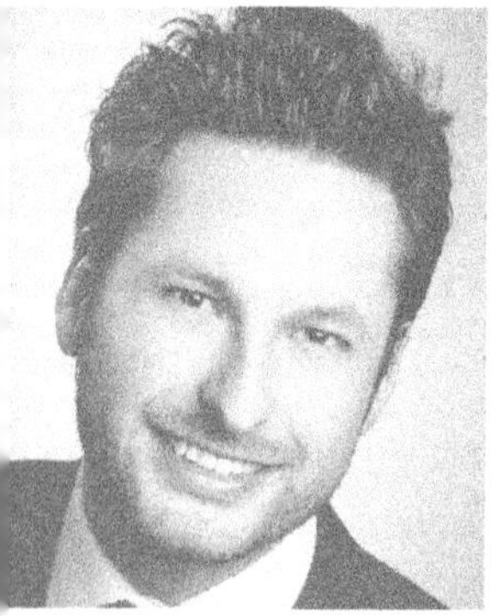
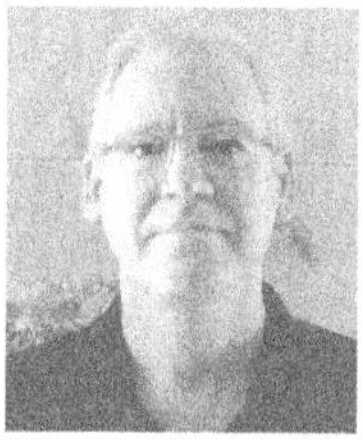

IntechOpen

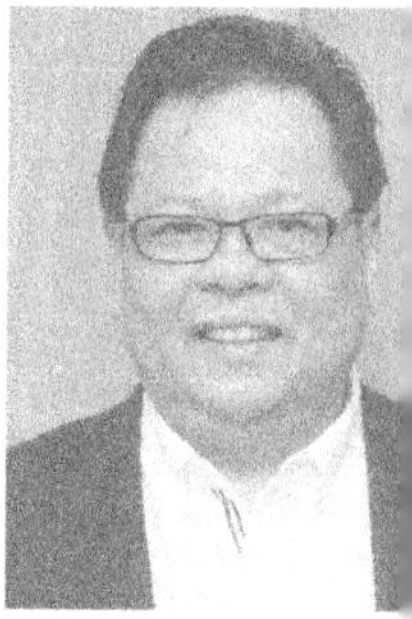
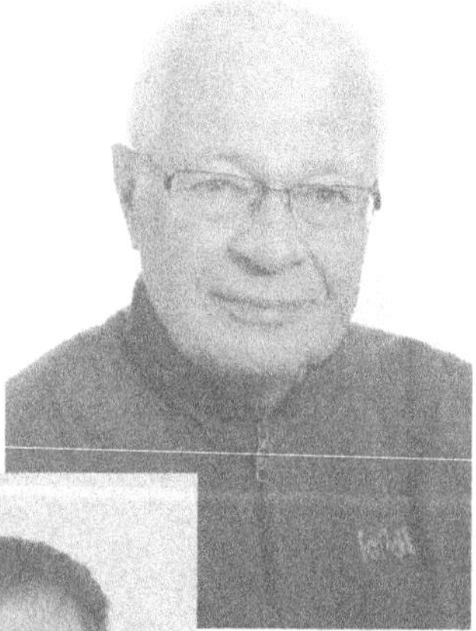
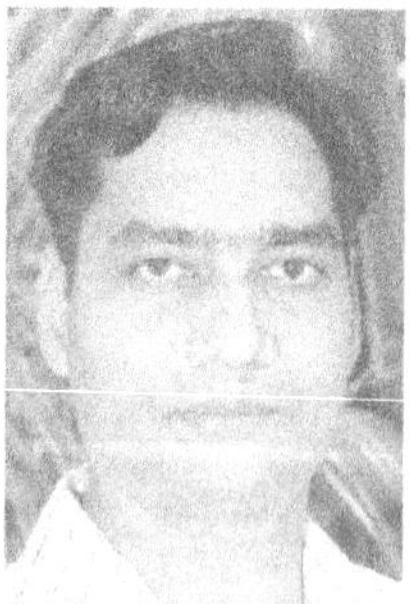
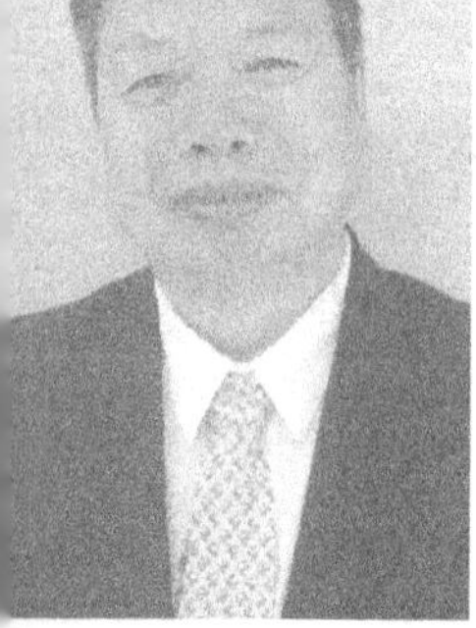
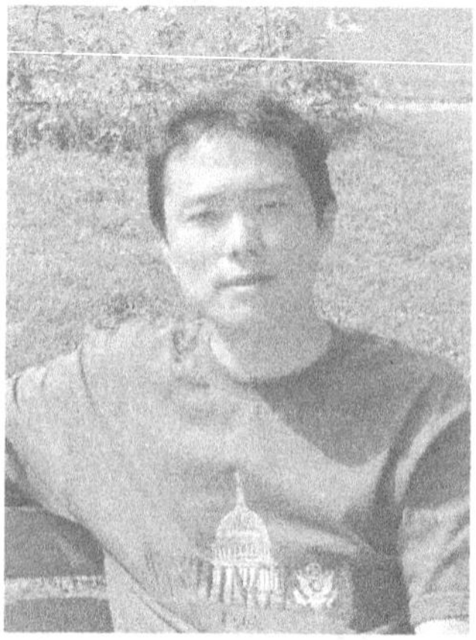
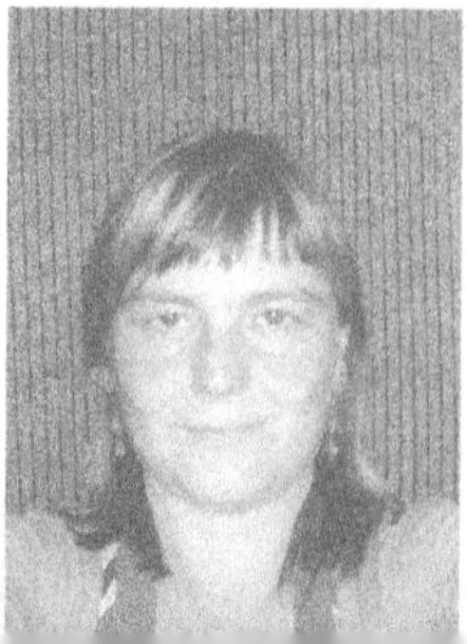

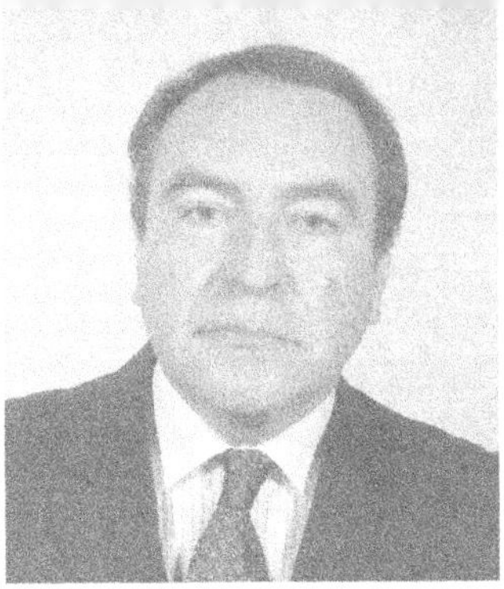
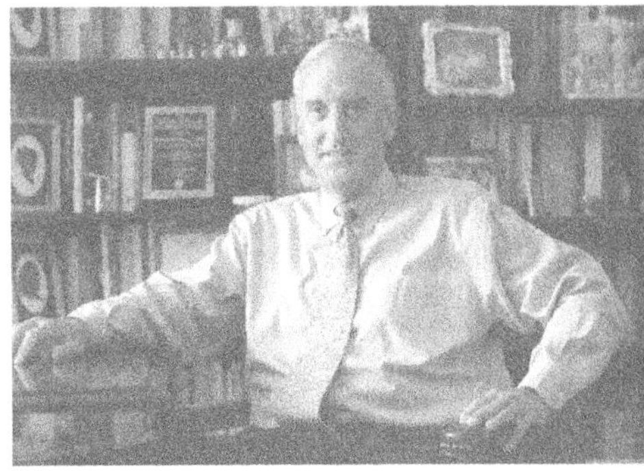
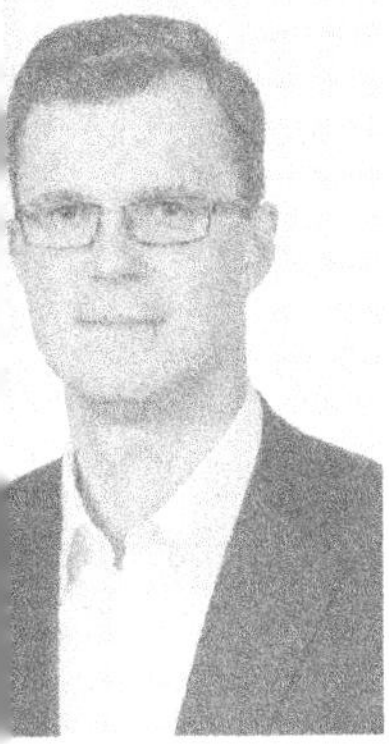
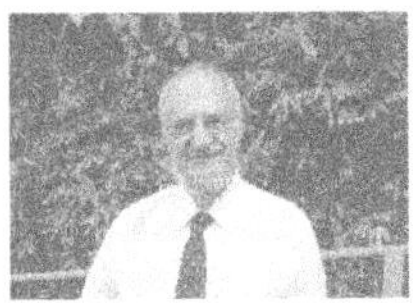
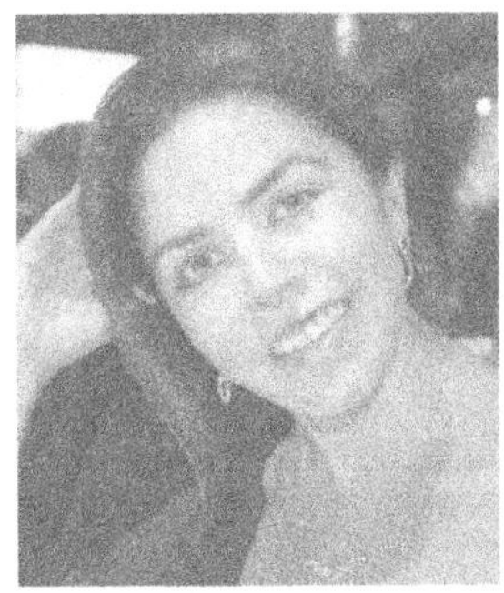

Supporting open minds since 2005

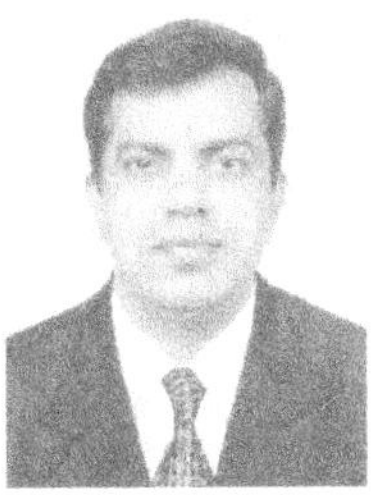
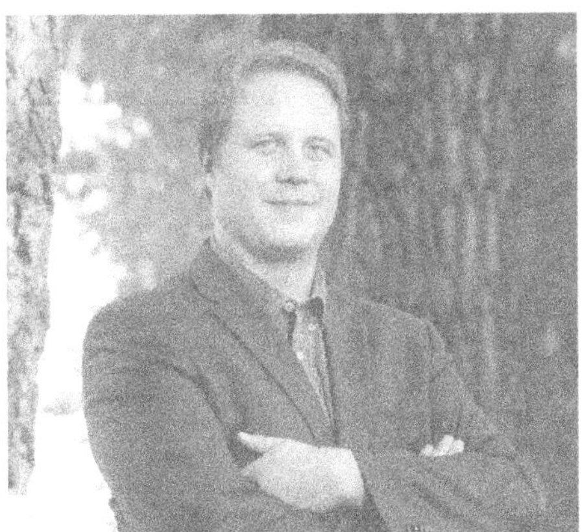
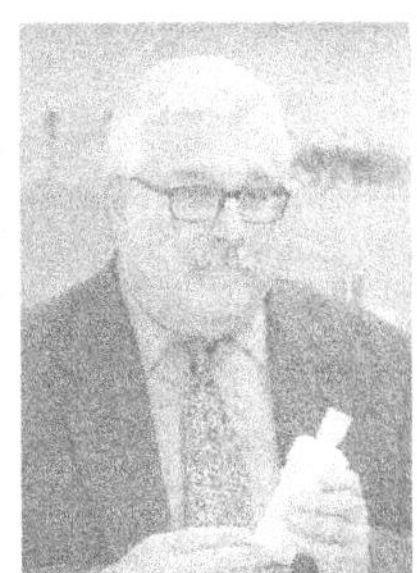
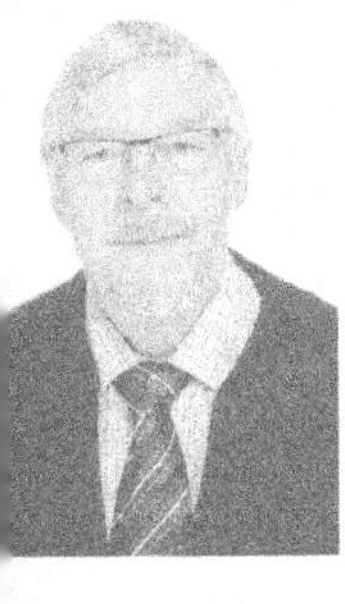
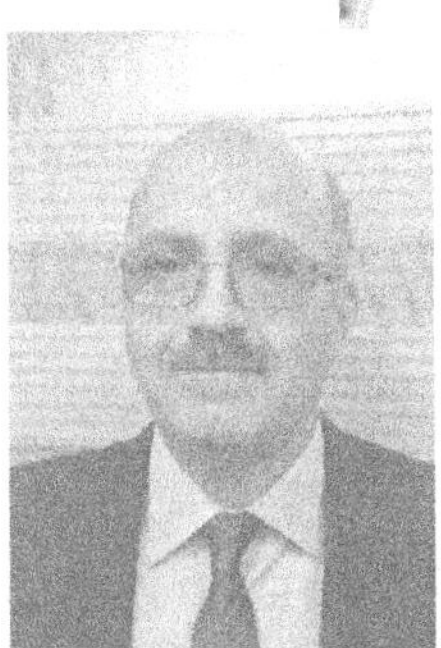
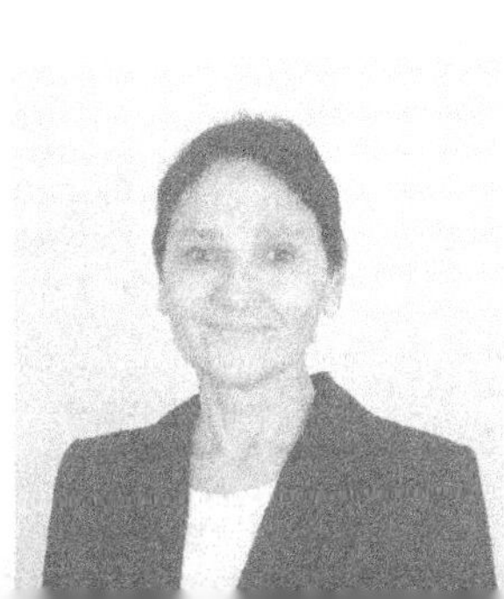
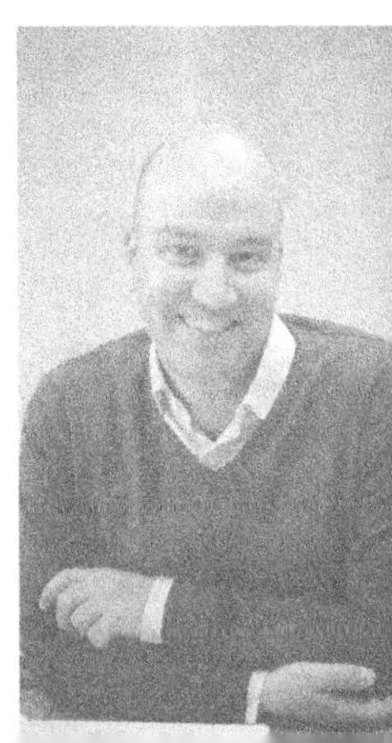

Arthroscopy
http://dx.doi.org/10.5772/intechopen.94681
Edited by Carlos Suarez-Ahedo

Contributors
Thun Itthipanichpong, Songthai Moonwong, Christian Konrads, Stefan Döbele, Matthew Brown, Anthony Scillia, Deepak Valjibhai Patel, Vincent McInerney, Jennifer Kurowicki, Iciar Davila Castrodad, Nuthan Jagadeesh, Sachindra Kapadi, Venkatesh Deva, Ankur Kariya, Adrian Góralczyk, Krzysztof Hermanowicz, Piotr Jancewicz, Uldis Krustins, Jānis Krustins

First published in London, United Kingdom, 2022 by IntechOpen
IntechOpen is the global imprint of INTECHOPEN LIMITED, registered in England and Wales, registration number: 11086078, 5 Princes Gate Court, London, SW7 2QJ, United Kingdom
Printed in Croatia

British Library Cataloguing-in-Publication Data
A catalogue record for this book is available from the British Library

Additional hard and PDF copies can be obtained from orders@intechopen.com

Arthroscopy
Edited by Carlos Suarez-Ahedo
p. cm.
Print ISBN 978-1-83969-478-3
Online ISBN 978-1-83969-479-0
eBook (PDF) ISBN 978-1-83969-480-6

Meet the editor

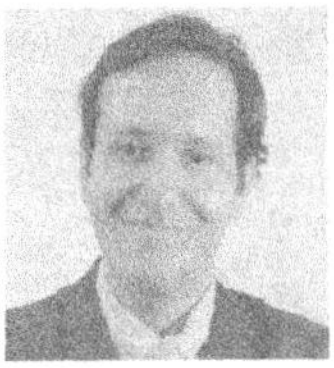

Dr. Carlos Suarez-Ahedo is a recognized orthopaedic surgeon specializing in minimally invasive total hip and total knee replacement, sports medicine, and arthroscopic surgery, providing superior knowledge and expertise to his patients. Dr. Suarez-Ahedo regularly gives lectures and teaches courses for orthopaedic surgeons around the world and is actively involved in the research and development of new techniques in joint replacement and arthroscopic surgery. He is also the author and co-author of several scientific publications in recognized international journals in the field of sports medicine, arthroscopic surgery, and hip pathology. Dr. Suarez-Ahedo graduated from La Salle University, Mexico. He completed his training in orthopedic surgery at the Spanish Hospital, Mexico City. His subspecialty training includes a fellowship in articular surgery, a fellowship in adult joint hip and knee reconstruction at the National Rehabilitation Institute of Mexico, and an additional fellowship in hip preservation surgery at the American Hip Institute, Chicago, USA. His professional affiliations include the American Academy of Orthopaedic Surgeons (AAOS), Arthroscopy Association of North America (AANA), International Society of Technology in Arthroplasty (ISTA), International Society for Hip Arthroscopy (ISHA), and Société Internationale de Chirurgie Orthopédique et de Traumatologie (SICOT).

Contents

Preface

This book provides a concise yet comprehensive introduction to some common articular pathologies and their arthroscopic treatment. Newer concepts continue to evolve and to keep abreast with these one should have a sound basic knowledge of the subject.

Every attempt has been made to narrate the concepts in a simplified manner keeping the originality. Wherever possible, illustrations have been used to help the reader to understand the subject. The target audience comprises orthopedic surgeons, either in practice or in training, as well as clinicians, radiologists, and physical therapists. The text is divided into three sections with short chapters providing a broad overview of anatomy, pathology, and treatment. Selected references are also provided without the claim of being exhaustive and with the aim of stimulating interest and discussion.

Many people helped make this book. I would like to acknowledge the medical publishing division of IntechOpen; a fantastic team of editors helped bring this book to fruition. I would also like to thank the extraordinary authors who contributed chapters to this volume.

Carlos Suarez-Ahedo
American Hip Institute,
United States of America

Section 1

Knee

Chapter 1

Medial Meniscus Root Tear: Current Update Review

Thun Itthipanichpong and Songthai Moonwong

Abstract

This chapter mainly focuses on medial meniscus posterior root tear which is the point of attention nowadays because it is the common degeneration process and can lead to early-onset osteoarthritis of the knee without treatment. The biomechanics of the medial meniscus root tear is similar to total meniscectomy. Hence, early detection and diagnosis will lead to better outcome. Most cases with medial meniscus root tear also have degenerative change of the knee. Meniscal extrusion is a common finding in magnetic resonance imaging (MRI) which represent impairing of hoop stress function of the meniscus. Patient selection and understanding of the natural history of the disease is a particularly important. Options for the treatment including conservative treatment, surgical treatment such as partial meniscectomy, meniscus root repair, or reduction of meniscal extrusion. Outcome of these treatments are variable depending on the condition of the patients. Long term outcome of surgical treatment revealed lower rate of knee replacement compared with conservative treatment.

Keywords: Meniscus root tear, Medial meniscus root tear, Medial meniscus tear, Meniscus extrusion

1. Introduction

Meniscus is a fibrocartilaginous structure which provides many functions to the knee joint such as distributing load to the knee, increased stability of the tibiofemoral articulation, lubrication, provides nutrient and a strong shock absorption. Without the meniscus, load to the articular cartilage will increase and progress to osteoarthritis. Meniscus root tear is one of the tear patterns which are increasingly important due to an increasing number of patients and the rapid progression of the osteoarthritis similar to total meniscectomy [1]. Hence, early detection and treatment may improve outcome of the patient.

1.1 Definition

The bone which avulsed from the attachment at tibial plateau which represent meniscus root tear, was first described in 1935 by Weaver by plain radiograph [2]. However, ligament or soft-tissue injury at the insertion site of meniscal root on tibial plateau was described later after the use of magnetic resonance imaging (MRI). In 1991, Pagnani reported a medial subluxation of the meniscus associated with an avulsion injury to the posterior horn medial meniscus in an athlete [3]. The modern definition commonly used for "meniscus root tear" is defined as avulsion of the meniscal attachments to the tibia or radial tears within 1 cm from the bony insertion [4].

1.2 Epidemiology

In the past, medial meniscus root tear has been neglected due to difficulties in diagnosis. The prevalence might be lower than it should be. With increasing recognition of the medial meniscus root tear, the prevalence is higher. In a study by Matheny et al., in 673 arthroscopic surgeries, they found 50 patients with meniscus root tear equivalent to 7% [5]. Another study by Ozkoc et al. found that prevalence of radial tear of the posterior horn of the medial meniscus in 7,148 patients who underwent partial menisectomy of the knee was about 10% (722 patients) [6]. The prevalence may be up to 15% in Asia which is a more common injury [7]. In case of traumatic knees, a study by Ho Jong Ra found 7 medial meniscus posterior root tear out of 51 patients who had multiple ligaments knee injury [8]. Most of the medial meniscus root tear were degenerative change. However, traumatic tear of the medial meniscus root is also common. The incidence of medial meniscus posterior root tear was up to 78% in patient underwent total knee arthroplasty. In addition, severity and varus deformity correlated with the root tear [9].

1.3 Natural history

As we know meniscus is a strong shock absorber. Without meniscal root attachment, hoop stress is lost and can lead to rapid progression of osteoarthritis [10]. Five-year follow up study of non-operative treatment in 52 patients with posterior meniscus root tear revealed association with low functional outcome and 31% of the patients need conversion to total knee arthroplasty [11]. In case of partial meniscectomy of the meniscus, long term follow up (5-8 years) also showed osteoarthritis progression about one-third of the patients [7]. The meniscus extrusion in a sign that showed impairment of the meniscus function and the degree of extrusion might be associated with severity of osteoarthritis [9, 12]. The longer the symptom, the degree of extrusion might be worse. According to a study by Furumatsu et al., in early period (<1 month) mean extrusion was 3.0 mm. In subacute (1-3 months) and chronic (3-12 months), the mean extrusion was 4.2 and 5.8 mm respectively [13]. The increasing rate of meniscus extrusion was studied by okazaki et al. which reviewed MRI of 33 patients who were diagnosed with medial meniscus posterior root tear and had done MRI twice at a mean interval of 48 days, the mean extrusion increased from 3.4 mm to 4.5 mm. The progression of the extrusion rate was 0.02 mm per day [14]. There is also an association between the presence of medial meniscus root tears and articular cartilage damage of the knee with an Outerbridge grade 2 or greater changes. Patients with a medial root tear were approximately five times more likely to also have an articular cartilage defect of the knee with an Outerbridge grade 2 score or higher [5]. In addition, osteonecrosis, bone contusion, and subchondral insufficiency fracture are commonly associated with the medial meniscus root tear [10, 15].

1.4 Biomechanics

As mentioned above, the complete medial meniscus posterior root tear had similar biomechanics with total meniscectomy due to impairment of hoop stress function of the meniscus (**Figure 1**). Normal load to the meniscus is about 50% of body weight and the other 50% transfers directly to the articular cartilage [16].

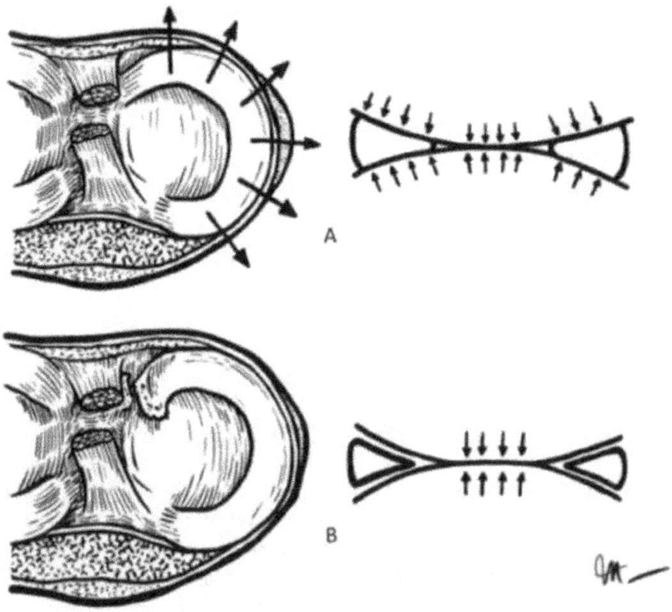

Figure 1.
Hoop stress function of meniscus. (A) Normal load distribution of meniscus with intact meniscal root. (B) With meniscal root tear, load is directly transferred to the articular cartilage.

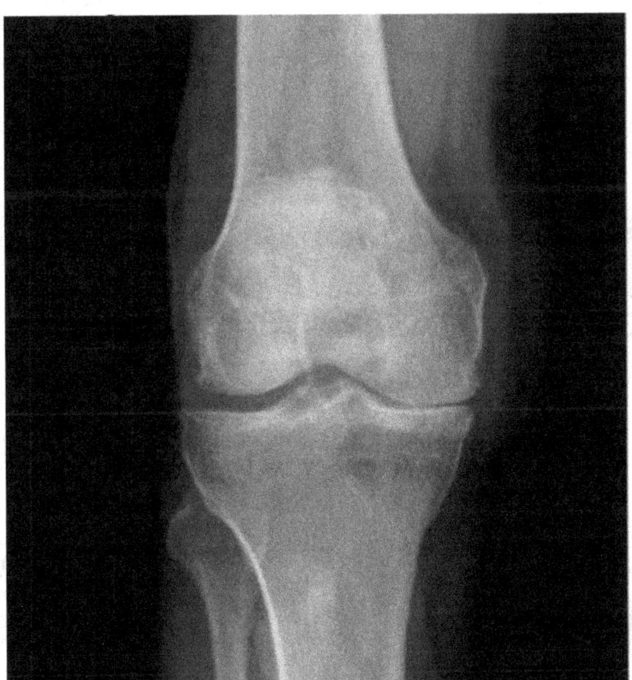

Figure 2.
Fairbank phenomenon after meniscectomy. Finding included narrowing of joint space, squaring of femoral condyle and antero-posterior osteophyte.

The body and posterior horn of the medial meniscus take most of the force applied to the medial compartment and are the least mobile parts. With knee flexion, the pressure to the posterior horn of meniscus is the highest this is due to the femoral roll back mechanism of the knee. That explains why posterior horn and posterior root injuries have been found to be more common compared to the anterior horn injury [17]. In case of torn medial meniscus posterior root or total menisectomy, the peak pressure to the medial articular cartilage increased 25% [1, 18]. Hence, this may lead to osteoarthritis change which was called "Fairbank's phenomenon" [19] (**Figure 2**). The biomechanics test of medial meniscus posterior root repair can restore the tibiofemoral contact pressure compared with intact meniscus knee [20, 21].

2. Anatomy

Medial Meniscus is a fibrocartilaginous structure composed of collagen fiber that orientates in radial and circumferential fiber. These fibers provided hoop stress function of the meniscus. The width of the medial meniscus being about 1 cm and bigger at the posterior part compared to the anterior part. The semi-lunar shape is divided into 3 segments: anterior horn, body, and posterior horn. In anatomical landmark, meniscus may divide into 5 anatomical zone; the anterior root (zone 1); the anteromedial zone (zone 2a and 2b); the medial zone (zone 3); the posterior zone (zone 4); and the posterior root (zone 5) [22]. The attachment of the medial meniscus to the tibia at the anterior horn and posterior horn are called "medial meniscus anterior root" and "medial meniscus posterior root" respectively. The root of the meniscus itself is not a fibrocartilaginous structure but more like a ligament which serves as an anchor to the tibia. The medial meniscus posterior root attaches to the posterior intercondylar fossa between the attachments of the posterior root of the lateral meniscus and posterior cruciate ligament. The attachment is about 9.6 mm posterior to the apex of medial tibial eminence and 3.5 mm lateral to medial tibial plateau articular cartilage (**Figure 3**) [23–25].

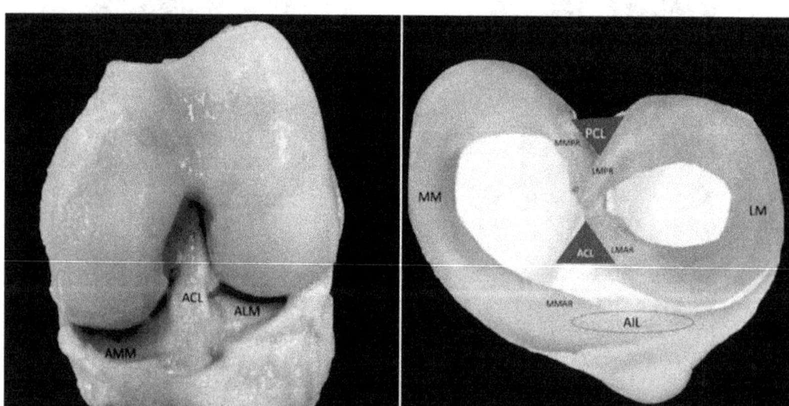

Figure 3.
Anatomy of left knee meniscus A: Intact ACL and meniscus knee. B: Drawing axial anatomy of meniscus. The red dot represented the apex of medial tibial spine. The MMPR attached behind this spot about 9.6 mm. ACL = anterior cruciate ligament, PCL = posterior cruciate ligament, AMM = anterior horn medial meniscus, ALM = anterior horn lateral meniscus, AIL = anterior intermeniscal ligament, MM = medial meniscus, LM = lateral meniscus, MMAR = medial meniscus anterior root, MMPR = medial meniscus posterior root, LMAR = lateral meniscus anterior root, LMPR = lateral meniscus posterior root.

3. Clinical presentation

There were 2 presentations of patients with meniscal root tear.

1. Traumatic event: In this group were younger patients who had major traumatic event such as a road traffic accident, or sports accidents. They were likely to have associated ligamentous injury [8].

2. Minor or non-traumatic event: Most of the patients with medial meniscus root tear especially medial meniscus posterior root tear fall in this group. Patients usually are in their fifth or sixth decade of life. Some patients had history of a "pop" sound while doing daily activity such as squatting and had sudden pain. The painful popping sound indicates a high chance of isolated medial meniscus posterior root injury [26]. Some patients had progressive medial knee pain without trauma history and the symptoms were similar to osteoarthritis [27].

Meniscus root tear's diagnoses is challenging. Patient might not have a problem of locking or catching knee. Medial knee pain and joint line tenderness are the most common symptom and sign especially at the posteromedial of the knee joint. Deep flexion of the knee might provoke the pain. Meniscus specific test such as Mcmurray's test was positive in 57%. Joint effusion presented in 14% [28]. Compared to other meniscus injuries, medial meniscus root tears are common in Asian populations, in particular, females and higher Body Mass Index (BMI > 30 kg/m^2 – 4.9 fold increase) patients. If patient had a varus mechanical axis, the risk of medial meniscus posterior root tear increased by 3.3-fold [29]. Generally, we recommend further investigation such as, an MRI in patients with progressive medial joint knee pain with no or mild osteoarthritis to rule out medial meniscus posterior root tear.

4. Imaging

The first imaging that detected medial meniscus root bony avulsion was in 1935 by plain radiograph [2]. We recommended to do plain radiograph in all patients suspected of medial meniscus root tear to evaluate degree of osteoarthritis change and axis deformity. The Kellgren and Lawrence (K-L) classification was a common and popular method to classify the severity of osteoarthritis change [30]. They classified 5 grades (**Figure 4**).

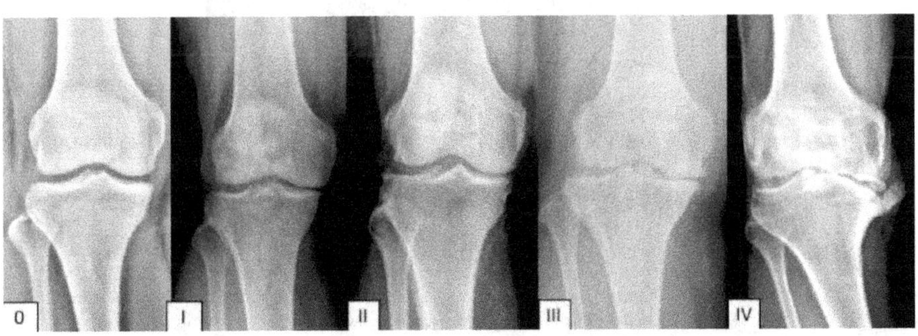

Figure 4.
Kellgren and Lawrence (K-L) classification, Grade 0 (none): definite absence of x-ray changes of osteoarthritis, Grade I (doubtful): doubtful joint space narrowing and possible osteophytes, Grade II (minimal): definite osteophytes and possible joint space narrowing, Grade III (moderate): moderate multiple osteophytes, definite narrowing of joint space and some sclerosis and possible deformity of bone ends, Grade IV (severe): large osteophytes, marked narrowing of joint space, severe sclerosis and definite deformity of bone ends.

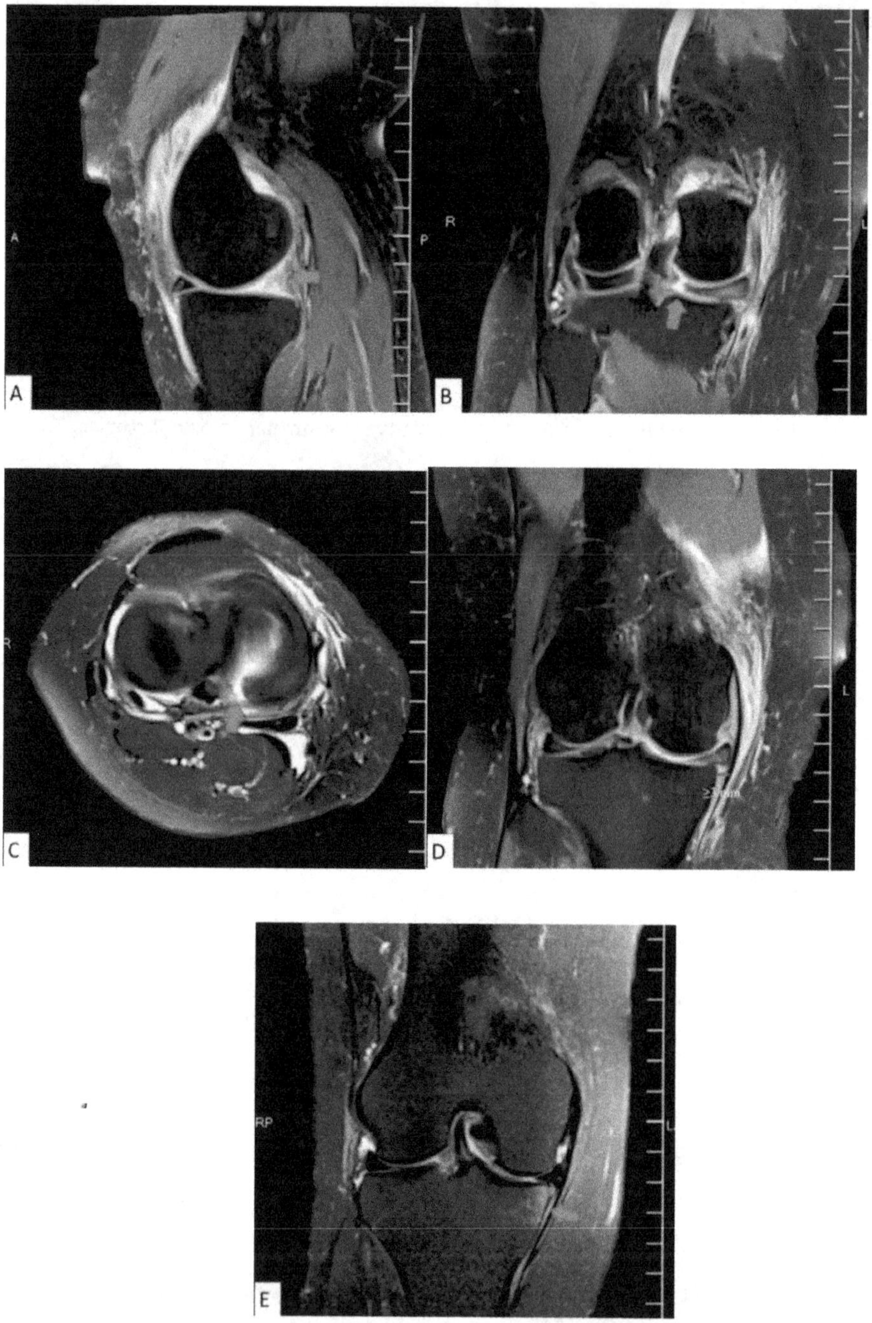

Figure 5.
MRI finding of meniscal root tear. A: Ghost sign (absent of posterior horn medial meniscus), B: Cleft sign (vertical linear defect on coronal images), C: Radial linear defect on axial image, D: Medial meniscus extrusion (≥3 mm), E: Bone contusion at the articular bearing area which is associated with medial meniscus root tear.

However, with popularize of MRI, soft tissue that avulsed from the attachment of the meniscus to the tibia could be easier to detect. Hence, MRI is now the goal standard in detecting medial meniscus root tear because of high sensitivity

(93.3%) and specificity (100%) [31]. Finding from MRI included absent of posterior horn meniscus called "ghost sign" on sagittal imaging adjacent to posterior cruciate ligament, vertical linear defect on coronal images called "cleft sign", radial linear defect on axial image, and medial meniscus extrusion (≥3 mm) on coronal image. Medial meniscus extrusion less than 3 mm could be found in general populations [32] (**Figure 5**). Medial meniscus that extruded usually larger and thicker than normal meniscus due to swelling and degeneration of meniscal tissue. The MRI study Okazaki showed that 3D MRI could estimate volume and thickness of extruded medial meniscus more precisely when compared to conventional 2D MRI [33].

Medial meniscus posterior root tear had an association with multiple findings including spontaneous osteonecrosis of the knee (SONK), subchondral insufficiency fracture, cartilage injury especially at the medial femoral condyle, and osteoarthritis change [34, 35].

5. Classification

There were many classifications for medial meniscus root tear mostly based on anatomic classification. For the medial meniscus anterior root attachment according to Berlet et al. there were four patterns of insertion of the anterior root [36].

Type I has the insertion located in the flat intercondylar region of the tibial plateau.
Type II (most common) has more medial insertion, closer to articular tibial surface.
Type III has a more anterior insertion, which is on the downslope of tibia.
Type IV shows no solid fixation.

For medial meniscus posterior root tear the most popular classification was classified by Laprade. The classification was based on the morphology of the tear and was classified into 5 types [37] (**Figure 6**).

Type I: partial stable root tear
Type II: complete radial tear within 9 mm from the bony root attachment.
Type III: bucket-handle tear with complete root detachment.
Type IV: complex oblique or longitudinal tear with complete root detachment.
Type V: bony avulsion fracture of the root attachment.

There was an arthroscopic classification by Bin et al. which developed a classification base on extrusion of the medial meniscus on MRI and finding of the torn site displacement. They were divided into 3 types; type A: non-displaced, type B: overlapped (the torn tissue overlap on each other), and type C: widely displaced [38] (**Figure 7**).

They found that the widely displaced group had a 4° greater varus deformity, and higher rates of meniscus extrusion, grade III or IV chondral wear in the medial femoral condyle and medial compartment osteoarthritis than did the nondisplaced or overlapped group.

Another classification by Kim et al. was made based on tear gap (**Figure 8**) of the medial meniscus posterior root in arthroscopic finding. The higher the tear type

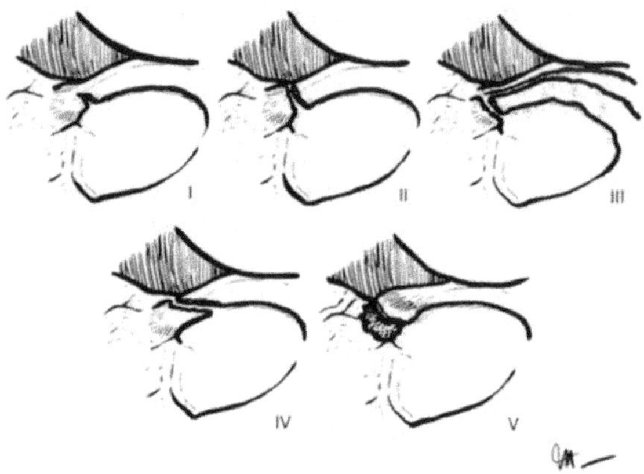

Figure 6.
Laprade's classification for medial meniscus root tear. Type I: Partial stable root tear. Type II: Complete radial tear within 9 mm from the bony root attachment. Type III: Bucket-handle tear with complete root detachment. Type IV: Complex oblique or longitudinal tear with complete root detachment. Type V: Bony avulsion fracture of the root attachment (redrawn from LaPrade et al. [37]).

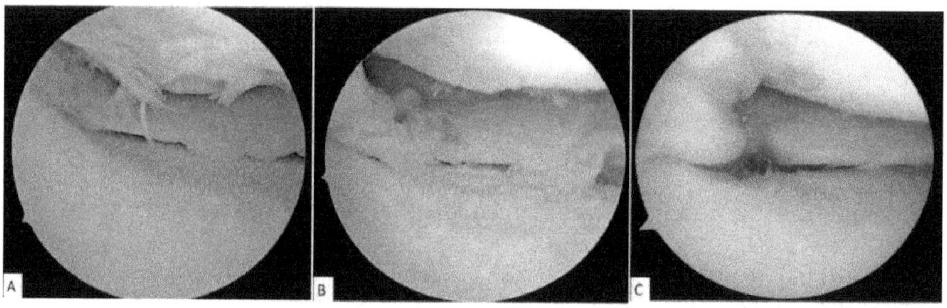

Figure 7.
A–C: Bin classification base on arthroscopic finding of meniscal tear and gap. A: Non-displaced, B: Overlapped and C: Widely displaced.

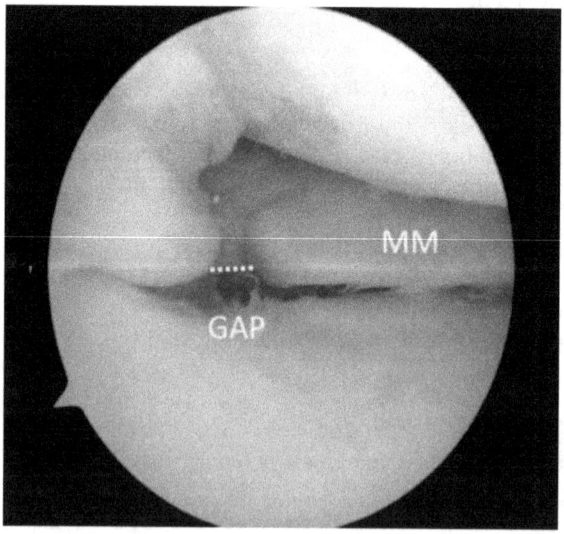

Figure 8.
Tear gap measurement from an arthroscopic view. MM = medial meniscus.

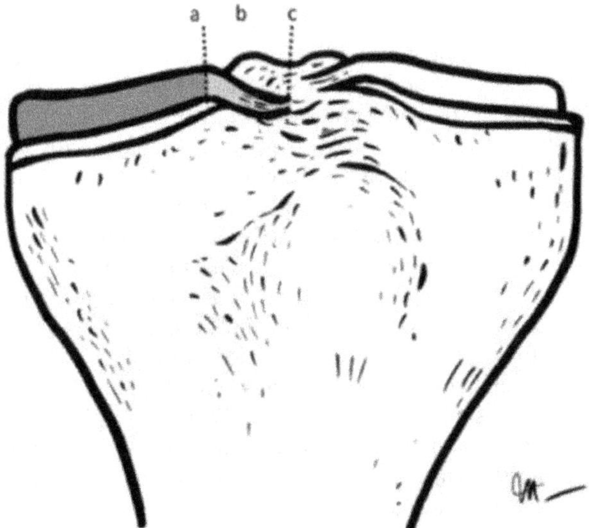

Figure 9.
Classification of medial meniscus posterior root tear based on MRI by Choi et al. posterior medial meniscus root ligament was defined as from tibial attachment point of root ligament to just lateral from articular cartilage inflection point of medial tibial plateau. Ligament was subcategorized into three zones: (a) transition to posterior horn of medial meniscus at junction between root and posterior horn, (b) midsubstance within root ligament proper, and (c) entheseal at tibial attachment point of root ligament (redrawn from Choi et al. [24]).

(increasing displacement of the tear gap in arthroscopic surgery), the higher association with degree of meniscal extrusion, chondral wear, and severity of arthritis. They were classified in to 5 types [39].

Type I: incomplete root tear.
Type 2: complete root tear with no gap or overlapped;
Type 3: complete root tear with gap measuring 1-3 mm.
Type 4: complete root tear with gap measuring 4-6 mm.
Type 5: complete root tear with gap measuring 7 mm.

There is an MRI classification based on the attachment of posterior medial meniscus root ligament. The term ligament is used because of the different of tissue component. This classification included both degenerative change and tear of the medial meniscus posterior root. They classified into 3 types; type a: Tear at transition to posterior horn of medial meniscus at junction between root and posterior horn, type b: Tear at midsubstance within root ligament proper, and type c: Tear at entheseal at tibial attachment point of root ligament [24] (**Figure 9**).

6. Treatment

According to the natural history of medial meniscus root tear, without proper treatment, there was a higher chance of progression of meniscal extrusion and osteoarthritis. Besides, the choice of treatment was still controversy because there were many factors which might lead to poor outcome. We divided the treatment into 2 categories: nonoperative and operative treatment.

6.1 Nonoperative treatment

The nonoperative treatment of medial meniscus posterior root tear was preserved for 1. Patients whose conditions were unfavorable for surgery. 2. Patients with advanced osteoarthritis of the knee (K-L grade III-IV) 3. Relieve pain before surgery. 4. Patients who could not follow the post-operative protocol. There were many methods of conservative treatment including taking non-steroidal anti-inflammatory drugs, cortisone injections, use of unloader knee brace, physical therapy, gait aid (cane or crutch) use, and orthotic use. We recommend using gait aid and hinge knee brace to prevent further damage to the meniscus and reduced the pain in acute setting. However, the use of cortisone injection should be avoided in patients who were planned for surgical repair of the meniscus due to the risk of infection and possibility of interference with the healing of the meniscal tissue. Nonoperative treatment provided symptomatic relief but could not prevent the progression of osteoarthritis in long term follow up [7, 40]. The physical therapy could improve functional score and reduce the pain especially from degenerative meniscal root tear [41]. From the meta-analysis by Faucett et al., the 10 years progression of osteoarthritis was about 95% and 45% conversion rate to knee replacement surgery [42]. Conversion to total knee replacement were also higher in nonoperative treatment compare with meniscus root repair in other studies [7, 43].

6.2 Operative treatment

The treatment choices might depend on many factors. The goal of the operative treatment was to: 1. Relieve pain, 2. Increase quality of life, 3. Prevent progression of osteoarthritis and 4. Restore function of meniscus. Before proceeding to the operation, physicians needed to talk to their patients about the goal of treatment and consequence after surgery. For example, a patient suffering an acute tear of the medial meniscus root, but the patient could not follow the post-operative protocol due to economic problem. Then, meniscus repair might not be a good choice for this patient. The choices of operative treatment are list below.

6.2.1 Meniscectomy

Meniscectomy was the majority of procedures that were done for the meniscus in the past. The procedure included removing some part of the meniscal tissue which preserved most of the meniscal tissue called "partial meniscectomy", or totally removed all the meniscal tissue called "total meniscectomy". The goal of this operation was to relive symptomatic pain from the unstable meniscus. The mechanical irritation from the unstable meniscal tear could be removed. However, the meniscectomy in medial meniscal root tear was different from other meniscal tears. Because, in other meniscal tear such as radial tear or vertical tear, if most of the meniscal tissue could be preserved, the hoop stress function of the meniscus remained. On the other hand, no matter how much meniscal tissue was preserved in medial meniscus root tear, the function of the meniscus still impaired and articular cartilage would play a major role in weight bearing which could lead to articular damage later. Thus, meniscectomy should be done in low demand patients, patients with advanced osteoarthritis and mechanical symptom meniscal tear, patients with partial root tear and the remaining attachment were more than 50%, or patients with poor meniscal tissue quality. The procedure could relieve symptomatic pain and swelling in short term result but in long term results the knee joint could deteriorate. From a study by Krych et al., the conversion rate to total knee replacement at a mean follow up of 5 years was 54% [44]. The rate of total knee replacement was quite similar to other studies [7, 42, 45].

6.2.2 Meniscus root repair

Meniscus root repair is getting more attention at present due to better long term outcome compared with non-repair treatment [46]. Meniscus root repair can restore the biomechanics of the knee joint. Hence, the distribution of the load was restored. Although the normal distribution load could not completely be restored due to the elongation of the suture after repair, the contact pressure and contact area could almost resemble an intact meniscus root knee [47, 48]. On the other hand, if non-anatomic repair was done, the distribution of the load might be abnormal. From a biomechanical study by Laprade in 2015, the mean and peak contact pressure were significantly increased after non-anatomic repair compared with normal and anatomic repair [49]. There were many techniques of repairing meniscus posterior root. All of them showed a significant improvement of functional outcome and reduced conversion rate to total knee replacement.

6.2.2.1 Transtibial pull out technique

This technique was the most popular technique for repairing medial meniscus posterior root due to familiarity and ease of assessment to the instruments. Many companies provided specific instruments for the transtibial repair. The technical step involved the used drill from the tibia to the root attachment at the posterior tibia, stitched the tear meniscus, pulled the meniscus to the drill hole with a knot tied on the tibia (**Figure 10**). The disadvantages of this technique were: 1. Bungee effect on the repair site, 2. The risk of neurovascular injury due to the drill misplaced 3. Transtibial tunnel can interfere with concomitant procedures 4. possibility of suture elongation and abrasion through bone tunnel [50, 51].

Most of the clinical studies of transtibial pull out technique showed good functional outcome, prevent progression of osteoarthritis and reduced conversion rate of total knee replacement. The 10-year conversion rate was much lower compared with partial meniscectomy and nonoperative treatment (33.5% vs. 51.5% vs. 45.5%) [42]. In younger patients (<50 years) the risk of re-operation were higher than older patients. The activities and demands of younger patients might be more compared with older patients. As a result, the strength of fixation might not be enough in younger patients [52]. Although transtibial pull out repair prevented the progression of osteoarthritis, this could not completely prevent the

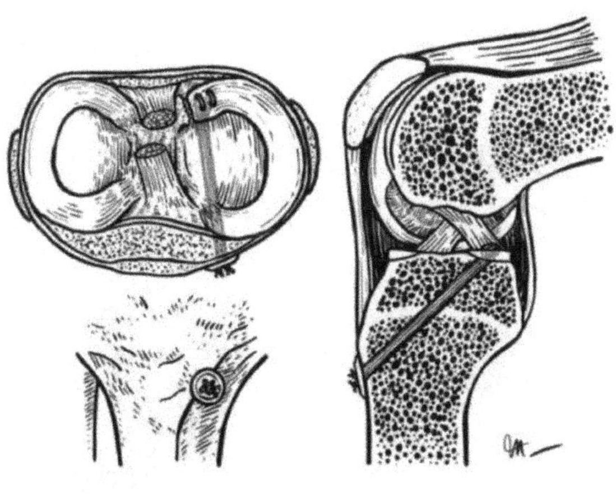

Figure 10.
Schematic drawing showed transtibial pull out repair of the medial meniscus root. The long tibial tunnel along with the "bungee effect" have the possibility of suture abrasion and elongation.

process. This helped only decelerate the process and most of the patients could not restore the meniscus extrusion [53, 54]. Healing of the repaired root and reduction of meniscal extrusion seem to be less predictable, being observed in two-third of the patients [55].

Stitches configuration might not play a major role for repairing the meniscal root. Modified Mason-Allen stitches had slightly better biomechanics in some studies but quite comparable to two simple stitches [56, 57]. There were no clinical different among repair configurations [58, 59].

6.2.2.2 Suture anchor technique

This technique was less popular when compared with transtibial technique due to the difficulty in placement of the anchor suture. This technical step involved the preparing the meniscal tissue and bed of the bone, placement of suture anchor, stitched the torn meniscal tissue, and tightened the knot (**Figure 11**).

The disadvantages of this technique were; 1. Difficult of suture anchor placement, 2. Potential cartilage irritation due to knots, 3. Fixation might loosen if anchor is not well placed, 4. Additional costs of suture anchor. To ease the placement of anchor suture, we proposed a technique to repair medial meniscus posterior root by using a curved sleeve soft anchor suture, made a far medial vertical portal, and flexed the knee while drilling the tibia for anchor suture placement (**Figure 12**) [60].

There were several methods to place anchor sutures proposed by several authors. Placing the anchor from the posteromedial portal was one option [61]. Also there was a technique which retrograde insertion of a soft anchor suture to the transtibial tunnel. So, additional portal for anchor placement was not required [62]. Functional outcome after repair showed a significant improvement. Complete healing rate form MRI was not different from transtibial repair. The meniscus extrusion was also not significantly reduced from pre-operative, similar to transtibial repair [27, 63].

Many comparison studies were made between transtibial technique and suture anchor technique because of their own advantages and disadvantages (**Table 1**).

In a biomechanics study by Feucht et al., Suture anchor provided lower displacement after cyclic loading and higher stiffness compared with the transtibial technique. However, both techniques did not reach the strength of the native tissue [57].

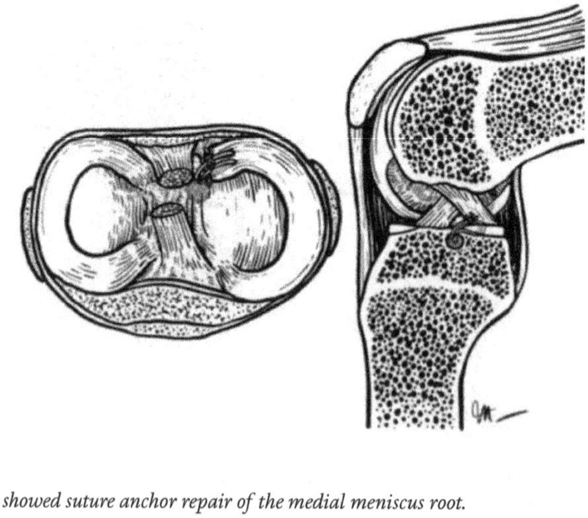

Figure 11.
Schematic drawing showed suture anchor repair of the medial meniscus root.

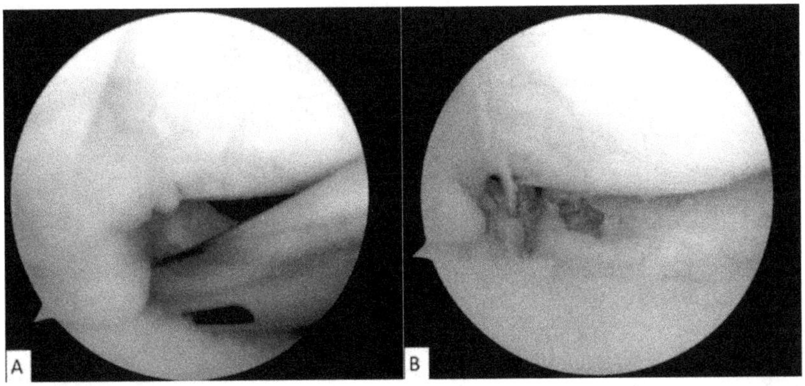

Figure 12.
Pictures of anchor suture repair for medial meniscus root tear. A: Placement of curved drill sleeve for soft anchor suture, B: After repair with 2 simple stitches.

	Transtibial technique	Suture anchor technique
Advantage	• Familiar to most surgeon • Technically easier than a suture anchor technique • Standard arthroscopic portals used • Fixation not rely on fixation device	• No Bungee effect • Not interfere with bone tunnel from other ligament reconstruction • Less elongation of suture • Low risk of neurovascular injury
Disadvantage	• Bungee effect on the repair site • The risk of neurovascular injury due to the drill misplaced • Transtibial tunnel can interfere with concomitant ligamentous procedures • Possibility of suture elongation and abrasion through bone tunnel.	• Difficult of suture anchor placement • Potential cartilage irritation due to knots • Fixation might loosen if anchor is not well placed • Additional costs of suture anchor

Table 1.
Advantages and disadvantages of transtibial technique compared with suture anchor technique.

In contrast, a study by Wu et al. showed that anchor suture had lower maximum load and stiffness compared with transtibial technique but the mean elongation was less. The reason might be because of the different techniques and the study was done with porcine knees which are different from human [64].

The mean meniscal extrusion, functional outcome, degree of cartilage loss and healing rate were comparable between these 2 techniques. The factor that significance effected the degree of cartilage loss was the healing status of the meniscal root. Complete healing showed significantly less cartilage loss compared with partial healing and no healing [27].

6.2.2.3 All inside technique (other than suture anchor)

This was another technique using for medial meniscus root repair. This technique was less popular when compared with other techniques because it depended on the condition of the meniscal tissue. This technical step was to suture the torn meniscus together with an all inside meniscus fixator device and may add a suture to the posterior capsule. This technique was suitable for tearing of the meniscus root which there was enough remnant for suturing and good tissue quality (**Figure 13**).

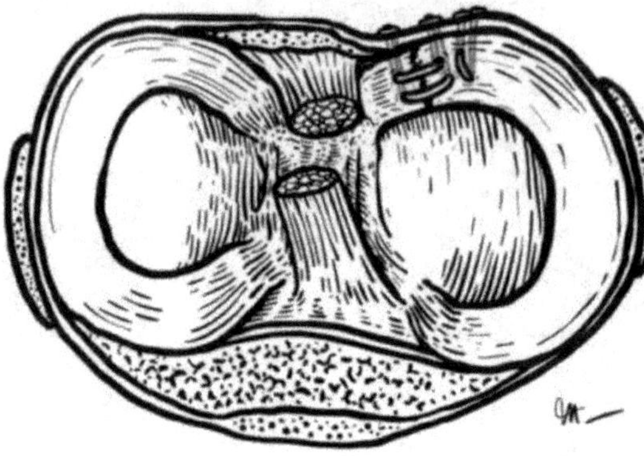

Figure 13.
Schematic drawing showed all-inside repair of the medial meniscus root with all-inside meniscal repair devices. Two horizontal stitches were used to repair the torn meniscal tissue together and one vertical stitch was used to repair the posterior capsule.

This technique provided a better functional outcome, lower progression rate of osteoarthritis, and lower conversion rate to total knee replacement compared with nonoperative treatment at a minimum of 2 years follow up [43].

Another all inside technique that was proposed by Zhu S., was using all the inside meniscus fixator device to non-anatomic repair the torn meniscus root to the posterior capsule. In contrast with previous biomechanics study, this non –anatomic repaired yielded an excellent outcome and a high rate of meniscus healing [65].

6.2.3 Reduction or centralization of medial meniscus extrusion

As mentioned above, the meniscal extrusion might not reduce after meniscal root repair regarding of technique. Thus, there were many techniques adding to the repair procedure to prevent meniscus displacement during flexion and extension of the knee [66–68]. There was a study of centralization the meniscus in rat knee by Ozeki et al. The study concluded that centralization improved the medial meniscus extrusion and delayed cartilage degeneration [69]. Centralization or reduction of extruded meniscus was still debatable. The mechanics and tension of the meniscus that changed might reflect pain and stiffness after doing the procedure.

From the available treatments mentioned above, the only treatment that could prevent the progression of the osteoarthritis and reduce the rate of knee replacement surgery was medial meniscus root repair [7, 42–46]. In addition, meniscal root repair had better long term functional outcome compare with nonoperative treatment and meniscectomy [42]. However, the result of the repair depended on multiple factors. To achieve the best result, all the necessary conditions must be presented. In systematic review from Jiang et al. in 2019, the bad prognostic factors for medial meniscus root repair were obesity, increasing age, advance osteoarthritis (KL III-IV), and varus malalignment >5° [70]. Therefore, the repair should preserve for patient who had medial meniscus posterior root tear without these conditions. For meniscectomy, the advantages of this procedure over the repair is the immediate pain relief, no need for special rehabilitation program, and could be done regardless of degree of osteoarthritis change. The present of a mechanical symptom such as "locking" was a good candidate for this procedure. The nonoperative treatment of medial meniscus posterior root tear was suitable for patients whose conditions were unfavorable for surgery and could not follow the post-operative protocol. The progression of osteoarthritis were high in both nonoperative and meniscectomy treatment [42].

The available treatments of medial meniscus posterior root tear with their advantages, disadvantages, and results concerning the development of osteoarthritis are summarized in **Table 2**.

6.3 Approach strategy for the treatment of medial meniscus posterior root tear

Due to many factors that alter the result of medial meniscus root repair. The significant factors were chronicity of tear, grading of osteoarthritis and mal-alignment (varus >5°). We developed a strategic approach for the treatment of medial meniscus posterior root tear (**Figure 14**).

Treatment	Advantages	Disadvantages	Results
Nonoperative	• symptomatic relief • less invasive • no surgical risks	• do not prevent OA progression • short term result	• 10 years - 95% progression of OA [42] • 10 years - 45% conversion to knee replacement surgery [7, 42–43]
Meniscectomy	• symptomatic relief • less complicated procedure • Immediate pain relief	• do not prevent OA progression • short term result	• 10 years - 99% progression of OA [42] • 5 years – 54% conversion to knee replacement surgery [44]
Meniscus root repair	• prevent OA progression • Good long term result	• reserve in none or mild OA change • technical demand • need rehabilitation	• 10 years - 53% progression of OA [42] • 10 years - 33% conversion to knee replacement surgery [42]

Table 2.
Advantages, disadvantages, and results of available treatment of medial meniscus posterior root tear.

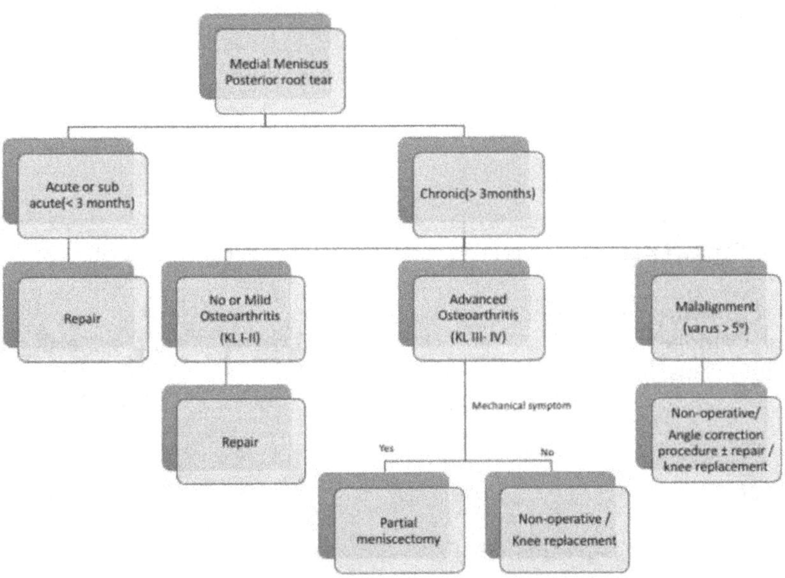

Figure 14.
Our strategic approach for symptomatic medial meniscus posterior root tear.

7. Post-operative protocol

In immediate post-operative period, the goal was to reduce pain and swelling. In one study, the continue passive motion machine was used immediately after surgery [71] but most of the studies would delay the motion after 4 weeks. Most of the repair protocol used cast or knee brace with locked flexion at first 4 weeks with the first 2 weeks in full extension and the other 2 weeks in 0-30° to prevent femoral roll back and injury to the repair meniscus [72]. Active range of motion exercise should be done after 4-6 weeks. Non-weight bearing or toe-touch weight bearing was used during the first 2 weeks after surgery. Then progressive weight bearing to full weight at 6-8 weeks after surgery. Isometric quadriceps exercise could start at the 1st post-operative day but active strengthening exercise should start at 8-12 weeks after surgery. In the majority of patients, full activity can be achieved by 4-6 months [23].

8. Conclusions

The number of medial meniscus root tear were found more often due to better understanding of the physicians and accessibility to the investigation tool such as MRI. The important aspect of meniscus root was the stability of the whole meniscus. With medial meniscus root tear, overall hoop stress function was impaired which will lead to early-onset osteoarthritis. Most of the tear occurred in adults through a minor trauma such as squatting or sitting. The pop sound is one of the significant happenings that is frequently found. Investigation of choice was the MRI because of its high sensitivity and specificity. Significance MRI finding included cleft sign, ghost sign, and medial meniscus extrusion. Diagnosis needed index of suspicious and confirmed by the investigation. Early detection would lead to better outcome of the treatment. The longer the duration, the worse the degree of meniscus extrusion and degree of cartilage damaged. Nonoperative treatment may relieve pain and swelling in the short term. We recommend meniscus root repair in case of acute tear, or mild degeneration of the knee. Early treatment may prevent the meniscal extrusion and reduce the rate of knee replacement conversion. Biologic treatments might have a role for enhancing repair and needing further study.

Acknowledgements

The author gratefully acknowledges the support of.

Prof. Somsak Kuptniratsaikul who is always a great teacher and teaches me many things.

Dr. Thanathep Tanpowpong who encourages me to do this work.

Thai Orthopedic Society for Sports Medicine (TOSSM) for supporting all the academic events.

Line group "Chamchuri Sports Medicine" for sharing cases and fun discussion.

Conflict of interest

The authors declare no conflict of interest.

Author details

Thun Itthipanichpong* and Songthai Moonwong
Department of Orthopaedics, Faculty of Medicine, Chulalongkorn University, King Chulalongkorn Memorial Hospital, Bangkok, Thailand

*Address all correspondence to: thunthedoc@gmail.com

References

[1] Allaire R, Muriuki M, Gilbertson L, Harner CD. Biomechanical consequences of a tear of the posterior root of the medial meniscus. Similar to total meniscectomy. J Bone Joint Surg Am. 2008 Sep;90(9):1922-1931.

[2] Weaver JB. Ossification of the internal semilunar cartilage. J Bone Joint Surg 1935; 17:195-198

[3] Pagnani MJ, Cooper DE, Warren RF. Extrusion of the medial meniscus. Arthroscopy. 1991;7(3):297-300.

[4] Petersen W, Forkel P, Feucht MJ, Zantop T, Imhoff AB, Brucker PU. Posterior root tear of the medial and lateral meniscus. Arch Orthop Trauma Surg. 2014 Feb;134(2):237-255.

[5] Matheny LM, Ockuly AC, Steadman JR, LaPrade RF. Posterior meniscus root tears: associated pathologies to assist as diagnostic tools. Knee Surg Sports Traumatol Arthrosc. 2015 Oct;23(10):3127-3131.

[6] Ozkoc G, Circi E, Gonc U, Irgit K, Pourbagher A, Tandogan RN. Radial tears in the root of the posterior horn of the medial meniscus. Knee Surg Sports Traumatol Arthrosc. 2008 Sep;16(9):849-854.

[7] Han SB, Shetty GM, Lee DH, Chae DJ, Seo SS, Wang KH, Yoo SH, Nha KW. Unfavorable results of partial meniscectomy for complete medial meniscus posterior root tear with early osteoarthritis: a 5- to 8-year follow-up study. Arthroscopy. 2010 Oct;26(10): 1326-1332. doi: 10.1016/j.arthro.2010. 01.032. Epub 2010 May 7. PMID: 20887931.

[8] Ra HJ, Ha JK, Jang HS, Kim JG. Traumatic posterior root tear of the medial meniscus in patients with severe medial instability of the knee. Knee Surg Sports Traumatol Arthrosc. 2015 Oct;23(10):3121-3126.

[9] Choi ES, Park SJ. Clinical Evaluation of the Root Tear of the Posterior Horn of the Medial Meniscus in Total Knee Arthroplasty for Osteoarthritis. Knee Surg Relat Res. 2015 Jun;27(2):90-94.

[10] Krych AJ, Johnson NR, Mohan R, Hevesi M, Stuart MJ, Littrell LA, Collins MS. Arthritis Progression on Serial MRIs Following Diagnosis of Medial Meniscal Posterior Horn Root Tear. J Knee Surg. 2018 Aug;31(7):698-704.

[11] Krych AJ, Reardon PJ, Johnson NR, Mohan R, Peter L, Levy BA, Stuart MJ. Non-operative management of medial meniscus posterior horn root tears is associated with worsening arthritis and poor clinical outcome at 5-year follow-up. Knee Surg Sports Traumatol Arthrosc. 2017 Feb;25(2):383-389.

[12] Gale DR, Chaisson CE, Totterman SM, Schwartz RK, Gale ME, Felson D. Meniscal subluxation: association with osteoarthritis and joint space narrowing. Osteoarthritis Cartilage. 1999 Nov;7(6):526-532.

[13] Furumatsu T, Kodama Y, Kamatsuki Y, Hino T, Okazaki Y, Ozaki T. Meniscal Extrusion Progresses Shortly after the Medial Meniscus Posterior Root Tear. Knee Surg Relat Res. 2017 Dec 1;29(4):295-301.

[14] Okazaki Y, Furumatsu T, Shimamura Y, Saiga K, Ohashi H, Uchino T, Kamatsuki Y, Okazaki Y, Ozaki T. Time-Dependent Increase in Medial Meniscus Extrusion after Medial Meniscus Posterior Root Tear Analyzed by Using Magnetic Resonance Imaging. Knee Surg Relat Res. 2019 Jun 1;31(2):120-125.

[15] Yamagami R, Taketomi S, Inui H, Tahara K, Tanaka S. The role of medial meniscus posterior root tear and proximal tibial morphology in the

development of spontaneous osteonecrosis and osteoarthritis of the knee. Knee. 2017 Mar;24(2):390-395.

[16] Jones RS, Keene GC, Learmonth DJ, Bickerstaff D, Nawana NS, Costi JJ, Pearcy MJ. Direct measurement of hoop strains in the intact and torn human meniscus. Clin Biomech 1996;11: 295e300.

[17] Johal P, Williams A, Wragg P, Hunt D, Gedroyc W. Tibio-femoral movement in the living knee. A study of weight bearing and non-weight bearing knee kinematics using 'interventional' MRI. J Biomech 2005; 38: 269e76.

[18] Krause WR, Pope MH, Johnson RJ, Wilder DG. Mechanical changes in the knee after meniscectomy. J Bone Joint Surg Am 1976;58:599e603

[19] FAIRBANK TJ. Knee joint changes after meniscectomy. J Bone Joint Surg Br. 1948 Nov;30B(4):664-670.

[20] Marzo JM, Gurske-DePerio J. Effects of medial meniscus posterior horn avulsion and repair on tibiofemoral contact area and peak contact pressure with clinical implications. Am J Sports Med. 2009 Jan;37(1):124-129.

[21] Kim JG, Lee YS, Bae TS, Ha JK, Lee DH, Kim YJ, Ra HJ. Tibiofemoral contact mechanics following posterior root of medial meniscus tear, repair, meniscectomy, and allograft transplantation. Knee Surg Sports Traumatol Arthrosc. 2013 Sep;21(9):2121-5. doi: 10.1007/s00167-012-2182-4. Epub 2012 Sep 7. PMID: 22955146.

[22] Śmigielski R, Becker R, Zdanowicz U, Ciszek B. Medial meniscus anatomy-from basic science to treatment. Knee Surg Sports Traumatol Arthrosc. 2015 Jan;23(1):8-14.

[23] Bhatia S, LaPrade CM, Ellman MB, LaPrade RF. Meniscal root tears: significance, diagnosis, and treatment. Am J Sports Med. 2014 Dec;42(12): 3016-3030.

[24] Choi JY, Chang EY, Cunha GM, Tafur M, Statum S, Chung CB. Posterior medial meniscus root ligament lesions: MRI classification and associated findings. AJR Am J Roentgenol. 2014 Dec;203(6):1286-1292. doi: 10.2214/AJR.14.12559. PMID: 25415707.

[25] Villegas DF, Donahue TL. Collagen morphology in human meniscal attachments: a SEM study. Connect Tissue Res. 2010 Oct;51(5):327-336.

[26] Bae JH, Paik NH, Park GW, Yoon JR, Chae DJ, Kwon JH, Kim JI, Nha KW. Predictive value of painful popping for a posterior root tear of the medial meniscus in middle-aged to older Asian patients. Arthroscopy. 2013 Mar;29(3):545-9. doi: 10.1016/j.arthro.2012.10.026. Epub 2013 Jan 29. PMID: 23375180.

[27] Kim JH, Chung JH, Lee DH, Lee YS, Kim JR, Ryu KJ. Arthroscopic suture anchor repair versus pullout suture repair in posterior root tear of the medial meniscus: a prospective comparison study. Arthroscopy. 2011 Dec;27(12):1644-1653.

[28] Lee JH, Lim YJ, Kim KB, Kim KH, Song JH. Arthroscopic pullout suture repair of posterior root tear of the medial meniscus: radiographic and clinical results with a 2-year follow-up. Arthroscopy. 2009 Sep;25(9):951-958.

[29] Hwang BY, Kim SJ, Lee SW, Lee HE, Lee CK, Hunter DJ, Jung KA. Risk factors for medial meniscus posterior root tear. Am J Sports Med. 2012 Jul;40(7):1606-1610.

[30] KELLGREN JH, LAWRENCE JS. Radiological assessment of osteo-arthrosis. Ann Rheum Dis. 1957 Dec;16(4):494-502.

[31] Choi SH, Bae S, Ji SK, Chang MJ. The MRI findings of meniscal root tear of the medial meniscus: emphasis on coronal, sagittal and axial images. Knee Surg Sports Traumatol Arthrosc. 2012 Oct;20(10):2098-2103.

[32] Lee YG, Shim JC, Choi YS, Kim JG, Lee GJ, Kim HK. Magnetic resonance imaging findings of surgically proven medial meniscus root tear: tear configuration and associated knee abnormalities. J Comput Assist Tomogr. 2008 May-Jun;32(3):452-457.

[33] Okazaki Y, Furumatsu T, Yamaguchi T, Kodama Y, Kamatsuki Y, Masuda S, Okazaki Y, Hiranaka T, Zhang X, Ozaki T. Medial meniscus posterior root tear causes swelling of the medial meniscus and expansion of the extruded meniscus: a comparative analysis between 2D and 3D MRI. Knee Surg Sports Traumatol Arthrosc. 2020 Nov;28(11):3405-3415.

[34] Yamagami R, Taketomi S, Inui H, Tahara K, Tanaka S. The role of medial meniscus posterior root tear and proximal tibial morphology in the development of spontaneous osteonecrosis and osteoarthritis of the knee. Knee. 2017 Mar;24(2):390-395.

[35] Guermazi A, Hayashi D, Jarraya M, Roemer FW, Zhang Y, Niu J, Crema MD, Englund M, Lynch JA, Nevitt MC, Torner JC, Lewis CE, Felson DT. Medial posterior meniscal root tears are associated with development or worsening of medial tibiofemoral cartilage damage: the multicenter osteoarthritis study. Radiology. 2013 Sep;268(3):814-821.

[36] Brown AA. The insertion of the anterior horn of the medial meniscus: an anatomic study. Muscles Ligaments Tendons J. 2013 Aug 11;3(3):210-212.

[37] LaPrade CM, James EW, Cram TR, Feagin JA, Engebretsen L, LaPrade RF. Meniscal root tears: a classification system based on tear morphology. Am J Sports Med. 2015 Feb;43(2):363-369.

[38] Bin SI, Jeong TW, Kim SJ, Lee DH. A new arthroscopic classification of degenerative medial meniscus root tear that correlates with meniscus extrusion on magnetic resonance imaging. Knee. 2016 Mar;23(2):246-250.

[39] Kim JY, Bin SI, Kim JM, Lee BS, Oh SM, Cho WJ. A Novel Arthroscopic Classification of Degenerative Medial Meniscus Posterior Root Tears Based on the Tear Gap. Orthop J Sports Med. 2019 Mar 18;7(3):2325967119827945.

[40] Lim HC, Bae JH, Wang JH, Seok CW, Kim MK. Non-operative treatment of degenerative posterior root tear of the medial meniscus. Knee Surg Sports Traumatol Arthrosc. 2010 Apr;18(4):535-539.

[41] Neogi DS, Kumar A, Rijal L, Yadav CS, Jaiman A, Nag HL. Role of nonoperative treatment in managing degenerative tears of the medial meniscus posterior root. J Orthop Traumatol. 2013 Sep;14(3):193-199.

[42] Faucett SC, Geisler BP, Chahla J, Krych AJ, Kurzweil PR, Garner AM, Liu S, LaPrade RF, Pietzsch JB. Meniscus Root Repair vs Meniscectomy or Nonoperative Management to Prevent Knee Osteoarthritis After Medial Meniscus Root Tears: Clinical and Economic Effectiveness. Am J Sports Med. 2019 Mar;47(3):762-769.

[43] Dragoo JL, Konopka JA, Guzman RA, Segovia N, Kandil A, Pappas GP. Outcomes of Arthroscopic All-Inside Repair Versus Observation in Older Patients With Meniscus Root Tears. Am J Sports Med. 2020 Apr;48(5):1127-1133.

[44] Krych AJ, Johnson NR, Mohan R, Dahm DL, Levy BA, Stuart MJ. Partial

meniscectomy provides no benefit for symptomatic degenerative medial meniscus posterior root tears. Knee Surg Sports Traumatol Arthrosc. 2018 Apr;26(4):1117-1122.

[45] Bernard CD, Kennedy NI, Tagliero AJ, Camp CL, Saris DBF, Levy BA, Stuart MJ, Krych AJ. Medial Meniscus Posterior Root Tear Treatment: A Matched Cohort Comparison of Nonoperative Management, Partial Meniscectomy, and Repair. Am J Sports Med. 2020 Jan;48(1):128-132.

[46] Lee JK, Jung M, Yang JH, Song SY, Shin YS, Cha M, Jung D, Seo YJ. Repair versus nonrepair of medial meniscus posterior root tear: A systematic review of patients' selection criteria, including clinical and radiographic outcomes. Medicine (Baltimore). 2020 Mar;99(10):e19499.

[47] Röpke EF, Kopf S, Drange S, Becker R, Lohmann CH, Stärke C. Biomechanical evaluation of meniscal root repair: a porcine study. Knee Surg Sports Traumatol Arthrosc. 2015 Jan;23(1):45-50.

[48] Padalecki JR, Jansson KS, Smith SD, Dornan GJ, Pierce CM, Wijdicks CA, Laprade RF. Biomechanical consequences of a complete radial tear adjacent to the medial meniscus posterior root attachment site: in situ pull-out repair restores derangement of joint mechanics. Am J Sports Med. 2014 Mar;42(3):699-707.

[49] LaPrade CM, Foad A, Smith SD, Turnbull TL, Dornan GJ, Engebretsen L, Wijdicks CA, LaPrade RF. Biomechanical consequences of a nonanatomic posterior medial meniscal root repair. Am J Sports Med. 2015 Apr;43(4):912-920.

[50] Cerminara AJ, LaPrade CM, Smith SD, Ellman MB, Wijdicks CA, LaPrade RF. Biomechanical evaluation of a transtibial pull-out meniscal root repair: challenging the bungee effect. Am J Sports Med. 2014 Dec;42(12): 2988-2995.

[51] Apivatgaroon A, Chernchujit B. A Medial Meniscal Root Pullout Repair With the Use of a Tibial Tunnel Suturing Technique. Arthrosc Tech. 2016 Jun 6;5(3):e595-e599.

[52] LaPrade RF, Matheny LM, Moulton SG, James EW, Dean CS. Posterior Meniscal Root Repairs: Outcomes of an Anatomic Transtibial Pull-Out Technique. Am J Sports Med. 2017 Mar;45(4):884-891.

[53] Kaplan DJ, Alaia EF, Dold AP, Meislin RJ, Strauss EJ, Jazrawi LM, Alaia MJ. Increased extrusion and ICRS grades at 2-year follow-up following transtibial medial meniscal root repair evaluated by MRI. Knee Surg Sports Traumatol Arthrosc. 2018 Sep;26(9):2826-2834.

[54] Kodama Y, Furumatsu T, Masuda S, Okazaki Y, Kamatsuki Y, Okazaki Y, Hiranaka T, Miyazawa S, Yasumitsu M, Ozaki T. Transtibial fixation for medial meniscus posterior root tear reduces posterior extrusion and physiological translation of the medial meniscus in middle-aged and elderly patients. Knee Surg Sports Traumatol Arthrosc. 2020 Nov;28(11):3416-3425.

[55] Feucht MJ, Kühle J, Bode G, Mehl J, Schmal H, Südkamp NP, Niemeyer P. Arthroscopic Transtibial Pullout Repair for Posterior Medial Meniscus Root Tears: A Systematic Review of Clinical, Radiographic, and Second-Look Arthroscopic Results. Arthroscopy. 2015 Sep;31(9):1808-1816.

[56] LaPrade RF, LaPrade CM, Ellman MB, Turnbull TL, Cerminara AJ, Wijdicks CA. Cyclic displacement after meniscal root repair fixation: a human

biomechanical evaluation. Am J Sports Med. 2015 Apr;43(4):892-898.

[57] Feucht MJ, Grande E, Brunhuber J, Burgkart R, Imhoff AB, Braun S. Biomechanical evaluation of different suture techniques for arthroscopic transtibial pull-out repair of posterior medial meniscus root tears. Am J Sports Med. 2013 Dec;41(12):2784-2790.

[58] Ulku TK, Kaya A, Kocaoglu B. Suture configuration techniques have no effect on mid-term clinical outcomes of arthroscopic meniscus root repairs. Knee. 2020 Jun;27(3):676-682.

[59] Lee DW, Kim MK, Jang HS, Ha JK, Kim JG. Clinical and radiologic evaluation of arthroscopic medial meniscus root tear refixation: comparison of the modified Mason-Allen stitch and simple stitches. Arthroscopy. 2014 Nov;30(11): 1439-1446.

[60] Kuptniratsaikul S, Itthipanichpong T, Kuptniratsaikul V. Arthroscopic Medial Meniscus Root Repair With Soft Suture Anchor Without Posterior Portal Technique. Arthrosc Tech. 2018 Apr 30;7(5):e553-e556.

[61] Lee SK, Yang BS, Park BM, Yeom JU, Kim JH, Yu JS. Medial Meniscal Root Repair Using Curved Guide and Soft Suture Anchor. Clin Orthop Surg. 2018 Mar;10(1):111-115.

[62] Balke M, Akoto R, Offerhaus C, Hoeher J. Suture Anchor Refixation of Meniscal Root Tears Without an Additional Portal. Arthrosc Tech. 2018 Apr 16;7(5):e511-e515.

[63] Jung YH, Choi NH, Oh JS, Victoroff BN. All-inside repair for a root tear of the medial meniscus using a suture anchor. Am J Sports Med. 2012 Jun;40(6):1406-1411.

[64] Wu SH, Yeh TT, Hsu WC, Wu ATH, Li G, Chen CH, Lee CH, Wu JL. Biomechanical comparison of four tibial fixation techniques for meniscal root sutures in posterior medial meniscus root repair: A porcine study. J Orthop Translat. 2020 Feb 17;24:144-149.

[65] Zhu S, Li X, Wu JL, Bao L, Wang P, Gu H, Wang C, Wang J. Non-anatomic repair of medial meniscus posterior root tears to the posterior capsule provided favourable outcomes in middle-aged and older patients. Knee Surg Sports Traumatol Arthrosc. 2021 Apr 9.

[66] Okazaki Y, Furumatsu T, Miyazawa S, Masuda S, Okazaki Y, Hiranaka T, Ozaki T. A novel suture technique to reduce the meniscus extrusion in the pullout repair for medial meniscus posterior root tears. Eur J Orthop Surg Traumatol. 2019 Dec;29(8):1805-1809.

[67] Koga H, Watanabe T, Horie M, Katagiri H, Otabe K, Ohara T, Katakura M, Sekiya I, Muneta T. Augmentation of the Pullout Repair of a Medial Meniscus Posterior Root Tear by Arthroscopic Centralization. Arthrosc Tech. 2017 Aug 21;6(4):e1335-e1339.

[68] Chernchujit B, Agrawal S. Arthroscopic All-Inside Medial Meniscus Extrusion Reduction. Arthrosc Tech. 2019 Apr 26;8(5):e495-e501.

[69] Ozeki N, Muneta T, Kawabata K, Koga H, Nakagawa Y, Saito R, Udo M, Yanagisawa K, Ohara T, Mochizuki T, Tsuji K, Saito T, Sekiya I. Centralization of extruded medial meniscus delays cartilage degeneration in rats. J Orthop Sci. 2017 May;22(3):542-548.

[70] Jiang EX, Abouljoud MM, Everhart JS, DiBartola AC, Kaeding CC, Magnussen RA, Flanigan DC. Clinical factors associated with successful meniscal root repairs: A systematic review. Knee. 2019 Mar;26(2):285-291.

[71] Vyas D, Harner CD. Meniscus root repair. Sports Med Arthrosc Rev. 2012 Jun;20(2):86-94.

[72] Papalia R, Vasta S, Franceschi F, D'Adamio S, Maffulli N, Denaro V. Meniscal root tears: from basic science to ultimate surgery. Br Med Bull. 2013;106:91-115.

Chapter 2

Injuries of the Posterolateral Corner of the Knee-Diagnosis and Treatment Options for Beginning and Advanced Arthroscopic Surgeons

Adrian Góralczyk, Piotr Jancewicz and Krzysztof Hermanowicz

Abstract

Injuries to the posterolateral corner (PLC) of the knee may have a devastating impact on whole joint. Posterolateral rotatory instability, despite getting more and more popular among orthopedic surgeons, still remains challenging to diagnose and even more challenging to treat. Available surgical techniques are demanding and require advanced surgical skills. In this chapter we are going to review the diagnostic tools which help to recognize posterolateral rotatory instability of the knee, to outline its importance and consequences of misdiagnosis as well as present arthroscopic popliteus tenodesis and arthroscopic-assisted posterolateral corner reconstruction which are our minimally invasive techniques used to treat this condition depending on PLC injury pattern and grading. Presented techniques are reproducible, safe and do not require advanced surgical skills being a useful alternative for available open PLC reconstructions.

Keywords: posterolateral corner of the knee, popliteus tendon, lateral collateral ligament, multiligament knee injury, popliteus tenodesis, arthroscopic posterolateral corner reconstruction

1. Introduction

When it comes to the traumatic soft tissue injury of the knee, the patient is always afraid of having a meniscus or cruciate ligament lesion. Despite the widespread disrepute of meniscal, cruciate ligaments or isolated collateral ligaments tears, the management and treatment options are well-established with scientifically proved good results. More challenging remain acute and chronic rotatory instabilities of the knee which require a high grade of suspicion to be recognized, a broad knowledge of anatomy and biomechanics to determine injured structures and properly addressed them and, finally, have a debilitating influence on the whole knee joint when left unrecognized [1–3].

One of the most common rotatory instability pattern is a posterolateral rotatory instability (PLRI), which is a consequence of injuries to the structures of so-called posterolateral corner (PLC) of the knee. This anatomical and functional region of the knee consists of many static and dynamic stabilizers from which the most important are three: fibular collateral ligament (FCL), popliteus tendon (PLT) and popliteofibular ligament (PFL). The others involve iliotibial band (ITB), biceps femoris tendon (BT), posterolateral knee capsule, fabello-fibular ligament [4, 5]. From three main stabilizers mentioned above, the FCL works as a primary restraint to varus stresses, especially close to knee extension, whereas PLT and PFL plays a crucial role in limitation of tibial external rotation. Furthermore, the PLT provides antero-posterior stability in 30° of knee flexion and, working as a dynamic stabilizer, actively rotates the knee internally [4, 6, 7].

Typical mechanisms of injury to the PLC involve knee hyperextension with varus deformation like for example direct hit to the anteromedial region of tibia, forced external rotation with the foot fixed on the ground, mostly during sport activities, but also motorbike or vehicle accidents as a part of complex knee injuries [4, 5, 8]. The PLC injuries account for 16% of all knee ligamentous injuries, but only 28% of them are isolated [5, 6]. Usually they are associated with anterior cruciate ligament (ACL) or posterior cruciate ligament (PCL) tears [5]. Non-recognition of PLRI concomitant with ACL or PCL tears may lead not only to unsatisfactory clinical results of surgical treatment, but also to reconstruction failures and further revision surgeries [9]. Thus, an adequate diagnosis and management of PLC injuries are essential for the knee joint well-being.

2. Diagnosis of posterolateral corner injury

Patient with PLRI of the knee may present with a history of knee sprain with hyperextension or direct hit to the anteromedial region of tibia, forced external rotation with the foot fixed on the ground during sport activities or motorbike accident. The patient usually complains on pain in posterolateral or lateral region of the knee, side-to-side instability close to full extension, difficulties in going up- and downstairs, inability to perform sports activities [4, 5].

In acute setting it is essential to rule out neuro-vascular injuries concomitant to PLC injury. Popliteal neuro-vascular bundle and common peroneal nerve are at risk during knee injuries leading to PLC tears. Moreover, it is very important to assess other intra- and extra-articular structures like ACL, PCL, menisci and exclude their lesions, because isolated PLC tears are rare [6].

The patient suspected for PLC tear should be assessed during gait, standing and lying on the examination table [4, 6, 8, 10]. Chronic PLRI may lead to so-called "triple-varus", which is an evolution from anatomical knee varus through weight-bearing varus to "varus thrust gait", when the knee developed excessive varus and hyperextension during the stance phase of gait [8]. Many clinical tests have been developed and are widely used to assess the structures of the PLC:

- Varus stress test in 0° and 30° of flexion
  This test is positive when applying a varus force to the knee leads to excessive opening of lateral joint space without firm endpoint. If positive in 30°, it suggests the FCL tear. If positive in both 0° and 30°, it suggests more complex lesion of PLC.

- Posterolateral drawer test and posterolateral external rotation test
  The test is performed in 30° and 90° of knee flexion. When applying posterolaterally directed force, excessive tibial translation and external rotation may be observed (**Figure 1**).

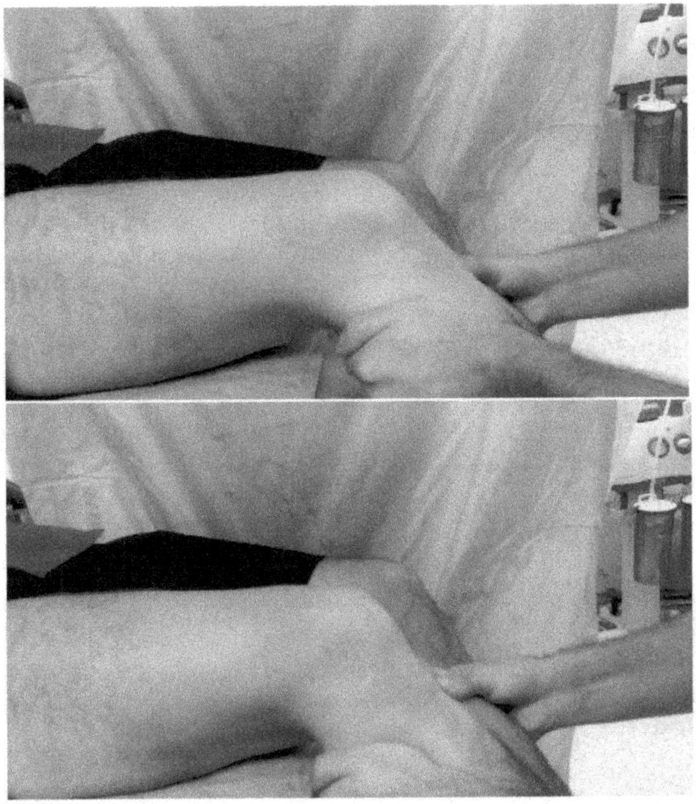

Figure 1.
Posterolateral drawer test performed in the right knee on the operating table. Upper image presents starting point and in the lower picture excessive posterolateral tibial translation with external rotation can be observed under loading.

- Dial test in 30° and 90° of flexion
  Having the patient lying prone, with stabilized thighs, passive tibial external rotation of both lower extremities is being compared considering feet positions. Asymmetric increased in external rotation in 30° suggests injury to the PLC, but asymmetric increased in external rotation in both 30° and 90° implies injury to the PLC and PCL.

- Reverse pivot-shift test
  Starting from from 90° of flexion, the knee is gradually extended with valgus and tibial external rotation applied. In case of PLC tear, posteriorly subluxed tibia is reduced in 30–40° of knee flexion by ITB, which changes its function from flexor to knee extensor.

- External rotation recurvatum test
  Having the patient lying supine, with stabilized thighs, both great toes are grasped and feet lifted by the physician. The knee with PLC injury presents hyperextension and varus deformity.

Other tests like Lachman test, anterior drawer test, posterior drawer test, valgus stress test, different meniscal tests are used to rule out concomitant lesions depending on examiners preferences and experience [4, 6, 8, 10].

Imaging studies are important in diagnosis of PLC injury. Classic anteroposterior and lateral X-rays are used to exclude fractures in acute setting and to assess any degenerative changes existence. Long-leg X-ray is necessary in chronic cases to rule out excessive varus deformity which may require correction before soft-tissue surgeries. Both knees stress X-rays performed in 20° of flexion may reveal asymmetric lateral joint space opening. Side-to-side difference in lateral gapping about 2.7 mm may indicate isolated FCL tear, whereas the difference above 4 mm represents complex PLC injury [11]. Magnetic resonance imaging (MRI) may be a useful technique to diagnose PLC injury in acute setting, but after 12 weeks from initial trauma only 26% of PLC tears are diagnosed this way [4]. Signs of PLC tears which may be observed on MRI scans are arcuate sign, which is an avulsion fracture of fibular head, avulsion or interstitial-type tear of ITB typically close to tibial attachment, BT tear close to fibula, FCL tear usually close to fibular or tibial attachment, rarely mid-substance, PLT injury usually localized on myotendinous junction [12]. It is worth noting that an abundant signal abnormality in the region of the posterior capsule is usually present in case of PLC tear [12]. **Figure 2** presents injury to the PLC of the knee on sagittal MRI scan. Furthermore, MRI allows to rule out other intra- and extra-articular pathologies like cruciate ligament and menisci tears or chondral lesions.

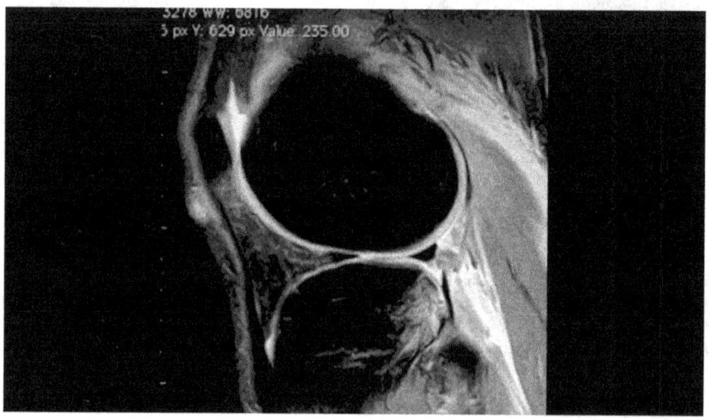

Figure 2.
Sagittal MRI scan of the right knee with PLC injury. Abnormal signal is observed in the region of posterior knee joint capsule.

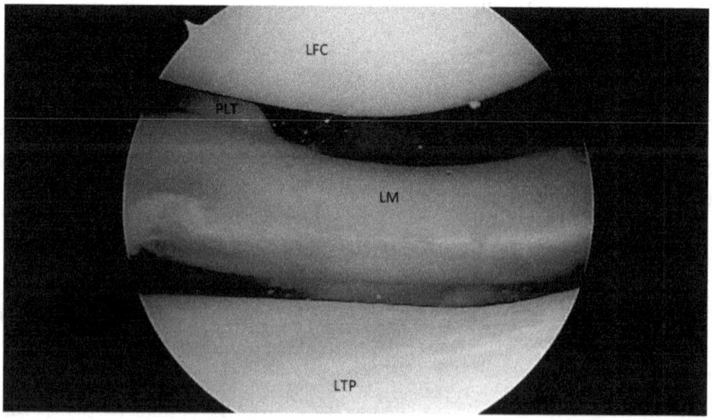

Figure 3.
Arthroscopic view from anterolateral portal in the right knee in figure-of-four position. "Drive-through sign" is visible. LM- lateral meniscus, LFC- lateral femoral condyle, LTP- lateral tibial plateau, PLT- popliteus tendon.

Arthroscopy is no longer only diagnostic procedure. Every surgeon who decided to scope the knee is obligated to treat recognized intra-articular lesions. The direct sign of PLC injury observed during diagnostic part of knee arthroscopy is so-called "drive-through sign" and involves lateral joint space widening with elevation of lateral meniscus (LM) in the figure-of-four position (**Figure 3**). In our practice this sign is very important in decision-making process. **Table 1** summarizes the pearls and pitfalls in diagnosis of PLC injuries.

There is a lack of comprehensive classification system which could cover all aspects of PLC injuries [10]. The most commonly used is classification developed by Fanelli and Larson which is presented in **Table 2** [13].

PLT- popliteus tendon, PFL- popliteofibular ligament, FCL- fibular collateral ligament, ER- external rotation.

Point of evaluation	Pearls	Pitfalls
Clinical exam		
Varus stress test	Perform in 0 and 30°. Positive indicates more complex PLC injury.	Patient may guard during examination. Try to eliminate muscle contraction.
Posterolateral drawer test Posterolateral external rotation test Dial test Reverse pivot-shift test External rotation recurvatum test	Always compare to the uninjured side. Choose 2–3 tests and train them. Dial test is useful to differentiate isolated PLC injury and concomitant PCL injury.	Tibial external rotation may be increased also in anteromedial rotatory instability.
Lachman test, anterior and posterior drawer, meniscal tests.	Rule out other ligamentous and meniscal lesions.	Lachman test may be positive due to PLT injury, anterior drawer may be false positive in complex PLC/PCL injuries.
Imaging		
X-ray Stress X-ray MRI	Rule out fractures. Segond, reverse Segond fracture and tibial head fracture are avulsion fractures due to pull of ligaments. Useful in assessing intra-articular pathologies.	X-ray does not directly assess soft tissue conditions. Stress X-rays difficult to perform in some countries. Poor sensitivity in diagnosis of PLC injuries especially > 12 weeks.
Arthroscopy	Look for "drive-through sign".	It is difficult to directly assess PLC injury.

Table 1.
Summarizes the pearls and pitfalls in diagnosis of PLC injury.

Grade	Injured structures	Instability pattern
A	PLT + PFL	Increased tibial ER
B	PLT + PFL FCL attenuation	Increased tibial ER Slightly increased lateral joint space opening
C	PLT + PFL FCL tear, capsule tear Commonly cruciate ligaments tear	Increased tibial ER Excessive lateral joint space opening Sagittal plane instability

Table 2.
Posterolateral corner injuries classification according to Fanelli and Larson [13].

3. Current surgical treatment options

Numbers of surgical techniques have been developed for treatment of PLC injuries what outlines that it is a very complex problem and no simple solution does exist [7, 9, 14–20]. Among them one can differentiate 3 types of procedures: tightening of injured structures, PLT bypass and anatomic reconstructions [9, 21]. Anatomic reconstructions, in turn, involve fibular-based and tibio-fibular based techniques [4]. Most anatomic techniques focus on reconstruction of three main stabilizers of the PLC: FCL, PLT and PFL. However, it has been emphasized that concerning surgical techniques, individual PLC structures should be reconstructed only if injured, avoiding reconstruction of that are not damaged [10]. Thus, a proper diagnosis of injured structures is a key to success in surgical treatment and Fanelli and Larson classification mentioned above may be a helpful tool in considering surgical approach. It is worth noting that in case of chronic PLC injury the success rate of surgical management is about 90% [21]. However, detailed description of each available technique for PLC tears treatment is far beyond the scope of this chapter. Interested readers we send to positions from literature [14–20].

When last two decades have provided a comprehensive knowledge about anatomy and anatomical reconstructions of PLC, especially due to studies of dr Laprade and his groups, last years brought a great development in arthroscopic surgery and shift from open to arthroscopic procedures based on previous assumptions [20]. The reasons of these changes were that open PLC reconstructions, despite their effectiveness, are very invasive procedures. They require a broad surgical approach with poor esthetic results, which some patients do not accept, and enforce less aggressive rehabilitation protocol. It causes a longer recovery after surgery. Moreover, common peroneal nerve neurolysis is obligatory [15]. Arthroscopic surgeries have many advantages including better visualization of anatomical landmarks, lower infection rates, lesser amount of scar tissue, less post-operative pain, faster rehabilitation, better protection of common peroneal nerve without obligatory neurolysis [21]. Another advantage of arthroscopic surgery for PLC injury is its proved reproducibility and high accuracy in tunnel placement during reconstructions [7]. However, most arthroscopic techniques require maneuvering in popliteal fossa and trans-septal portal placement, what puts at risk popliteal neuro-vascular bundle. Thus, these techniques are reserved for very experienced arthroscopic surgeons.

Following sections of these chapter will present arthroscopic popliteus tenodesis and minimally invasive arthroscopic-assisted PLC reconstructions which are techniques for PLC injuries developed and used with success for many years by senior authors (K.H, P.J) [22, 23]. Indications, contraindications, advantages, disadvantages and surgical details will be explained.

4. Arthroscopic posterolateral corner stabilization with popliteus tenodesis

4.1 Indications and contraindications

Indication for this procedure is a posterolateral rotatory instability of the knee grade A according to Fanelli and Larson classification (**Table 2**) [22]. It can also be used in grade B and C PLRI as a part of combined procedure with reconstruction of other structures of the PLC. The main purpose of this technique is to prevent excessive tibial external rotation. Secondly, it allows to reduce posterior tibial subluxation caused by PLC injury.

The contraindications are: damaged femoral attachment of PLT, complete mid-substance PLT tear without scar formation, excessive varus deformity of the knee, advanced osteoarthritis, rheumatoid arthritis.

4.2 Rationale for using arthroscopic PLT tenodesis

The rationale for using arthroscopic PLT tenodesis are facts that most popliteus tears are extra-articular, involving usually the muscle or myotendinous portion and in chronic cases sulcus popliteus is usually covered by popliteus tendon and/or scar tissue [7, 12]. Thus, the PLT is still presented in its anatomical location, despite losing its function. Moreover, it has been proved that anatomic reconstruction of the passive part of PLT significantly restores proper range of tibial external rotation [24].

Presented technique does not require advanced skills in arthroscopic surgery, is safe and reproducible, does not exhaust other surgical options.

4.3 Arthroscopic PLT tenodesis-surgical technique

The patient is positioned supine with a thigh tourniquet applied on operated leg, which is placed in a leg holder. The procedure is performed using standard anterolateral (AL) and anteromedial (AM) portals. After arthroscopic inspection of whole knee joint and excluding other intra-articular pathologies, the arthroscope is inserted to the lateral knee recess and PLT unit is visualized (**Figure 4**). With the knee in full extension an additional mid-lateral portal is placed 1,5 cm above the fibular head, just anterior or posterior to FCL depending on better angle of attack determined with a marking needle (**Figure 5**). It is important to stay anterior to BT to avoid common peroneal nerve injury. Then, under visual control, Pean's forceps with fastened one end of suture tape (FiberTape, Arthrex, GmBH Munich, Germany) are inserted behind the PLT to the posterolateral knee recess, the tape is introduced to lateral knee compartment using an arthroscopic grasper and then it is pulled out the joint through mid-lateral portal with Pean's forceps making a ring around the PLT at the level of planned place for tenodesis (**Figure 6**). The ideal point for PLT fixation is the crossing of the horizontal line at the tip of fibular head with vertical line at the medial edge of fibular head, 1 cm below the joint line [7].

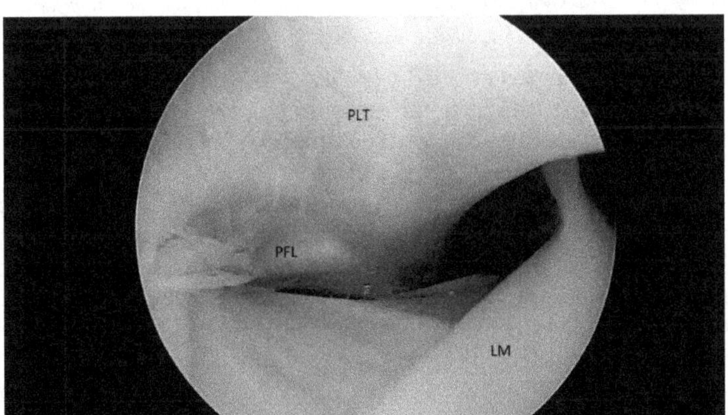

Figure 4.
Arthroscopic view from anterolateral viewing portal in the right knee with the arthroscope in lateral knee recess. Popliteus muscle-tendon unit may be observed. PLT- popliteus tendon, PFL- popliteofibular ligament, LM- lateral meniscus.

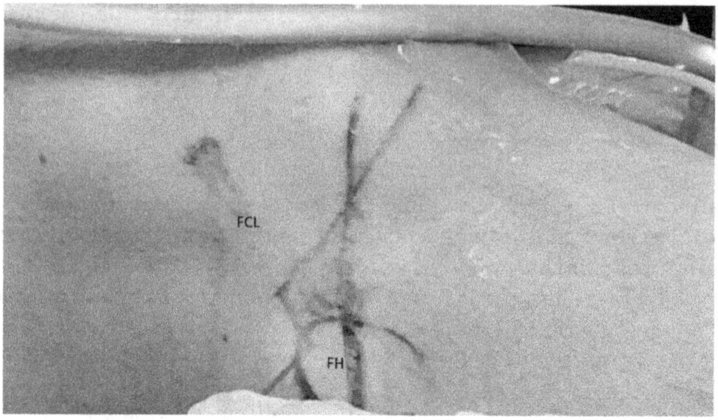

Figure 5.
A marking needle is used to determine the proper place for mid-lateral portal placement in the right knee. FH-fibular head, FCL- fibular collateral ligament.

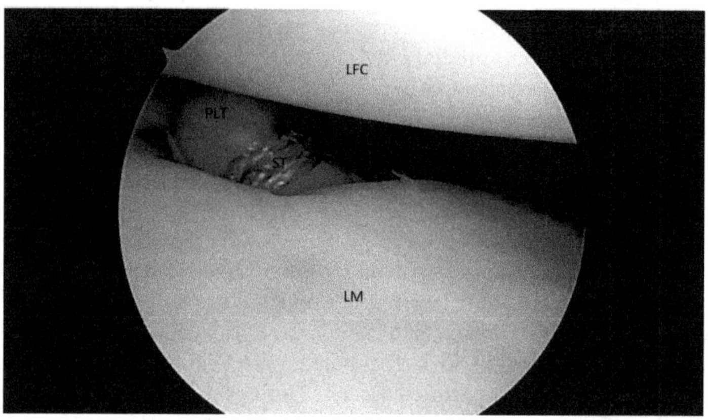

Figure 6.
Arthroscopic view from anterolateral viewing portal in the right knee. Suture tape (ST) rounded the popliteus tendon (PLT) right before making a tenodesis. LFC- lateral femoral condyle, LM- lateral meniscus.

In this place the proximal part of tibial popliteus aiming guide (senior author K. H prototype) is fixed and the distal part is positioned on the anteromedial tibial cortex, just below the pes anserinus where a small skin incision is made. Both parts of the aiming guide are connected and the eyelet pin is drilled through tibia (**Figure 7**). For advanced arthroscopic surgeons it is possible to drill the tibia with an eyelet pin using a free-hand technique after positioning the tip of pin in the proper place for PLT fixation which was previously described. Then, using a 6 mm drill, a 2-cm depth bone sockets are formed in the posterolateral and anteromedial cortex of the tibia. After that, free ends of suture tape rounding PLT are passed through the eye in an eyelet pin and the pin is pulled-out through the anteromedial tibial cortex introducing the PLT into bone socket. Free ends of suture tape are tied on the cortical button placed in the socket on the anteromedial tibial cortex. The tension of tenodesis is regulated by twisting the cortical button with Pean's forceps under arthroscopic control until the drive-through sign and lateral meniscus elevation are eliminated in the figure-of-four position (**Figures 8** and **9**).

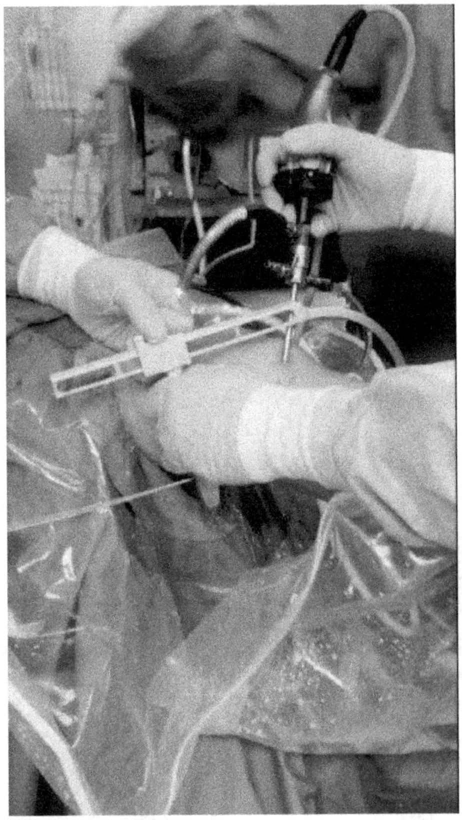

Figure 7.
The right knee. The tibial popliteus aiming guide (K.H prototype) is positioned from posterolateral to anteromedial tibial cortex and the eyelet pin is being used to drill the tunnel.

4.4 Postoperative rehabilitation

After surgery the knee is immobilized in a brace with limited knee extension (30–90°) for 6 weeks. Passive knee motion starts from the second day after surgery. Walking on crutches is recommended for 6 weeks after surgery. Supervised rehabilitation program with experienced physiotherapist is advised. The rehabilitation protocol is similar to this widely-accepted for PCL reconstructions.

4.5 Advantages and disadvantages of PLT tenodesis

The main advantage of arthroscopic PLT tenodesis is that this is a minimal invasive technique utilizing native, vascularized material present in the joint. It does not require harvesting grafts and does not exhaust other treatment options. It allows to restore static PLT function. Presented technique does not demand advanced arthroscopic skills and may be useful for beginning arthroscopic surgeons treating PLRI with dominant external rotation component. Following described technique it is a safe procedure because is performed far from common peroneal nerve and does not require maneuvering in the posterior knee close to the popliteal neuro-vascular bundle. Positioning the tunnel in the tibia from posterolateral to anteromedial facilitates utilizing this surgery without special instruments making it a cost-effective procedure.

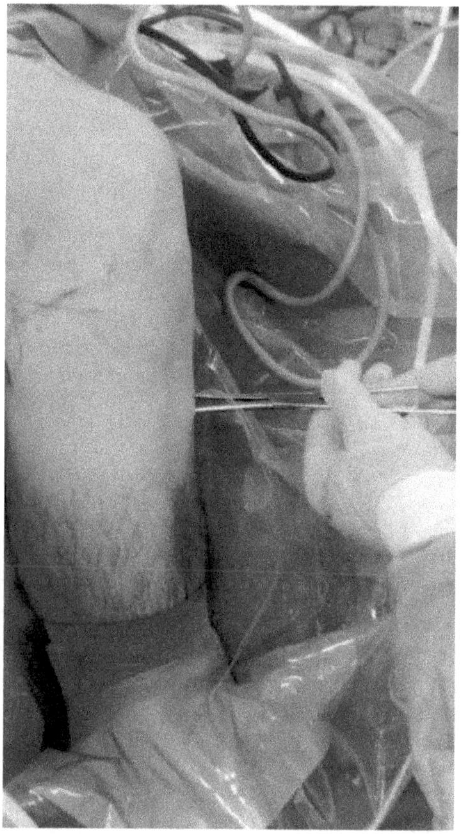

Figure 8.
Tensioning of the tenodesis by twisting the cortex button with Pean's forceps until the drive-through sign is eliminated.

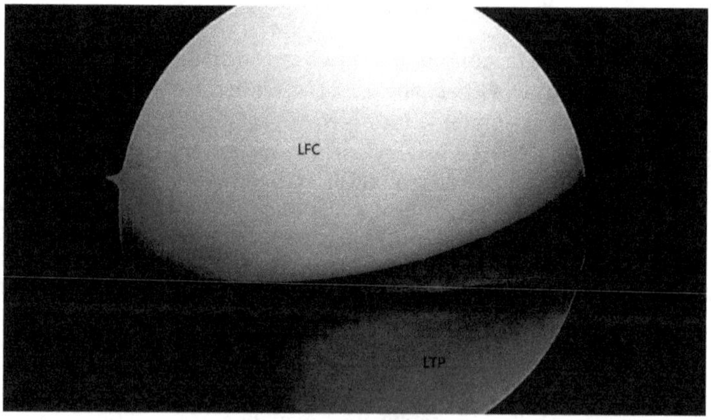

Figure 9.
Eliminated drive-through sign. LFC- lateral femoral condyle, LM- lateral meniscus, LTP- lateral tibial plateau.

Main disadvantage of presented technique is that it is limited to grade A PLRI and higher grades with varus instability require additional FCL reconstruction. Moreover, reconstruction of PFL is not possible. Being focused on static PLT function, its dynamic function may be lost. Furthermore, there is a risk of PLT or LM injury during mid-lateral portal formation. It is also worth noting that knee extension deficit may exclude applying this technique.

5. Arthroscopic-assisted anatomic PLC reconstruction

5.1 Indications and contraindications

The indications for this complex procedure are grade B and C PLC injuries according to Fanelli and Larson classification, especially when varus instability requiring FCL reconstruction is presented and excessive tibial external rotation which cannot be treated with PLT tenodesis is observed [23].

The contraindications are excessive varus deformity, poor bone quality, advanced degenerative joint disease, rheumatoid arthritis, limited range of motion.

5.2 Rationale for using arthroscopic-assisted anatomic PLC reconstruction

The rationale for using presented technique is a scientifically proved efficacy of anatomic PLC reconstructions in treatment of PLRI. Presented technique allows for a stepwise approach and management only this structure which has been damaged-PLT or FCL, or both. Whereas FCL reconstruction is obligatory in case of chronic lateral instability, in many patients the external rotation component of PLRI may be addressed with PLT tenodesis. However, when PLT femoral attachment is damaged or complete mid-substance tear occurs, anatomic PLT reconstruction is necessary.

5.3 Arthroscopic-assisted anatomic PLT reconstruction-surgical technique

The patient is positioned supine with a thigh tourniquet applied on operated leg, which is placed in a leg holder. The procedure is performed using standard anterolateral (AL) and anteromedial (AM) portals. When the diagnosis of PLC injury is confirmed, semitendinosus tendon (ST-T) is harvested, prepared as a graft and double folded on the suspensory fixation device. Then, additional arthroscopic portals are created: mid-lateral, which was described in the section about PLT tenodesis, and high mid-lateral portal, which is situated at the level of PLT femoral attachment. A retraction suture may be placed on PLT to facilitate maneuvering. With the knee in full extension tibial popliteus aiming guide (K.H prototype) or an ACL tibial aiming guide is used to create tibial tunnel for PLT reconstruction. Senior author prototype allows to drill the tunnel from posterolateral to anteromedial direction without the risk of uncontrolled common peroneal nerve injury, whereas an ACL aiming guide enforces the surgeon to drill in anteromedial-posterolateral direction. The tibial tunnel should be positioned as it was previously described for PLT tenodesis. The drill matched to the size of the graft is used to create the tunnel. Then the knee is flexed to 90°. An eyelet pin introduced through high mid-lateral portal is placed in the PLT femoral attachment and used as an aiming guide to direct the femoral tunnel to the point just above the medial femoral epicondyle. Then the drill matched to the size of the ST-T graft is used to create the tunnel. A passing suture is passed through the eye in the eyelet pin and the pin is pushed medially to introduce the passing suture into the femoral tunnel. The second passing suture is grasped with an arthroscopic grasper inserted through tibial tunnel and pulled out through tibial tunnel outside the joint. It is important to have both passing sutures in mid-lateral portal without tissue bridges between them. At first, the ST-T graft is passed with passing suture through tibial tunnel, then passed below the skin and introduced with the second passing suture to femoral tunnel. The graft is fixed on medial femoral cortex with suspensory cortical device and on the anteromedial tibial cortex with cortical button (**Figure 10**). In this way an anatomic PLT reconstruction was performed.

5.4 Minimally invasive anatomic FCL reconstruction-surgical technique

The procedure starts from harvesting gracilis tendon (GT-T). The graft is prepared and double folded on the suspensory cortex device. Then, with the knee in 90° of flexion, a 4–5 cm horizontal skin incision is done above the femoral FCL attachment and 3 cm vertical skin incision is made above the fibular head. Subcutaneous tissues are dissected to bony landmarks. An eyelet pin is placed in the native FCL femoral attachment just proximal and posterior to the lateral femoral epicondyle and used to direct the femoral tunnel toward the point above the medial femoral epicondyle. The drill matched to the size of GT-T graft is used to create femoral tunnel. Then, the eyelet pin is used to introduce the passing suture into the femoral tunnel. In the second step, the eyelet pin is placed in the middle of fibular head and used to position the fibulo-tibial tunnel from this point toward the point just below the MCL tibial insertion (**Figure 11**). The drill matched to the

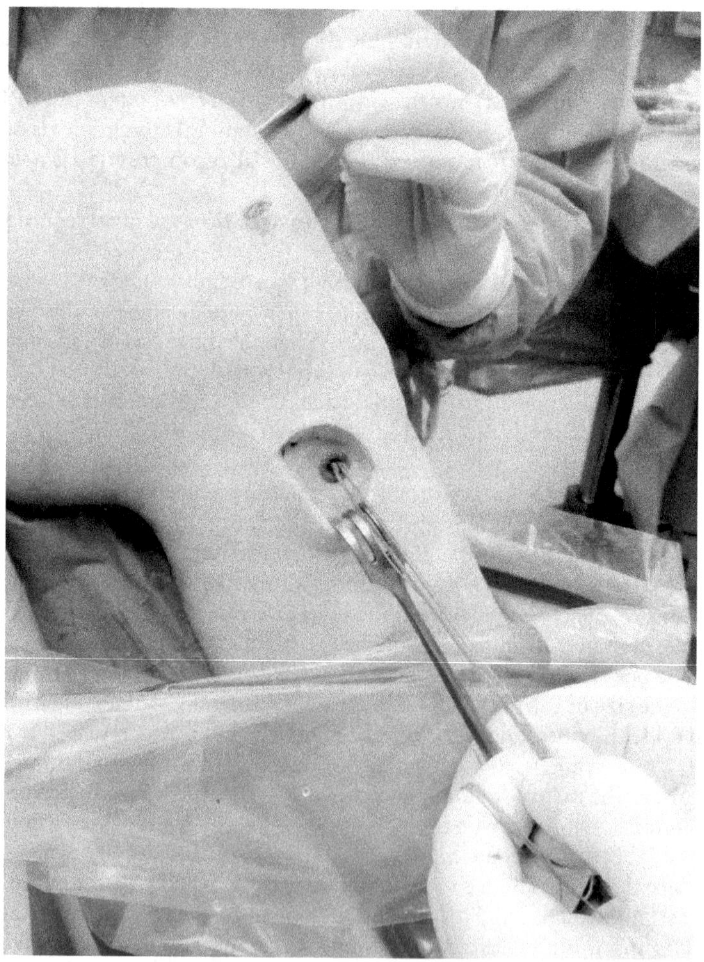

Figure 10.
Politeus tendon graft fixed on the anteromedial tibial cortex with cortical button.

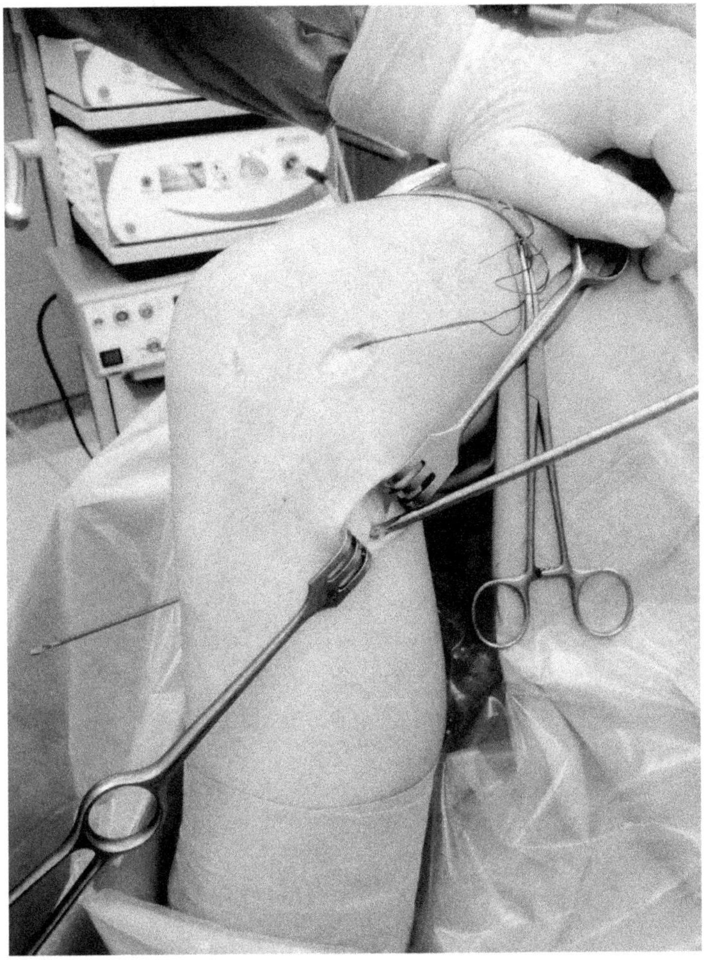

Figure 11.
Minimally invasive approach to fibular collateral ligament reconstruction. An eyelet pin and drill guide matched to the size of the graft are used to create tibial tunnel. Passing suture introduced to femoral tunnel may be observed.

size of the GT-T graft is used to create the tunnel and an eyelet pin is utilized to pass the second passing suture through the fibulo-tibial tunnel. The GT-T graft is passed through fibulo-tibial tunnel from medial to lateral, then passed below the skin and ITB using Pean's forceps and finally introduced into femoral tunnel using the first passing suture (**Figure 12**). The graft is fixed on medial femoral cortex with suspensory device, in the femoral FCL attachment and fibular head using 2 interference screws and additionally on the anteromedial tibial cortex using cortical button (**Figure 13**). In this way the FCL reconstruction is performed.

5.5 Postoperative rehabilitation

Postoperative rehabilitation protocol is similar to this described previously for arthroscopic PLT tenodesis.

5.6 Advantages and disadvantages

The main advantage of presented technique is that this is an anatomic reconstruction of the most important PLC structures with limited invasiveness and faster

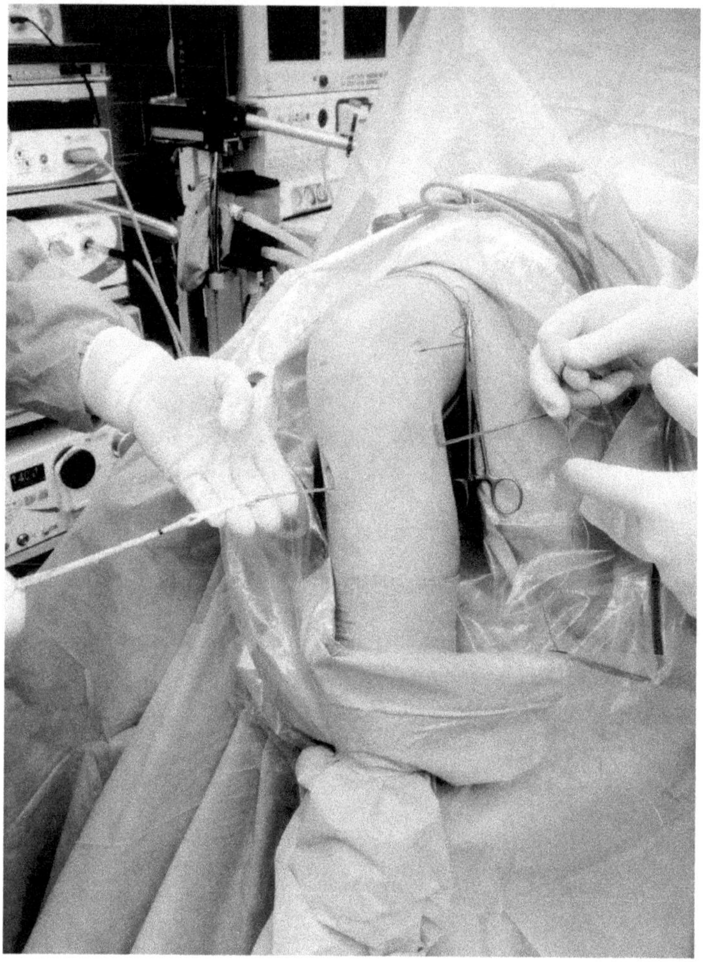

Figure 12.
The gracilis tendon graft is passed through tibial tunnel from medial to lateral, then passed below the skin and ITB and introduced to femoral tunnel using passing suture.

recovery in comparison to classic open surgeries. Both procedures can be performed as isolated surgeries. Moreover, fibular part of this technique may be used to stabilize the proximal tibio-fibular joint in case of instability. An another asset of this procedure is that there is no need for maneuvering in posterior knee compartment.

Despite its efficacy and many advantages, presented technique has also some disadvantages. Firstly, there is no possibly to reconstruct PFL in presented way. Secondly, more advanced surgical skills and some experience are required to perform it properly. Moreover, graft harvesting is required what can lead to donor-site morbidity. Improper tunnel positioning may lead to MCL symptoms as well as tunnel convergence during cruciate ligaments reconstructions in the future. Finally, in opposition to arthroscopic PLT tenodesis it is a costly procedure.

6. Discussion

More and more orthopedic surgeons are familiar with treatment of multi-ligament knee injuries [25]. Last two decades brought a great development in

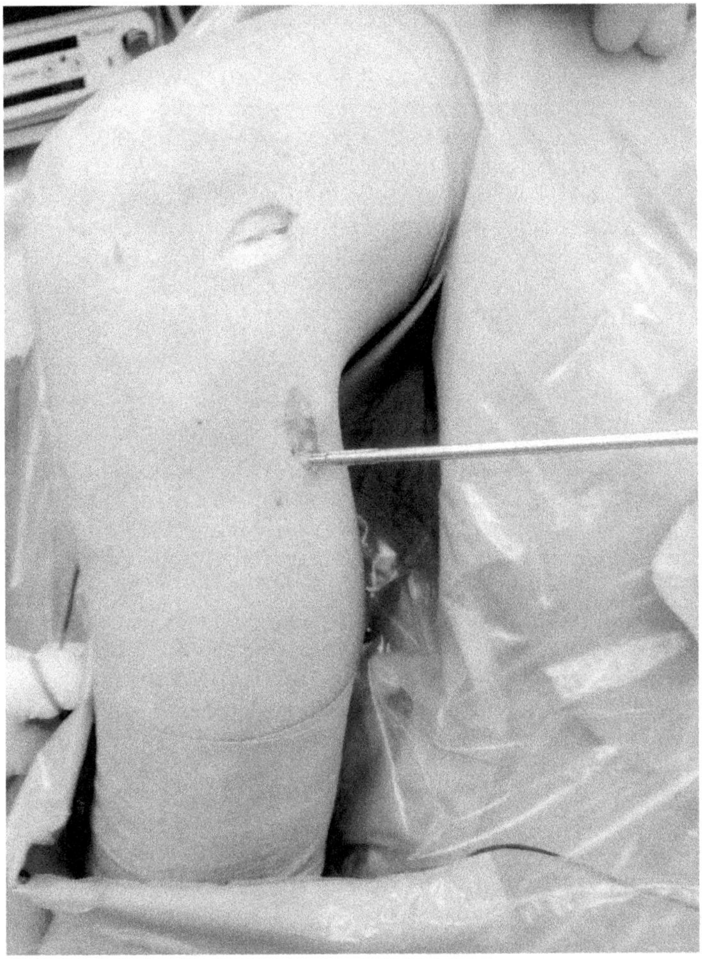

Figure 13.
Fixation of gracilis tendon graft in fibular head using interference screw.

understanding of anatomy, function and biomechanics not only of central knee structures like ACL, PCL and menisci, but also for so-called "knee corners" including PLC and PMC. That has put more interest on rotatory instabilities of the knee and caused introduction of many surgical techniques to address them [1–25]. A lot of surgical techniques were published, however only few presented results, what outlines the fact that objective measurement of rotatory knee stability remains difficult. Currently, reported results include patient subjective outcome scores, clinical examination findings and stress X-ray findings [21]. Each study presented significant increase in Lysholm score and International Knee Documentation Committee score and improvement in clinical exam after surgery [21]. However, it is worth noting that all these factors are subjective and at risk of bias. More objective factor, a stress X-ray, which allows to measure lateral joint line opening or posterior tibial translation, may be useful, but only in more complicated PLC injury patterns, usually with concomitant injuries. The "gray-zone" remain an isolated grade A or B posterolateral rotatory instabilities, where reporting of objective results is difficult. The solution may be a biomechanical cadaveric study. However, as it was previously said, overall success rate in PLC reconstructions may reach about 90% [21]. It depends, among others, on indications and techniques, which were applied. In cases of any doubt, expert consensus statement from 2019 is helpful to make a proper decision about treatment.

Most advantages and disadvantages of open and arthroscopic procedures were explained earlier in this chapter. A shift toward arthroscopic procedures was also outlined. Previously described reasons inspired senior authors (K.H, P.J) to develop arthroscopic PLT tenodesis and arthroscopic-assisted PLC reconstruction, which have been used by our team for many years. Indications, advantages and disadvantages of presented technique were described in detail. These methods meet with high patients satisfaction rate, significant improvement in clinical examination may be observed, thus in our opinions they are effective in treatment of PLRI, however studies on objective results lasts.

7. Conclusions

Posterolateral rotatory instability of the knee (PLRI), which is a consequence of injury to the structures of PLC, is a serious condition causing clinical symptoms and biomechanical changes which may lead to early osteoarthritis development and cruciate ligament reconstructions failures. Many clinical tests and imaging modalities are available for making a proper diagnosis and differentiate injured structures. It is widely accepted that only injured structures should be addressed, whereas reconstructions of structures which are not damaged should be avoided. Surgical treatment remains a gold-standard for high-grade PLC injuries. Arthroscopic popliteus tenodesis and minimally invasive arthroscopic-assisted PLC reconstruction are another surgical procedures which may be useful in hands of arthroscopic surgeons involved in the treatment of instabilities around the knee.

Conflict of interest

The authors declare no conflict of interest.

Author details

Adrian Góralczyk[1*], Piotr Jancewicz[2] and Krzysztof Hermanowicz[2]

1 Department of Orthopaedics and Traumatology, Hospital of Ministry of Internal Affairs and Administration in Bialystok, Bialystok, Poland

2 Ortim Orthopaedic Clinic, Bialystok, Poland

*Address all correspondence to: adriangoralczyk1@yahoo.com

References

[1] Hughes JD, Rauer T, Gibbs CM, Musahl V. Diagnosis and treatment of rotatory knee instability. J Exp Orthop. 2019 Dec 21;6(1):48. doi: 10.1186/s40634-019-0217-1.

[2] Engebretsen L, Lind M. Antero-medial rotatory laxity. Knee Surg Sports Traumatol Arthrosc. 2015 Oct;23(10):2797-2804. doi: 10.1007/s00167-015-3675-8.

[3] Chen FS, Rokito AS, Pitman MI. Acute and chronic posterolateral rotatory instability of the knee. J Am Acad Orthop Surg. 2000 Mar-Apr;8(2):97-110. Doi: 10.5435/00124635-200003000-00004.

[4] Shon OJ, Park JW, Kim BJ. Current concepts of Posterolateral corner injuries of the knee. Knee Surg Relat Res. 2017 Dec 1;29(4):256-268. doi: 10.5792/ksrr.16.029.

[5] Chahla J, Moatshe G, Dean CS, LaPrade RF. Posterolateral corner of the knee: Current concepts. Arch Bone Jt Surg. 2016 Apr;4(2):97-103.

[6] Crespo B, James EW, Metsavaht L, LaPrade RF. Injuries to posterolateral corner of the knee: A comprehensive review from anatomy to surgical treatment. Rev Bras Ortop. 2014 Dec 24;50(4):363-370. doi: 10.1016/j.rboe.2014.12.008.

[7] Frosch KH, Akoto R, Heitmann M, Enderle E, Giannakos A, Preiss A. Arthroscopic reconstruction of the popliteus complex: accuracy and reproducibility of a new surgical technique. Knee Surg Sports Traumatol Arthrosc. 2015 Oct;23(10):3114-20. doi: 10.1007/s00167-014-3000-y. Epub 2014 Apr 22. Erratum in: Knee Surg Sports Traumatol Arthrosc. 2016 Nov;24(11):3693.

[8] Nannaparaju M, Mortada S, Wiik A, Khan W, Alam M. Posterolateral corner injuries: Epidemiology, anatomy, biomechanics and diagnosis. Injury. 2018 Jun;49(6):1024-1031. doi: 10.1016/j.injury.2017.10.008.

[9] Djian P. Posterolateral knee reconstruction. Orthop Traumatol Surg Res. 2015 Feb;101(1 Suppl):S159-S170. doi: 10.1016/j.otsr.2014.07.032.

[10] Chahla J, Murray IR, Robinson J, Lagae K, Margheritini F, Fritsch B, Leyes M, Barenius B, Pujol N, Engebretsen L, Lind M, Cohen M, Maestu R, Getgood A, Ferrer G, Villascusa S, Uchida S, Levy BA, Von Bormann R, Brown C, Menetrey J, Hantes M, Lording T, Samuelsson K, Frosch KH, Monllau JC, Parker D, LaPrade RF, Gelber PE. Posterolateral corner of the knee: an expert consensus statement on diagnosis, classification, treatment, and rehabilitation. Knee Surg Sports Traumatol Arthrosc. 2019 Aug;27(8):2520-2529. doi: 10.1007/s00167-018-5260-4.

[11] James EW, Williams BT, LaPrade RF. Stress radiography for the diagnosis of knee ligament injuries: A systematic review. Clin Orthop Relat Res. 2014;472(9):2644-2657. doi:10.1007/s11999-014-3470-8

[12] Porrino J, Sharp JW, Ashimolowo T, Dunham G. An update and comprehensive review of the Posterolateral corner of the knee. Radiol Clin North Am. 2018 Nov;56(6):935-951. doi: 10.1016/j.rcl.2018.06.006.

[13] Fanelli GC, Larson RV. Practical management of posterolateral instability of the knee. Arthroscopy. 2002 Feb;18(2 Suppl 1):1-8. doi: 10.1053/jars.2002.31779.

[14] Frosch KH, Akoto R, Drenck T, Heitmann M, Pahl C, Preiss A. Arthroscopic popliteus bypass graft for posterolateral instabilities of the

knee: A new surgical technique. Oper Orthop Traumatol. 2016 Jun;28(3):193-203. doi: 10.1007/s00064-015-0432-6.

[15] Serra Cruz R, Mitchell JJ, Dean CS, Chahla J, Moatshe G, LaPrade RF. Anatomic Posterolateral corner reconstruction. Arthrosc Tech. 2016 Jun 6;5(3):e563-e572. doi: 10.1016/j.eats.2016.02.006.

[16] Zantop T, Petersen W. Posterolaterale Rekonstruktion des Kniegelenks nach Larson [Modified Larson technique for posterolateral corner reconstruction of the knee]. Oper Orthop Traumatol. 2010 Oct;22(4):373-86. German. doi: 10.1007/s00064-010-9030-9.

[17] Murgier J, Boisrenoult P, Steltzlen C, Beaufils P, Pujol N. Anatomical knee postero-lateral corner reconstruction: The "Versailles" technique. Orthop Traumatol Surg Res. 2017 Nov;103(7):1031-1034. doi: 10.1016/j.otsr.2017.05.026.

[18] Ohnishi Y, Pascual-Garrido C, Kumagae H, Sakai A, Uchida S. Arthroscopic technique for isolated Posterolateral rotational instability of the knee. Arthrosc Tech. 2017 Mar 6;6(2):e291-e295. doi: 10.1016/j.eats.2016.09.033.

[19] Frings J, Kolb JP, Drenck TC, Krause M, Alm L, Akoto R, Frosch KH. Anatomic reconstruction of the Posterolateral corner: An all-arthroscopic technique. Arthrosc Tech. 2019 Jan 21;8(2):e153-e161. doi: 10.1016/j.eats.2018.10.010.

[20] Weiss S, Krause M, Frosch KH. Posterolateral corner of the knee: A systematic literature review of current concepts of arthroscopic reconstruction. Arch Orthop Trauma Surg. 2020 Dec;140(12):2003-2012. doi: 10.1007/s00402-020-03607-z.

[21] Moulton SG, Geeslin AG, LaPrade RF. A systematic review of the outcomes of Posterolateral corner knee injuries, part 2: Surgical treatment of chronic injuries. Am J Sports Med. 2016 Jun;44(6):1616-1623. Doi: 10.1177/0363546515593950.

[22] Hermanowicz K, Góralczyk A, Malinowski K, Jancewicz P. Arthroscopic Posterolateral corner stabilization with Popliteus Tenodesis. Arthrosc Tech. 2018 May 28;7(6):e669-e674. doi: 10.1016/j.eats.2018.02.015.

[23] Hermanowicz K, Malinowski K, Góralczyk A, Guszczyn T, LaPrade RF. Minimally Invasive, Arthroscopic-assisted, Anatomic Posterolateral Corner Reconstruction. Arthrosc Tech. 2019 Feb 11;8(3):e251-e257. doi: 10.1016/j.eats.2018.10.021.

[24] Krause M, Akoto R, Drenck TC, Frosch KH, Preiss A. Posterolateral rotatory knee instability-MRI evaluation of anatomic landmarks for Tibial drill tunnel placement in open and arthroscopic Popliteus tendon reconstruction. J Knee Surg. 2019 Jul;32(7):667-672. doi: 10.1055/s-0038-1666832.

[25] Ng JWG, Myint Y, Ali FM. Management of multiligament knee injuries. EFORT Open Rev. 2020 Mar 2;5(3):145-155. doi: 10.1302/2058-5241.5.190012. PMID: 32296548; PMCID: PMC7144894.

Chapter 3

Risk Factors of ACL Injury

Nuthan Jagadeesh, Sachindra Kapadi, Venkatesh Deva and Ankur Kariya

Abstract

An anterior cruciate ligament(ACL) is one of the major stabilizers of the knee joint, injury to which can be quite dreadful even ending many sports careers if not properly treated. Knowledge of the risk factors contributing to ACL injury will help in identifying at-risk individuals and develop preventive strategies. The factors contributing to ACL injury are multi-factorial involving biomechanical, anatomical, hormonal, neuromuscular factors etc; and can be broadly classified as Intrinsic and Extrinsic factors. Intrinsic factors are mostly non-modifiable risk factors may be subdivided into anatomical, genetic, gender, previous ACL Injuries etc. Whereas Extrinsic factors are mostly modifiable risk factors include environmental factors, characteristic of surface and shoe, BMI and others. Anatomical risk factors can divided into tibial parameters like posterior tibial slope, medial tibial plateau depth etc; femoral parameters like notch width, notch index etc.

Keywords: risk factors of ACL injury, Notch index, posterior tibial slope, prevention of ACL injury

1. Introduction

The Anterior Cruciate ligament (ACL) is said to be one of the most important stabilisers of the knee preventing the anterior translation of the tibia over the femur. Injuries to the anterior Cruciate ligament commonly occur during sports and are caused usually by sudden stops or change in direction while running, jumping and landing [1–4]. These injuries are quite disabling and take a significant amount of time to recover and rehabilitate despite the surgery. Moreover, people with these injuries tend to end up with increased articular wear with time and end up with early post-traumatic arthritis even with the best of surgeries [5].

ACL injuries have been increasingly common in elite athletes who have ramifications in terms of contract/scholastic obligations, sponsorships and revenue-generating potential. Though the number of people returning to sports post ACL reconstruction has increased, most professional sportsperson face challenges of returning to preinjury level and performances expected of them. As most of them, do not return to a high level of performance, many careers have ended or shortened because of ACL injury when compared to those without the injury [6, 7]. Consequently, it's important to identify the risk factors which might lead to an increased probability of ACL injury so that preventive measures can be taken.

Risk factors of ACL injury could be divided into two major categories like intrinsic and extrinsic [8]. Intrinsic factors include those which are innate to the individual and are usually non-modifiable. These include factors such as anatomic factors (Notch parameters, posterior tibial slope, lower extremity alignment etc.), neuromuscular factors, genetic factors, hormonal milieus and cognitive function. Extrinsic factors are those which surround the athlete and may include level and intensity of games or activity, playing surface and environmental conditions, as well as equipment used [9–12]. In this chapter, we have attempted to create a comprehensive yet exhaustive list of the risk factors contributing to ACL injury.

2. Material and methods

In this review of literature, the authors have used Pubmed database to search for various studies that factors that may contribute to ACL injury. The authors used the keywords anterior cruciate ligament, risk factors, extrinsic risk factors, intrinsic risk factors to search for articles. After eliminating the duplicates, the authors identified the trends and patterns in the risk factors and have summarised the findings in this article to create a concise review for readers and students.

3. Discussion

3.1 Intrinsic factors

3.1.1 Anatomical factors

The anatomic factors have been studied thoroughly these days as these factors could be picked up easily by investigations pertaining to the diagnosis of ACL injuries like knee radiographs and MRI. Establishing correlation with these anatomic factors could help us in establishing a reliable tool in screening individuals at risk of ACL injury. Variations in these anatomical features are well documented in individuals especially between men and women which may explain why women are maybe at more risk of ACL injury than men. Various anatomic factors commonly studied include those related to knee geometry, alignment of the lower extremity, knee laxity, and body mass index [12, 13]. Factors related to knee geometry can be divided into a) tibial parameters like posterior tibial slope, depth of medial tibial plateau b) femoral/ notch parameters like notch width, bicondylar width, notch width index.

3.1.1.1 Notch parameters

Notch parameters have been one of the widely researched risk factors related to an ACL injury but there are wide differences in the way these parameters are measured. The femoral attachment of ACL is in the medial aspect of lateral femoral condyle over lateral intercondylar ridge [14, 15]. It is observed that impinging of ACL at various knee positions are well documented especially in those with narrow notch width. But controversy exists whether it's due to geometry and size of notch itself, or due to volume of ACL or amalgamation of these characteristics [16]. It's proven that women are known to have smaller notches when compared to males and that the people with smaller notches tend to have thinner and weaker ACL compared to those with wider notch [17–19]. The stenotic notches cause ACL impingement over the lateral femoral condyle and if the knee is subjected to any anterior shear force or tibial rotational forces causing rupture of ACL ligament [20–23].

LaPrade et all demonstrated that there is an increased risk of ACL injury in people with a narrow intercondylar notch [24, 25]. Souryal et all in their study on bilateral ACL injuries found narrow notch width to be associated but they used only the plain radiographs to calculate the Notch width. The major drawback of these studies was that they were done on plain radiographs where errors due to magnification were common. A notch width index was thus used to overcome these issues. Notch width index (NWI) can be measured using tunnel view radiographs or Coronal section MRI. The NWI was identified as the ratio of the width of the intercondylar notch to the width of the distal femur at the level of the popliteal groove. Souryal et al. used a tunnel view of radiographs and compared patients with unilateral and bilateral ACL injuries and found that patient with bilateral ACL ruptures have significantly smaller notch and NWI when compared to those with unilateral ACL ruptures. Moreover, they found no difference in NWI of unilateral ACL ruptures when compared to those with normal knees. Furthermore, they conducted a cohort study and reported that men athlete had higher NWI compared to female athletes who suffered ACL injuries when compared to those uninjured ones [26, 27]. S.M. Fahim et all in their randomised control study used MRI for the calculation for NWI, reported that there were no differences in NWI in either sex and the NWI was significantly lower in those with ACL injury [28]. Ashwini et al., in their MRI based comparative study, demonstrated that people with ACL injury had NWI of 0.29 ± 0.02 or lesser compared to those without an ACL injury, whereas Bhasukala et al., postulated the cutoff of NWI to be 0.28 ± 0.06.21. S.M. Fahim Et all reported cut off value of 0.29 with a sensitivity of 90% and specificity of 86.7%. However, Gormeli CA et al. In their study on bilateral knees with ACL injury demonstrated cut-off values of NWI of 0.22 ± 0.008 in bilateral injured knees and 0.24 ± 0.01 in the unilateral injured knee [29–31]. So the cut off varies depending on the ethnicity and the exact cutoff values are still controversial but most authors have concluded the critical value NWI ranging from 0.19 to 0.26.

The shape of the intercondylar notch is another parameter frequently studied with regards to the notch shape that is most associated with an ACL injury [32–34]. We could use a semi-quantitative approach to classify the various intercondylar notch shapes. It is classified into three shapes i.e. A, Inverse U, and Omega (U). Two parameters are calculated to ascertain the notch shape viz. notch width at the level of the popliteal groove(NWP) and notch width at the joint line(NWJ). If NWP equal to or near equal to NWJ, then the notch is of "U" shape. If NWP < NWJ then the notch is of "A" shape.If the NWP > NWJ then the notch shape is of Omega shape. 'A' shaped femoral notch is commonly associated with ACL injury whereas an inverted U shaped notch is more favourable to prevent ACL injury [29, 30, 35].

Overall, most authors found a positive relationship with an ACL injury and narrow notch and smaller NWI increased the risk of ACL injury I.e as intercondylar notch width decreases, an increase in ACL injury risk is observed.

3.1.1.2 Posterior tibial slope

Several studies related to proven multiple times that the Posterior tibial slope could be the major factor contributing to the stability of the knee joint [35, 36]. Cadaveric studies have shown that an increased posterior tibial slope has resulted in an increased anterior translation of tibia over the femur, thus increasing stresses on the ACL ligament especially during active gait [37, 38]. The posterior tibial slope is traditionally measured on lateral knee radiograph, the tibial axis is to be drawn connecting midpoints of lines connecting anterior and posterior cortex 4-5 cm apart as caudally as possible from the joint line. The angle between tangent connecting anterior and posterior cortex at joint and line perpendicular to the tibial axis corresponds posterior tibial slope in lateral knee radiograph. But again controversies regarding errors due to magnification or lack of true lateral radiographs and inability to measure lateral posterior tibial slope(LPTS) and medial Posterior tibial slope(MPTS) have resulted in calculating these parameters in an MRI. To measure the medial and lateral posterior tibial slope on MRI first is to determine the tibial axis. For this, a sagittal section at the centre of the knee which contains intercondylar eminence and PCL attachment is selected. Two lines joining anterior and posterior cortices was drawn approximately 4-5 cm apart as caudally as possible from the joint line, the line joining the midpoint of the above two lines corresponds to the tibial axis. (**Figure 1**) Now the sagittal section of the centre of the lateral tibial plateau is identified, a tangent connecting the anterosuperior cortex to the posteroinferior cortex is drawn. The angle between the above tangent and the line perpendicular to the tibial axis corresponds to the medial posterior tibial slope. A similar technique is to be used to measure Lateral posterior tibial slope by drawing tangent at the centre of the lateral tibial plateau (**Figures 2** and **3**). A detailed view of MRI have found lateral posterior tibial slope(LPTS) to be more involved with ACL injury than medial Posterior tibial slope(MPTS) [39] but a meta-analysis has shown that ACL injury was associated with

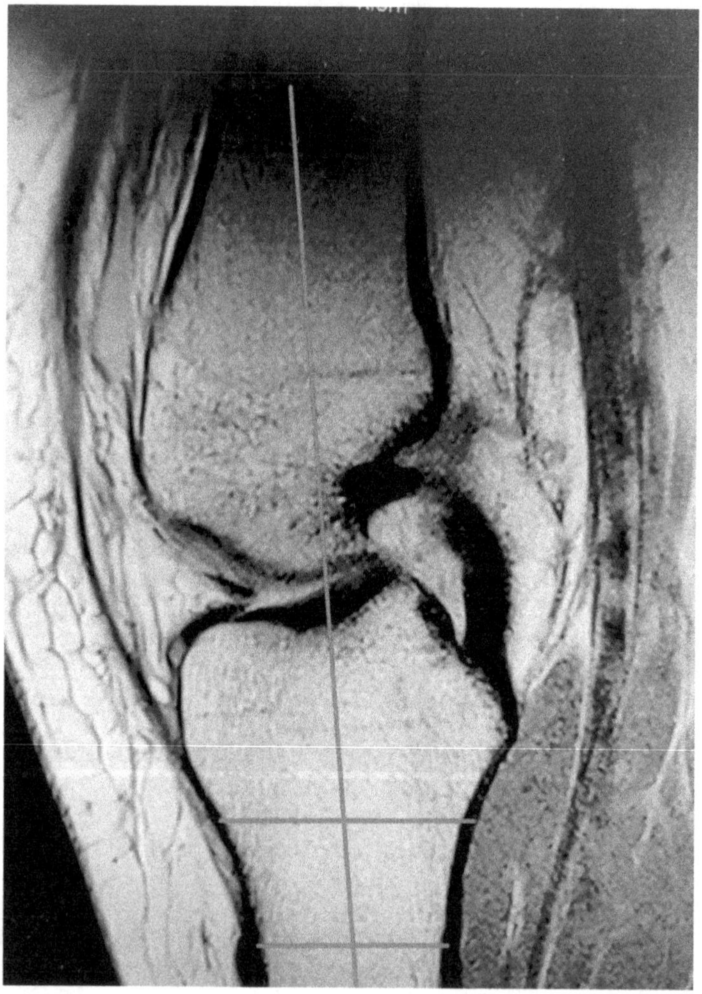

Figure 1.
MRI picture depicting calculation of Tibial Axis.

medial and lateral PTS [40]. Hashemi et all [41], in their study of 104 patients, both MTPS and LTPS were increased, injured group. Though females had higher LTPS than males they concluded that increased lateral posterior-directed tibial plateau slope is one of the major risk factor irrespective of gender. Whereas MPTS was significantly increased only in men. Stijak et all, in their utilised both knee radiographs and the MRI, to determine the correlation between PTS and lateral plateau and concluded that increased lateral PTS was seen among the ACL injury cohort compared to the ACL intact cohort but they found increased MPTS in the uninjured group when compared to the injured cohort. They suggested that an increase in LTPS would influence the rotation of the knee joint causing pivoting of the knee. In our study, Both MPTS and LTPS had a positive correlation with ACL injury they were significantly increased in the ACL tear group when compared to uninjured group irrespective of the gender. Females had higher MPTS and LTPS when compared to males in both groups but the difference was statistically significant in either sex.

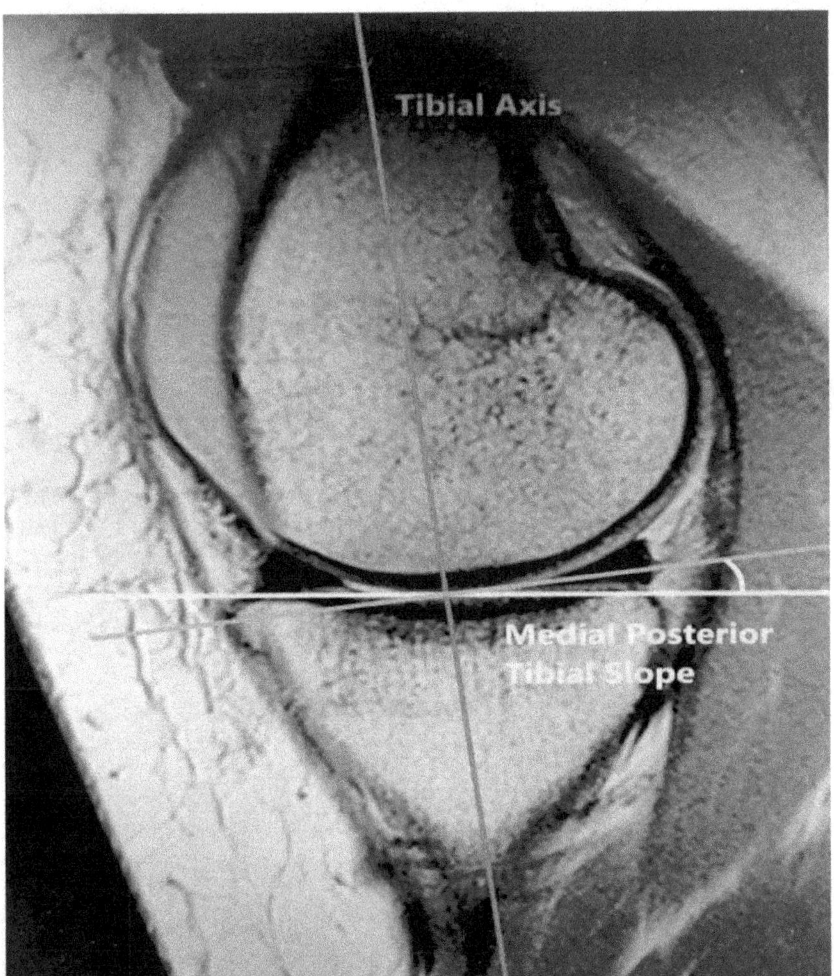

Figure 2.
MRI picture depicting calculation of medial posterior Tibial slope(MPTS).

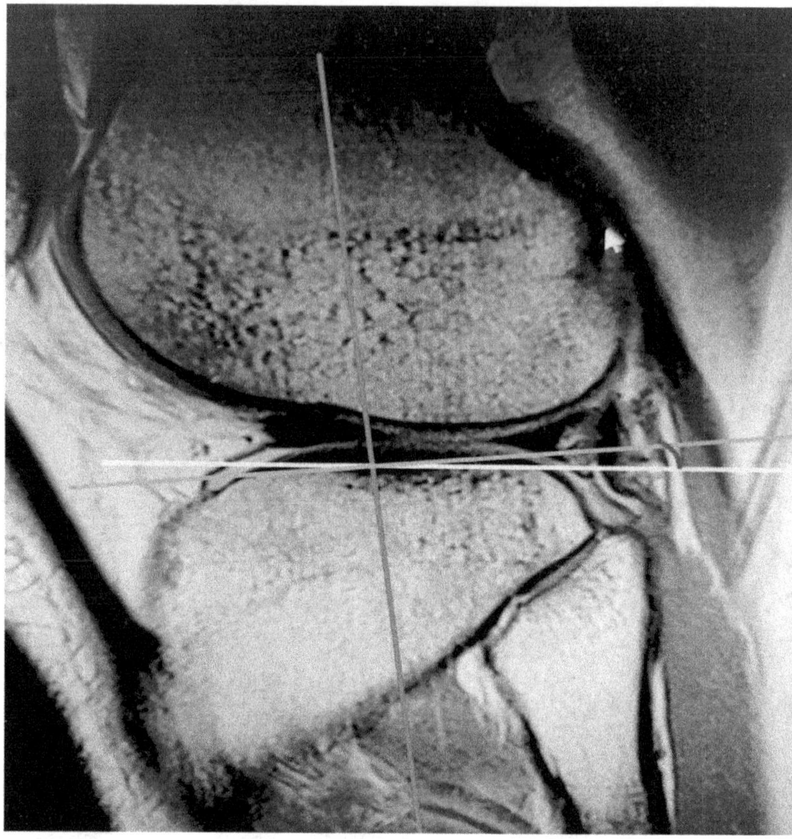

Figure 3.
MRI picture depicting calculation of lateral posterior Tibial slope(MPTS).

3.1.1.3 Medial tibial plateau depth

Other tibial medial parameters assessed are with the correlation of medial and lateral tibial plateau depth with an ACL injury but the evidence in this regard is very limited. It is measured with two parallel lines line drawn, one connecting the highest point of anterior and posterior points of the medial tibial plateau and the other line is tangent drawn at the deepest point of the medial tibial plateau, the distance between these two lines corresponds to medial tibial plateau depth. Hashemi et al. suggested that deepening of the surface of the medial tibial plateau leads to better joint congruity and prevents anterior translation of the tibia. In their study, they concluded that decreased MTD is associated with a greater risk of ACL injury. They found MTD to be a bigger risk factor than LPTS or MPTS whereas Blanke F et all suggested there is no correlation of medial tibial plateau death with an ACL injury [41–44]. More research in this area is required to come to a proper consensus on the influence of MTPD in ACL injury.

3.1.1.4 Other factors

Other parameters said to be associated with ACL injury are subtalar pronation, knee recurvatum, quadricep angle but the mechanism of how these parameters affect and evidence regarding its association is very limited.

3.1.2 Neuromuscular risk factors

In Contrast to anatomical risk factors which non-modifiable without surgical intervention, neuromuscular deficit are often modifiable risk factors. Intervention could reduce the risk of ACL injuries. Better control over the core body and improved proprioceptive control over the lower extremity have said to be associated with reduced risk of ACL injury. Proprioceptive performance can be improved by exercises improving muscle strength, synergistic coordination etc. which in turn help to reduce the risk of ACL injury. The mechanism of ACL injury occurs when the athlete takes off from valgus positioned knee, during which the knee is typically in 10–30° of flexion and tries to internally rotate the externally rotated foot aiming to suddenly change the direction.

There is a greater risk of injury to ACL injury when the knee is in abduction, there are intersegmental abduction movements and increased ground reaction force with decreased stance time. A study by Hewett et al. showed that when landing from jump in double leg stance, increased knee abduction angle and intersegmental forces, greater ground reaction force and shorter stance time caused increased ACL injuries [44–48].

A small knee flexion angle coupled with strong quadriceps contraction during sports activity will cause increased posterior loading on the knee. As a result, this increases ACL injury risk.

In female athletes, while landing from heigh during a jump, they perform cutting and pivoting manoeuvres with less knee flexion and hip flexion, increased valgus at the knee, increased internal rotation of the hip coupled with increased external rotation of the tibia and increased quadriceps muscle activation caused increased ACL injury due to increased strain on the knee.

Females have poor neuromuscular control of hamstrings and weaker gluteus medius strength, weaker hip abductors which coupled with poor landing mechanism increases the risk of ACL injury.

Balance training, core strengthening, jump training, dynamic joint stability and plyometric exercises training increased core stability and improved proprioception, which reduced the risk of ACL injury.

When the knee is in valgus loading the medial collateral ligament becomes taut and lateral compression occurs. This as well as the anterior force vector caused by quadriceps contraction causes the lateral femoral condyle to shift posteriorly and the tibia shifts anteriorly and internally rotates, resulting in ACL rupture.

3.1.3 Sex differences

Anterior cruciate ligament tears vary in incidence by gender being more common among women. In fact, studies have shown that the rate of ACL tears could be 9 times more common in women as compared to men [49]. Many studies have tried to study the exact reason for this sex-based discrepancy in ACL injuries. Though the exact reason still remains unclear, it appears there are various intercalated intrinsic factors that lead to this. The possible factors could be due to their unique effects of sex hormones, anatomic differences in the female ACL s and/or neuromuscular control variations among the sexes [50].

Female athletes have been found to have different movement and muscle activation patterns [51, 52]. Females while jumping, due to their increased quadriceps activation coupled with decreased hip and knee flexion increases the load on the ACL, thus injuring it [53]. A study conducted by Anderson et al. have found that the lack of stiffness and strength in the quadriceps and hamstrings in females along with anatomically smaller ACLs predispose them to injuries [52]. Furthermore, female athletes displayed greater knee laxity values as compared to their male counterparts [54].

Anthropometric studies on ACL have shown Intercondylar notch is an anatomic factor that has links to the risk of ACL injuries [55, 56]. Subjects with a narrow/ stenotic intercondylar notch have a higher incidence of ACL injury. Therefore, females by the virtue of having smaller intercondylar notch and notch width index, have an increased likelihood of sustaining an ACL injury [57].

3.1.4 Hormonal risk factors

There is wide variations in hormonal milieu over the course of menstrual in females. The occurrence of ACL injuries has been found to have an association with the menstrual cycle phase. The reason for this may be because of the presence of progesterone and oestrogen receptor sites on the ACL [58–60]. However, all the studies on this have been either in vitro or in animal models and the presence of these receptors on human ACLs have not been proved. The hypothesis is that oestrogen has an effect on the synthesis and breakdown of the matrix components of ACL. The rate of occurrence of ACL injuries is more during the ovulatory phase of the menstrual cycle, which is hallmarked by high concentrations of serum oestrogen [58, 59]. What's perplexing about these injuries in women is that they have been found to occur during non-contact event usually due to deceleration or a change of direction manoeuvre rather than a direct impact injury [61]. Oestrogen decreases the rate of proliferation of fibroblast and synthesis of types I procollagen whilst progesterone promotes the same [62]. Hence this variation in the concentration of oestrogen and progesterone in the various phases of menstruation influence the materialistic properties of ACL. Thus, ACL injuries in women are more common during the pre-ovulatory phase of menstruation, when the serum oestrogen levels are high [63].

3.1.5 Familial predisposition

There is some evidence to prove that ACL injuries do have a familial predisposition. A study conducted by Flynn et al. showed that people with anterior cruciate ligament tear were twice as likely to have a relative who has an anterior cruciate ligament tear as compared to the controls [64]. They concluded from this study that there is a familial predisposition to an anterior cruciate ligament tear. Another study by Harner et al. found that the incidence of anterior cruciate ligament tear was higher in the patients who have had a family history of ACL injury [65]. However, these studies have not looked into the similarities between the patients and their family. A study by Goshima et al. looked into the mechanism, situation and the types of sports played between patients and their family members to avoid bias [66]. They found that there was a strong familial predisposition to ACL injuries. Furthermore, individuals with FH of ACL injury had an increased risk of repeat ACL injuries and thus require prevention programs.

3.1.6 Genetic risk factors

Mutation in the specific genetic sequence variants of genes that code for the extracellular matric of the ACL are found to predispose such individuals to ACL injury. These genes include COL1A1, COL5A1 and COL12A1. The COL1A1 gene codes for the primary subunit of type 1 collagen which I the primary constituent of the ACL matrix. The TT genotype of the COL1A1 gene was found to be underrepresented in patients with ACL ruptures as compared to those with control. These studies concluded that individuals with TT genotype of COL1A1 gene are less prone to ACL tears [67]. The COL5A1 gene codes for a major subunit of type V collagen which is a minor constituent of the ACL. A recent study showed that mutation of this gene was associated with ACL ruptures in these individuals [68]. The COL12A1 gene codes for collagen XII which is involved in the fibrillogenesis of ACL. In a recent study by Posthumus et al., it was found that COL12A1 AluI RFLP was found to be associated with ACL ruptures [69].

Matrix metalloproteins that are physiological mediators of collagen cleavage and removal are located on chromosome 11q22. A study done by Posthumus et al. this found that underrepresentation of the AG and GG genotypes caused an increased incidence of ACL injuries [70]. However, these factors are usually associated with other intrinsic and extrinsic factors and their independent association is difficult to determine. It is important that genetic variants be determined in various at-risk population and their phenotypes identified.

3.1.7 Cognitive function risk factor

Neurocognitive performance is one risk factor that has been understudied, though it is potentially a modifiable risk factor. Researchers have been looking into the association of loss of neuromuscular control and noncontact ACL injuries. They hypothesised that reduced baseline neurocognitive functions predispose an individual to ACL injuries. Athletes who had suffered ACL injuries were demonstrated significantly slower reaction time and processing speed. Furthermore, they performed poorly on visual and verbal memory composite scores as compared to the controls. Poor neurocognitive performance is associated with reduced neuromuscular control and coordination issues thereby causing ACL injuries [71].

3.1.8 Previous injury

Previous ACL injury and reconstruction is in itself a risk factor for injury of the contralateral ACL and reinjury of the reconstructed ACL as well [72]. It was found that football players with an old ACL injury and/or reconstruction were predisposed to an ACL injury in either the contralateral knee ACL or the reconstructed ACL graft [73]. Patients who have had ACL reconstruction in the past 12 months have 11 times the risk of sustaining a new / re-injury of the ACL. Some researchers have looked into the incidence of ACL injury in patients who have had other musculoskeletal injuries. It was seen that previous ankle injuries had a correlation to the likelihood of sustaining an ACL injury [74]. However, the site of previous injury and the recovery from the same dictates the risk of having an ACL injury. For example, patients with injuries of the lower limb and trunk have a greater predilection of sustaining an ACL injury as compared to those of the upper limb. Rehabilitation from the injury to pre-injury levels also reduces the risk of sustaining an ACL injury in the future.

4. Extrinsic risk factors

Extrinsic risk factors are the environmental factors, which predispose a person to ACL injury [75–79]. Firstly, weather plays a role wet and rainy days have an increased risk of Anterior cruciate ligament injury as they decrease friction in-between shoes and field. As a result, there is a greater risk of ACL injury. In addition, there is more risk of ACL injury in hot weather as heat increases ligament extensibility predisposing the patent to ACL injury. Orchard et al. prospective study showed increased risk with hot climate for ACL injury [76–79].

Secondly, the type of Cleats on shoes play a role in ACL injury. Cleats that have higher torsion such as edge cleats have higher resistance and will increase the risk of Anterior cruciate injury. Lampson et al. prospective study showed that cleats with higher torsional resistance have a significant risk of ACL injury. Their study was conducted on 3119 athletes which showed that 42 Athletes with edge cleats had ACL injuries which showed a higher predisposition to ACL injury with Edge cleats. Cleats design such as flat cleats, small cleats and fewer cleats had a fewer ACL injury [75].

Another factor that can contribute to the risk of ACL injury is the surface of the field. The field which has Bermuda grass have a higher risk of ACL injury compared to the field with Ryegrass due to cleats getting trapped in Bermuda grass. Orchard et al. prospective study show an increased risk of trapping in Bermuda grass compared to the field with Ryegrass, but this study did not take into account the different cleats used by the players [76–79].

Another study by Olsen Et al, compared ACL injuries in handball players in synthetic and wooden courts. They have found that the incidence of ACL injuries was 2.35 times higher in synthetic courts compared to the wooden courts [49]. There is usually an interplay between the foot ware and surface of which indoor games take place which increases the ACL injury risk and similar interplay could play in outdoor activities as well in combination with the weather conditions.

5. Conclusion

Several intrinsic and extrinsic risk factors contribute to ACL injury. Focus must be on modifiable risk factors in order to mitigate the risk of ACL tears. In depth knowledge and understanding of these risk fators can help surgeons and physiotherapists to educate patients and sportspersons on prevention of ACL tears.and identify at risk individual (**Table 1**).

Intrinsic risk factors		
Anatomical risk factors		
Tibial Parameters		
Posterior tibial slope	Increased posterior tibial slope associated with increased translation of tibia over femur	
Medial tibial plateau depth	Increased MTD prevents tibial translation. Increased congruence of tibial plateau reduces the risk of ACL tear	
Notch parameters		
Notch width index	Narrow notch area associated with thinner ACLs Stenotic notch is associated with impingement of ACL	Notch width index <0.29 associated with high risk
Shape of intercondylar notch	Three shapes based on notch width at the level of patellar groove (NWP) and at the level of joint line (NWJ)	'A' shaped femoral notch is commonly associated with ACL injury
Other factors	subtalar pronation knee recurvatum quadricep angle, neuromuscular factors	

Intrinsic risk factors	
Gender	More common in females Hormonal effects Anatomical variations in ACL Neuromuscular variation Differences in movements and muscle activation patterns Greater knee laxity Smaller intercondylar notch
Hormonal risk factors	ACL injury more common in pre- ovulatory phase due to high oestrogen
Familial and genetic risk factors	Two times higher risk with family history Mutations in COL1A1, COL5A1 and COL12A1 chromosome 11q22
Cognitive function	Poor neurocognitive performance is associated with reduced neuromuscular control and coordination issues thereby causing ACL injurie
Previous injury	11 times higher risk of ACL injury on same side after reconstruction or opposite side Previous ankle injury
Extrinsic risk factors	
Weather	Wet and rainy days – reduced friction with surface Hot weather – increased ligament extensibility
Type of cleat on shoes	Edge cleats – higher risk of torsion – higher risk of injury
Type of grass	Higher risk with Bermuda grass as compared to ryegrass due to trapping of cleats in Bermuda grass
Type of courts	2.35 times higher in synthetic courts compared to the wooden courts.

Table 1.
Summary of all the risk factors of ACL injury.

Author details

Nuthan Jagadeesh*, Sachindra Kapadi, Venkatesh Deva and Ankur Kariya
Wrightington Wigan and Leigh NHS Foundation Trust, Wigan, United Kingdom

*Address all correspondence to: nuthanjagadeesh@yahoo.com

References

[1] Kobayashi H, Kanamura T, Koshida S, et al (2010) Mechanisms of the anterior cruciate ligament injury in sports activities: a twenty-year clinical research of 1,700 athletes. J Sports Sci Med 9(4):669-675 PubMed PubMed Central Google Scholar

[2] Brophy RH, Stepan JG, Silvers HJ, Mandelbaum BR (2015) Defending puts the anterior cruciate ligament at risk during soccer: a gender-based analysis. Sports Health 7(3):244-249.

[3] Walden M, Krosshaug T, Bjorneboe J, Andersen TE, Faul O, Hagglund M (2015) Three distinct mechanisms predominate in non-contact anterior cruciate ligament injuries in male professional football players: a systematic video analysis of 39 cases. Br J Sports Med 49(22):1452-1460

[4] Shimokochi Y, Shultz SJ (2008) Mechanisms of noncontact anterior cruciate ligament injury. J Athl Train 43(4):396-408

[5] Lohmander LS, Ostenberg A, Englund M, Roos H. High prevalence of knee osteoarthritis, pain, and functional limitations in female soccer players twelve years after anterior cruciate ligament injury. Arthritis Rheum. 2004;50:3145-3152.

[6] Mihata LCS, Beutler AI, Boden BP. Comparing the incidence of anterior cruciate ligament injury in collegiate lacrosse, soccer, and basketball players: implications for anterior cruciate ligament mechanism and prevention. Am J Sports Med. 2006;34:899-904.

[7] Buerba RA, Zaffagnini S, Kuroda R, et al. ACL reconstruction in the professional or elite athlete: state of the art Journal of ISAKOS: Joint Disorders & Orthopaedic Sports Medicine Published Online First: 16 February 2021. doi: 10.1136/jisakos-2020-000456

[8] Williams JPG. Aetiologic classification of sports injuries. Br J Sports Med. 1971;4:228-230.

[9] Hudek R, Schmutz S, Regenfelder F, Fuchs B, Koch PP. Novel Measurement Technique of the Tibial Slope on Conventional MRI. Clin Orthop Relat Res. 2009 Aug;467(8):2066-72. DOI: 10.1007/s11999-009-0711-3

[10] Canale ST, Beaty JH, Campbell WC, Daugherty K, Burns B. Campbell's operative orthopedics: get full access and more at ExpertConsult.com. 12. ed., internet. ed. Philadelphia, Pa: Elsevier, Mosby; 2013. ISBN: 978-0-8089-2430-2 978-0-323-07243-4

[11] Shelbourne KD, Facibene WA, Hunt JJ. Radiographic and intraoperative intercondylar notch width measurements in men and women with unilateral and bilateral anterior cruciate ligament tears. Knee Surg Sports Traumatol Arthrosc. 1997 Oct 21;5(4):229-33. DOI: 10.1007/s001670050055

[12] Shultz SJ, Schmitz RJ, Nguyen AD, et al. ACL Research Retreat V: an update on ACL injury risk and prevention, March 25-27, 2010, Greensboro, NC. J AthlTrain. 2010;45:499-508.

[13] Griffin LY, Agel J, Albohm M, Arendt EA, et al. Noncontact anterior cruciate ligament injuries: risk factors and prevention strategies. J Am Acad Orthop Surg. 2000;8:141-150.

[14] Sasaki N, Ishibashi Y, Tsuda E, et al. The femoral insertion of the anterior cruciate ligament: discrepancy between macroscopic and histological observations. Arthroscopy. 2012;28: 1135-1146.

[15] Amis AA, Dawkins GP (1991) Functional anatomy of the anterior cruciate ligament. Fibre bundle actions

related to ligament replacements and injuries. J Bone Joint Surg Br 73(2):260-267

[16] Griffin LY, Albohm M, Agel J, et al. Understanding and preventing noncontact anterior cruciate ligament injuries: a review of the Hunt Valley II Meeting, January 2005. Am J Sports Med. 2006;34:1512-1532.

[17] Muneta T, Takakuda K, Yamamoto H. Intercondylar Notch Width and Its Relation to the Configuration and Cross-Sectional Area of the Anterior Cruciate Ligament: A Cadaveric Knee Study. Am J Sports Med. 1997 Jan;25(1):69-72. DOI: 10.1177/036354659702500113

[18] Olsen O-E, Myklebust G, Engebretsen L, Bahr R. Injury Mechanisms for Anterior Cruciate Ligament Injuries in Team Handball: A Systematic Video Analysis. Am J Sports Med. 2004 Jun;32(4):1002-12. DOI : 10.1177/0363546503261724

[19] Petersen W, Tillmann B. Structure and vascularization of the cruciate ligaments of the human knee joint. Anat Embryol (Berl). 1999 Sep;200(3):325-34. DOI: 10.1007/s004290050283

[20] Kennedy JC, Weinberg HW, Wilson AS. The anatomy and function of the anterior cruciate ligament. As determined by clinical and morphological studies. J Bone Joint Surg Am. 1974 Mar;56(2):223-35. PMID: 4452683

[21] Stijak L, Nikolic V, Malis M, Maksimovic R, Aksic M, Filipovic B. The influence of the morphometric parameters of the intercondylar notch on rupture of the anterior cruciate ligament. Vojnosanit Pregl. 2012;69(7):576-80. DOI : 10.2298/VSP101224012S

[22] Anderson AF, Dome DC, Gautam S, Awh MH, Rennirt GW. Correlation of Anthropometric Measurements, Strength, Anterior Cruciate Ligament Size, and Intercondylar Notch Characteristics to Sex Differences in Anterior Cruciate Ligament Tear Rates. Am J Sports Med. 2001 Jan;29(1):58-66. DOI: 10.1177/03635465010290011501

[23] Domzalski M, Grzelak P, Gabos P. Risk factors for Anterior Cruciate Ligament injury in skeletally immature patients: analysis of intercondylar notch width using Magnetic Resonance Imaging. Int Orthop. 2010 Jun;34(5):703-7. DOI: 10.1007/s00264-010-0987-7

[24] LaPrade RF, Burnett QM. Femoral Intercondylar Notch Stenosis and Correlation to Anterior Cruciate Ligament Injuries: A Prospective Study. Am J Sports Med. 1994 Mar;22(2):198-203. DOI: 10.1177/036354659402200208

[25] Lund-Hanssen H, Gannon J, Engebretson L, et al. Intercondylar notch width and the risk for anterior cruciate ligament rupture: a case-control study in 46 female handball players. Acta Orthop Scand. 1994;65(5):529-532.

[26] Souryal TO, Freeman TR. Intercondylar notch size and anterior cruciate ligament injuries in athletes. Am J Sports Med. 1993;21:535-539.

[27] Souryal TO, Moore HA, Evans JP. Bilaterality in anterior cruciate ligament injuries. Am J Sports Med. 1988;16:449-454.

[28] Sheik Mohammed Fahim , Tushar Dhawan , Nuthan Jagadeesh, Yogesh Ashwathnarayan.The relationship of anterior cruciate ligament injuries with MRI based calculation of femoral notch width, notch width index, notch shape - A randomized control study. Journal of Clinical Orthopaedics and Trauma 17 (2021) 5-10. https://doi.org/10.1016/j.jcot.2021.01.006

[29] Ashwini T, Jain Aditi. MRI correlation of anterior cruciate ligament

injuries with femoral intercondylar notch, posterior tibial slopes and medial tibial plateau depth in the Indian population. Int J Anat Radiol Surg. July, 2018;7(3). https:// doi.org/10.7860/ IJARS/2018/36086:2397. RO01e6.

[30] Basukala B, Joshi A, Pradhan I. The effect of the intercondylar notch shape and notch width index on anterior cruciate ligament injuries. J Nepal Health Res Counc. 2020 Jan 21;17(4):532e536. https://doi. org/10.33314/jnhrc.v17i4.1858.

[31] Gormeli CA, Gormeli G, Oztürk BY, et al. The effect of the intercondylar notch width index on anterior cruciate ligament injuries: a study on groups with unilateral and bilateral ACL injury. Acta Orthop Belg. 2015 Jun;81(2): 240e244. PMID: 26280962.

[32] Hoteya K, Kato Y, Motojima S, et al. Association between intercondylar notch narrowing and bilateral anterior cruciate ligament injuries in athletes. Arch Orthop Trauma Surg. 2011 Mar;131(3):371e376. https://doi. org/10.1007/ s00402-010-1254-5.

[33] Uhorchak JM, Scoville CR, Williams GN, Arciero RA, Pierre PSt, Taylor DC. Risk factors associated with noncontact injury of the anterior cruciate ligament. Am J Sports Med. 2003 Nov;31(6):831e842. https://doi. org/10.1177/ 03635465030310061801.

[34] Al-Saeed O, Brown M, Athyal R, Sheikh M. Association of femoral intercondylar notch morphology, width index and the risk of anterior cruciate ligament injury. Knee Surg Sports Traumatol Arthrosc. 2013 Mar;21(3):678e682. https:// doi. org/10.1007/s00167-012-2038-y.

[35] Dejour H, Bonnin M. Tibial translation after anterior cruciate ligament rupture: two radiological tests compared. J Bone Joint Surg Br. 1994; 76:745-749.

[36] MAJ Micheal S.Todd et al. The relationship between posterior tibial slope and anterior cruciate ligament injuries, the American Journal of sports Medicine; 2010;38:63

[37] Galway HR, Macintosh DL. The lateral pivot shift: a symptom and signof anterior cruciate ligament insufficiency. C/in Orthop 1980;147;45-50.

[38] Dejour H, Neyret P, Eberhard P, Walch G. [Bilateral congenital absence of the anterior cruciate ligament and the internal menisci of the knee. A case report]. Revue de Chirurgie Orthopedique et Reparatrice de L'appareil Moteur. 1990;76(5):329-332

[39] Alana Waiwaiole, Ajay Gurbani, Kambiz Motamedi, Leanne Seeger, Myung Shin Sim, DrPH, Patricia Nwajuaku,and Sharon L. Hame. Relationship of ACL Injury and Posterior Tibial Slope With Patient Age, Sex, and Race.The Orthopaedic Journal of Sports Medicine, 4(11), 2325967116672852. DOI:10.1177/ 2325967116672852

[40] Zeng C, Cheng L, Wei J, et al. The influence of the tibial plateau slopes on injury of the anterior cruciate ligament: a meta-analysis. Knee Surg Sports Traumatol Arthrosc. 2014;22:53-65.

[41] Hashemi J, Chandrashekar N, Gill B, Beynnon BD, Slauterbeck JR, Schutt RC Jr, et al. The geometry of the tibial plateau and its influence on the biomechanics of the tibiofemoral joint. J Bone Joint Surg Am. 2008;90(12): 2724-34.

[42] Stijak L, Herzog RF, Schai P. Is there an influence of the tibial slope of the lateral condyle on the ACL lesion? A case-control study. Knee Surg Sports Traumatol Arthrosc. 2008;16:112-117.

[43] Louboutin H, Debarge R, Richou J, et al. Osteoarthritis in patients with anterior cruciate ligament rupture: a

review of risk factors. Knee. 2009;16: 239-244.

[44] Blanke F, Kiapour AM, Haenle M, Fischer J, Majewski M, Vogt S, Camathias C. Risk of Noncontact Anterior Cruciate Ligament Injuries Is Not Associated With Slope and Concavity of the Tibial Plateau in Recreational Alpine Skiers: A Magnetic Resonance Imaging-Based Case-Control Study of 121 Patients. Am J Sports Med. 2016 Jun;44(6):1508-14. doi: 10.1177/0363546516632332. Epub 2016 Mar 8. PMID: 26957218.

[45] Hashemi, J, Breighner, R, Chandrashekar, N. Hip extension, knee flexion paradox: a new mechanism for non-contact ACL injury. J Biomech. 2011;44:577-585. Google Scholar | Crossref | Medline | ISI

[46] Hewett, TE, Myer, GD, Ford, KR. Biomechanical measures of neuromuscular control and valgus loading of the knee predict anterior cruciate ligament injury risk in female athletes: a prospective study. Am J Sports Med. 2005;33:492-501. Google Scholar | SAGE Journals | ISI

[47] Hewett, TE, Stroupe, AL, Nance, TA, Noyes, FR. Plyometric training in female athletes. Decreased impact forces and increased hamstring torques. Am J Sports Med. 1996;24:765-773. Google Scholar | SAGE Journals | ISI

[48] Hewett, TE, Torg, JS, Boden, BP. Video analysis of trunk and knee motion during non-contact anterior cruciate ligament injury in female athletes: lateral trunk and knee abduction motion are combined components of the injury mechanism. Br J Sports Med. 2009;43:417-422. Google Scholar | Crossref | Medline | ISI

[49] Prodromos CC, Han Y, Rogowski J, Joyce B, Shi K. A meta-analysis of the incidence of anterior cruciate ligament tears as a function of gender, sport,and a knee injury-reduction regimen. Arthroscopy. 2007;23:1320-1325.

[50] Wojtys EM, Huston LJ, Schock HJ, Boylan AP, Ashton-Miller JA. Gender differences in muscular protection of the knee in torsion in size-matched athletes. J Bone Joint Surg Am. 2003;85(5):782-789.

[51] Chappell JD, Creighton RA, Giuliani C, Yu B, Garrett WE. Kinematics and electromyography of landing preparation in vertical stop-jump: risks for noncontact anterior cruciate ligament injury. Am J Sports Med. 2007;35(2):235-241.

[52] Anderson AF, Dome DC, Gautam S, Awh MH, Rennirt GW. Correlation of anthropometric measurements, strength, anterior cruciate ligament size, and intercondylar notch characteristics to sex differences in anterior cruciate ligament tear rates. Am J Sports Med. 2001;29:58-66.

[53] Chandrashekar N, Mansour JM, Slauterbeck J, Hashemi J. Sex-based differences in the tensile properties of the human anterior cruciate ligament. J Biomech. 2006;39(16):2943-2950.

[54] Scerpella TA, Stayer TJ, Makhuli BZ. Ligamentous laxity and non-contact anterior cruciate ligament tears: a gender based comparison. Orthopedics. 2005;28(7):656-660.

[55] Souryal TO, Freeman TR. Intercondylar notch size and anterior cruciate ligament injuries in athletes. A prospective study. Am J Sports Med. 1993 Jul-Aug;21(4):535-9. doi: 10.1177/036354659302100410. Erratum in: Am J Sports Med 1993 Sep-Oct;21(5):723. PMID: 8368414.

[56] LaPrade RF, Burnett QM 2nd. Femoral intercondylar notch stenosis and correlation to anterior cruciate ligament injuries. A prospective study. Am J Sports Med. 1994

Mar-Apr;22(2):198-202; discussion 203. doi: 10.1177/036354659402200208. PMID: 8198187.

[57] Fayad, L.M., Rosenthal, E.H., Morrison, W.B. and Carrino, J.A. (2008), Anterior cruciate ligament volume: Analysis of gender differences. J. Magn. Reson. Imaging, 27: 218-223

[58] Arendt EA, Bershadsky B, Agel J. Periodicity of noncontact anterior cruciate ligament injuries during the menstrual cycle. The Journal of Gender-specific Medicine : JGSM : the Official Journal of the Partnership for Women's Health at Columbia. 2002 Mar-Apr;5(2):19-26.

[59] Adachi N, Nawata K, Maeta M, Kurozawa Y. Relationship of the menstrual cycle phase to anterior cruciate ligament injuries in teenaged female athletes. Arch Orthop Trauma Surg. 2008 May;128(5):473-8. doi: 10.1007/s00402-007-0461-1. Epub 2007 Oct 2. PMID: 17909824.

[60] Faryniarz DA, Bhargava M, Lajam C, Attia ET, Hannafin JA. Quantitation of estrogen receptors and relaxin binding in human anterior cruciate ligament fibroblasts. In Vitro Cell Dev Biol Anim. 2006 Jul-Aug;42(7):176-81. doi: 10.1290/0512089.1. PMID: 16948498.

[61] Renstrom P, Ljungqvist A, Arendt E, et al. Non-contact ACL injuries in female athletes: an International Olympic Committee current concepts statement. Br J Sports Med. 2008;42(6):394-412. doi:10.1136/bjsm.2008.048934

[62] Yu WD, Liu SH, Hatch JD, Panossian V, Finerman GA. Effect of estrogen on cellular metabolism of the human anterior cruciate ligament. Clin Orthop Relat Res. 1999 Sep;(366): 229-38. doi: 10.1097/00003086-199909000-00030. PMID: 10627740.

[63] Wojtys EM, Huston LJ, Boynton MD, Spindler KP, Lindenfeld TN. The effect of the menstrual cycle on anterior cruciate ligament injuries in women as determined by hormone levels. Am J Sports Med. 2002 Mar-Apr;30(2):182-8. doi: 10.1177/03635465020300020601. PMID: 11912085.

[64] Flynn RK, Pederson CL, Birmingham TB, Kirkley A, Jackowski D, Fowler PJ. The familial predisposition toward tearing the anterior cruciate ligament: a case-control study. Am J Sports Med. 2005;33:23-28.

[65] Harner CD, Paulos LE, Greenwald AE, Rosenberg TD, Cooley VC. Detailed analysis of patients with bilateral anterior cruciate ligament injuries. Am J Sports Med. 1994;22: 37-43.

[66] Kenichi Goshima, Katsuhiko Kitaoka, Junsuke Nakase, Hiroyuki Tsuchiya, Familial predisposition to anterior cruciate ligament injury, Asia-Pacific Journal of Sports Medicine, Arthroscopy, Rehabilitation and Technology, Volume 1, Issue 2, 2014, Pages 62-66.

[67] Khoschnau S, Melhus H, Jacobson A, Rahme H, Bengtsson H, Ribom E, Grundberg E, Mallmin H, Michaëlsson K. Type I collagen alpha1 Sp1 polymorphism and the risk of cruciate ligament ruptures or shoulder dislocations. Am J Sports Med. 2008 Dec;36(12):2432-6. doi: 10.1177/0363546508320805. Epub 2008 Jul 31. PMID: 18669982.

[68] Posthumus M, September AV, O'Cuinneagain D, van der Merwe W, Schwellnus MP, Collins M. The COL5A1 gene is associated with increased risk of anterior cruciate ligament ruptures in female participants. Am J Sports Med. 2009 Nov;37(11):2234-40. doi: 10.1177/0363546509338266. Epub 2009 Aug 4. PMID: 19654427.

[69] Posthumus M, September AV, O'Cuinneagain D, van der Merwe W, Schwellnus MP, Collins M. The association between the COL12A1 gene and anterior cruciate ligament ruptures. Br J Sports Med. 2010;44(16):1160-1165.

[70] Posthumus M, Collins M, van der Merwe L, O'Cuinneagain D, et al. Matrix metalloproteinase genes on chromosome 11q22 and the risk of anterior cruciate ligament (ACL) rupture [published online ahead of print March 16,Scand J Med Sci Sports

[71] Swanik CB, Covassin T, Stearne DJ, Schatz P. The relationship between neurocognitive function and noncontact anterior cruciate ligament injuries. Am J Sports Med. 2007 Jun;35(6):943-8. doi: 10.1177/0363546507299532. Epub 2007 Mar 16. PMID: 17369562

[72] Orchard J, Seward H, McGivern J, Hood S. Intrinsic and extrinsic risk factors for anterior cruciate ligament injury in Australian footballers. Am J Sports Med. 2001;29:196-200.

[73] Walden M, Hagglund M, Ekstrand J. High risk of new knee injury in elite footballers with previous anterior cruciate ligament injury. Am J Sports Med. 2006;40:158-162.

[74] Kramer LC, Denegar CR, Buckley WE, Hertel J. Factors associated with anterior cruciate ligament injury: history in female athletes. J Sports Med Phys Fitness. 2007;47:446-454.

[75] Olsen OE, Myklebust G, Engebretson L, Holme I, Bahr R. Relationship between floor type and risk of ACL injury in team handball. Scand J Med Sci Sports. 2003;13:299-304.

[76] Orchard J, Seward H, McGivern J, Hood S. Intrinsic and extrinsic risk factors for anterior cruciate ligament injury in Australian footballers. Am J Sports Med. 2001;29:196-200.

[77] Orchard J, Seward H, McGivern J, Hood S. Rainfall, evaporation and the risk of non-contact anterior cruciate ligament injury in the Australian Football League. Med J Aust. 1999;170:304-306.

[78] Orchard JW, Chivers I, Aldous D, Bennell K, Seward H. Rye grass is associated with fewer non-contact anterior cruciate ligament injuries than Bermuda grass. Br J Sports Med. 2005;39:704-709.

[79] Orchard JW, Powell JW. Risk of knee and ankle sprains under various weather conditions in American football. Med Sci Sports Exerc. 2003;35(7):1118-1123.

Chapter 4

Patellofemoral Instability

Deepak V. Patel, Iciar M. Dávila Castrodad, Jennifer Kurowicki, Vincent K. McInerney and Anthony J. Scillia

Abstract

Recurrent patellofemoral instability is a common cause of knee pain and functional disability in adolescent and young adult patients, resulting in loss of time from work and sports. There are numerous factors that contribute to recurrent patellofemoral instability; these factors include tear of the medial patellofemoral ligament (MPFL), weakening or hypoplasia of the vastus medialis obliquus (VMO), trochlear dysplasia, increased tibial tuberosity-trochlear groove (TT-TG) distance (>20 mm), valgus malalignment, increased Q angle, malrotation secondary to internal femoral or external tibial torsion, patella alta, and generalized ligamentous laxity. A detailed history and a thorough physical examination are crucial to clinch an early, accurate diagnosis. Imaging studies play an important role to confirm the clinical diagnosis and also help to identify concomitant intra-articular pathologies. Initially, nonoperative management (including the use of physical therapy, patellar taping or brace) is offered to patients with acute, first-time patellar dislocations and most patients respond well to this mode of treatment. Surgical treatment is indicated for patients who have post-trauma osteochondral fracture or loose body; predisposing anatomical risk factors; recurrent, symptomatic instability; and who have failed an adequate trial of nonoperative management. Surgical treatments include MPFL reconstruction, proximal or distal realignment procedures, and trochleoplasty. Lateral release is often performed in combination with other procedures and seldom performed as an isolated procedure. An individualized case-by-case approach is recommended based on the underlying anatomical risk factors and radiographic abnormality.

Keywords: Knee, Patellofemoral instability, Patellar subluxation or dislocation, Nonoperative management, Surgical treatment, Medial patellofemoral ligament reconstruction, Tibial tuberosity transfer, Trochlear dysplasia, Trochleoplasty

1. Introduction

This chapter is divided into 2 major sections. Section 2 provides a brief overview of acute dislocation of the patella. In Section 3, we discuss the soft tissue and osseous anatomy, clinical presentation and physical examination, radiographic studies, nonoperative management, surgical treatment, and authors' preferred method of medial patellofemoral ligament (MPFL) reconstruction for patients with recurrent patellofemoral instability.

2. Patellofemoral instability: acute dislocation of the patella

Acute dislocation of the patella is an orthopedic disorder of the knee that frequently affects adolescent and young adult population (peak age of 10 to 20 years). Acute patellar dislocation accounts for 2–3% of all knee injuries. It has been reported that there is a 17–49% risk of redislocation following first-time, acute patellar dislocation [1]. The risk increases to 44–71% following a second-time dislocation [2]. Acute traumatic patellar dislocation (with or without associated osteochondral fracture) is the second most frequent cause of traumatic hemarthrosis of the knee, after anterior cruciate ligament tear. The patella usually dislocates laterally, causing ruptures of the MPFL in about 90% of the cases.

2.1 Studies on the natural history of acute dislocation of the patella

Hawkins et al. [1] have reported on the natural history of acute patellar dislocations. The authors of this study reviewed 27 patients who sustained primary dislocations of the patellae. Of these 27 patients, 20 were treated with immobilization and subsequent physical therapy (including nine patients who underwent arthroscopy) and seven with immediate surgical stabilization and lateral release. In this study, the patients with predisposing factors such as patellofemoral malalignment, abnormal patellar configuration, and a history of prior symptoms of patellofemoral instability were more prone to recurrent dislocation and may benefit from operative intervention. These authors noted that at least 30–50% of all patients having sustained a primary patellar dislocation will continue to have symptoms of instability and/or anterior knee pain.

Atkin et al. [3] prospectively studied the characteristics and early recovery of an unselected population of patients who had acute, first-time lateral dislocation of the patella. Seventy-four patients (average age 20 years) met the enrollment criteria. A standardized rehabilitation program was utilized, emphasizing range of motion, muscle strength, and return of function. Patients returned to stressful activities (including sports) as tolerated when they regained a full passive range of motion in the knee, had no joint effusion, and when quadriceps muscle strength was at least 80% as compared with the opposite, non-injured extremity. Sports participation remained significantly reduced throughout the first 6 months after injury, with the greatest limitations in kneeling and squatting. The patients who had acute primary patellar dislocation were young and active, and most injuries occurred during sports.

Fithian et al. [4] published a prospective cohort study to define the epidemiology and natural history of acute dislocation of the patella, and to identify risk factors for subsequent patellofemoral instability episodes. These authors prospectively followed 189 patients for a period of 2 to 5 years. The overall annual risk for a first-time patellar dislocation was 5.8 per 100,000 members, with 61% of injuries occurring during sports. There was an increasingly higher incidence of patellar dislocation in younger and female patients. The annual risk for patients with a previous history of patellar subluxation or dislocation was 3.8 per 100,000 members, with a statistically higher proportion of older and female patients.

2.2 Anatomy

Warren and Marshall [5] have delineated the anatomy of the medial aspect of the knee. These authors dissected 154 fresh human knee joints and found a consistent three-layered pattern with condensations between the tissue planes.

The fibers of MPFL were transversely oriented within layer II, superficial to the joint capsule and deep to the vastus medialis. Since then, various studies have been reported on the anatomy of the MPFL [6–21]. Schottle and associates [22], in their landmark cadaveric study, defined a radiographic point representing the femoral attachment of the MPFL. This was described on a true lateral radiograph of the knee (with both posterior condyles projected in the same plane), as 2 mm anterior to the posterior cortex extension line, 2.5 mm distal to the posterior origin of the medial femoral condyle, and proximal to the level of the posterior-most point of the Blumensaat's line.

In earlier anatomical dissection studies, the MPFL has been defined as a pure ligament spanning from the medial femoral condyle to the medial border of the patella. However, recent advances in the surgical anatomy of the MPFL have revealed that there are fibers that insert onto the deep, undersurface of the quadriceps tendon as well as the patella, thus earning the name "medial patellofemoral complex" to allow for the variability in its anatomy [23]. The medial patellofemoral complex (MPFC) has been more recently identified as a broad, fan-shaped structure with both bony and soft tissue insertions [24, 25]. The MPFC origin is generally accepted to originate within a triangular saddle of bony landmarks on the medial condyle of the femur, formed by the medial gastrocnemius tubercle, the medial femoral epicondyle, and the adductor tubercle [17, 24, 25]. The insertion of the MPFC is more variable; about 57% of its fibers attach to the patella and the remaining 43% attach to the undersurface of the quadriceps tendon [26]. Fulkerson has described this quadriceps portion of the MPFC as the medial quadriceps tendon-femoral ligament (MQTFL) [27]. The length of the MPFL ranges from 45 mm to 64 mm, and its width is slightly greater at its patellar insertion than its femoral origin [11, 13]. The midpoint of the 30.4-mm-wide insertion of the MPFC has been reproducibly found at the junction of the medial border of the quadriceps tendon with the articular surface of the patella [24, 26].

Tanaka [26] undertook a cadaveric study to describe and quantify the variability of the attachments of the MPFL. In his study, 33 cadaveric knees were dissected, and the MPFL was identified from the articular side after anterior reflection of the extensor mechanism and removal of the synovium. The mean width of the MPFL was 10.7 ± 1.8 mm at the femoral origin and 30.4 ± 5.5 mm at the patellar attachment. Tanaka [26] concluded that MPFL fibers vary in their width and percentage of attachments to the patella and quadriceps tendon. Further research is required to identify the appropriate fixation points to recreate the anatomy and isometry of the MPFL during patellar stabilization surgery for patients with patellofemoral instability.

Aframian et al. [17] conducted a systematic review of anatomical dissections and imaging studies to identify the true anatomical origin and insertion of the MPFL. After screening and review of 2045 papers, a total of 67 studies investigating the relevant anatomy were included. The authors found that the origin of the MPFL appears to be from an area rather than a single point (as previously reported) on the medial femoral condyle. The weighted average length of the MPFL was 56 mm with an 'hourglass' shape, fanning out at both ends of the ligament. The MPFL is an hourglass-shaped structure running from a triangular space between the adductor tubercle, medial femoral epicondyle and gastrocnemius tubercle, and inserts onto the superomedial aspect of the patella. **Figure 1** shows the diagram summarizing the femoral and patellar attachment areas of the MPFL. Awareness of anatomy is essential for accurate placement of the graft while performing MPFL reconstruction for patellofemoral instability.

The MPFL has been regarded as the major medial soft tissue stabilizer of the patella (particularly in early knee flexion), originating from the medial femoral

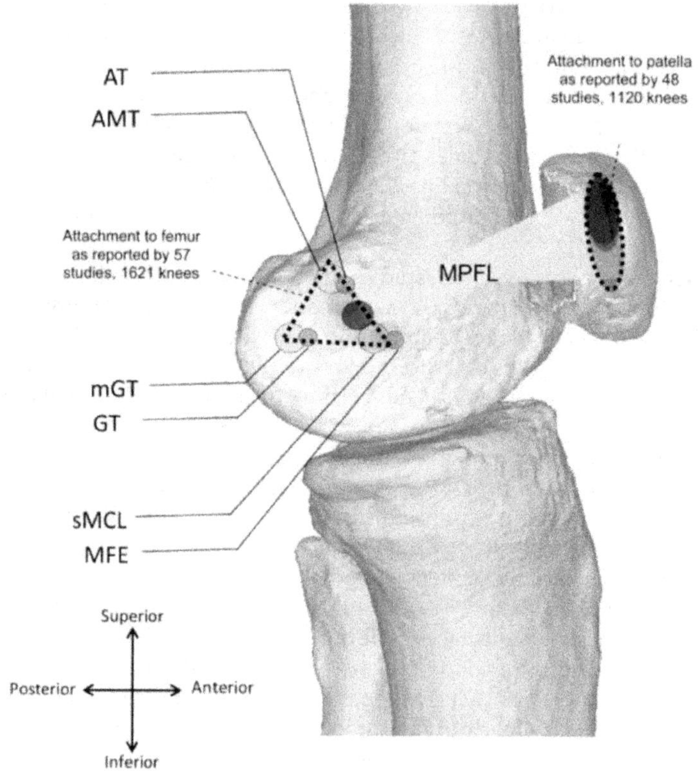

Figure 1.
Diagram summarizing the MPFL attachment areas. Darker shading represents study concordance. AT - adductor tubercle; AMT - adductor magnus tendon; GT - gastrocnemius tubercle; mGT - medial gastrocnemius tendon; sMCL – superficial medial collateral ligament; MFE – medial femoral epicondyle. Reprinted with permission from: Aframian et al. [17]. Copyright © The Author(s) 2016. Creative Commons Attribution 4.0 International License (http://creativecommons.org/licenses/by/4.0/). No changes we made.

condyle and inserting onto the proximal two-thirds of the medial border of the patella. The MPFL acts as a primary static checkrein to resist lateral translation of the patella, providing approximately 208 N of mean tensile strength before rupture [6, 28, 29]. Conlan et al. [6], based on their landmark cadaveric study of the knees, reported that the MPFL is the major medial soft tissue restraint that prevents lateral displacement of the distal knee-extensor mechanism, contributing an average of 53% of the total force. The patellomeniscal ligament and associated retinacular fibers in the deep capsular layer of the knee (which were previously thought to be functionally unimportant) in the stabilization of the patella, contributed an average of 22% of the total force. The patellotibial band and the medial patellotibial ligament are less important restraints to lateral translation of the patella. The quadriceps functions as a dynamic stabilizer of the patella.

A number of anatomic risk factors have been associated with acute dislocation of the patella (**Table 1**). These risk factors become increasingly important when evaluating patients with recurrent patellofemoral instability.

2.3 Clinical presentation

Most acute patellar dislocations occur during sport. Sporting injuries account for 61–72% of acute patellar dislocations [3, 4]. Acute dislocation of the patella can

1. Genu valgum
2. Increased Q angle
3. Increased femoral anterversion; internal femoral torsion
4. External tibial torsion
5. Lateralized tibial tuberosity
6. Lateral patellar tilt
7. Patella alta
8. Generalized ligamentous laxity
9. Weakening or hypoplasia of the vastus medialis obliquus (VMO)
10. Trochlear dysplasia or hypoplasia
11. Pes planus (Flat foot)

Table 1.
Anatomic Risk Factors Associated with Acute Dislocation of the Patella.

occur either by a direct blow to the knee or indirectly, as the body rotates around a planted foot. The player may sense that "kneecap is out of place", but often the patella will dislocate and spontaneously reduce. If the patella remains dislocated, it may be palpable over the lateral aspect of the femur, and the medial femoral condyle appears prominent. The indirect mechanism of injury is more common than a direct blow. This mechanism is noncontact and occurs with the knee in slight flexion and valgus as the tibia externally rotates relative to the femur. It can occur on a planted foot as the femur and body rotate internally, such as the hind leg of a baseball player swinging hard at a pitch. Alternatively, the free foot can be forced into external rotation, such as a soccer player whose instep kick is met with excessive resistance, or a snow skier whose ski acts as an offending lever arm [30]. Patellar dislocation can occur in various sports, such as American football, soccer, baseball, basketball, ice hockey, gymnastics, wrestling, tennis and golf. **Figure 2** demonstrates the indirect (noncontact) and direct (contact) mechanisms of injury that can result in acute dislocation of the patella.

2.4 Physical examination

Most patients present to the outpatient clinic in the subacute phase after their injury. Physical examination at this stage may be difficult due to presence of pain and swelling. In select cases, aspiration of a tense joint effusion may be required to relieve pain, and to allow better physical examination and radiographic evaluation. The appearance of the joint aspirate may provide important diagnostic clue. Lipohemarthrosis indicates presence of a concomitant osteochondral fracture.

A complete examination of the injured lower extremity should be undertaken. The astute clinician should look for limb malalignment (especially genu valgum), patella alta, and rotational abnormality, such as excessive anteversion of the femoral neck (internal femoral torsion) and external tibial torsion. A comprehensive ligamentous examination of the injured knee should be performed to rule out associated injury to the cruciate and/or collateral ligaments. Joint-line tenderness and a positive McMurray's test may indicate presence of concomitant meniscal injury. Generalized ligamentous hyperlaxity should be noted by examining finger metacarpophalangeal joint hyperextension, thumb-to-forearm apposition, knee hyperextension, and elbow hyperextension. A complete neurovascular examination of the limb should be performed.

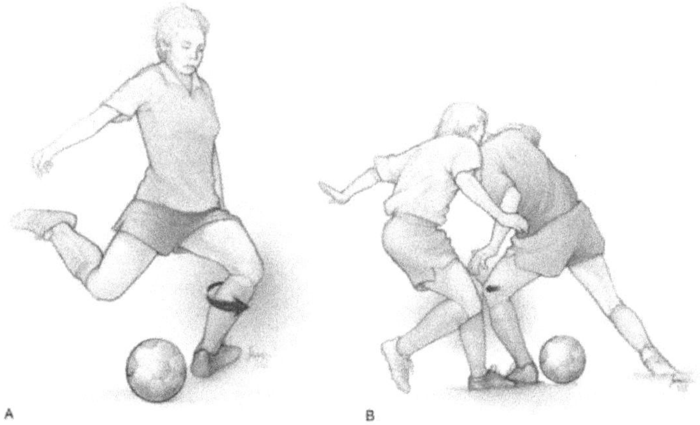

Figure 2.
Mechanisms of acute patellar dislocation: (A) A noncontact dislocation occurs by external rotation of the lower leg relative to the body. (B) Contact injury is caused by a direct blow to the medial aspect of the knee. Adapted from Steiner and Parker [30]. Reprinted with permission of The Cleveland Center for Medical Art & Photography © 2008. All Rights Reserved.

The knee should be specifically palpated for areas of localized, maximal tenderness. There is tenderness along the medial border of the patella and also over the injured or torn medial patellar retinaculum. In some cases, a palpable defect in the medial retinaculum is noted. There may be localized tenderness at the origin, at the insertion, or along the course of the MPFL. Tenderness at the medial border of the patella or along the lateral femoral condyle may suggest osteochondral injury. Tenderness or asymmetry at the distal portion of the vastus medialis obliquus (VMO) may suggest significant disruption of its tendinous insertion. The patellar apprehension test should be performed to determine patellar instability. The apprehension test is performed by applying a laterally directed force along the medial border of the patella with the knee in 20 to 30 degrees of flexion (**Figure 3**). A positive finding occurs when the patient has a sense of pain and impending subluxation or dislocation. In addition to apprehension, there may be increased translation of the patella when compared with the uninjured knee.

2.5 Associated injuries

The most common findings associated with acute dislocation of the patella are chondral and osteochondral injuries. Stefancin and Parker [31] systematically reviewed the literature on patients who had had first-time patellar dislocation. The average age of the patients was 21.5 years. In their compilation of 70 articles, the incidence of osteochondral fracture (confirmed by open surgery, arthroscopy, or MRI) ranged from 0% to 73%, with an overall incidence of 24%. Osteochondral injuries resulting from lateral patellar dislocation have a characteristic pattern; there is an injury to the medial facet of the patella and the lateral femoral condyle. The osteochondral fragments may remain attached, may become loose in the joint, or may be retained in the peripatellar retinacular tissue [30].

2.6 Radiographic studies

The radiographic evaluation of patients with patellar dislocation include plain radiographs and MRI of the knee.

The plain radiograph series of the knee should include standing anterior–posterior view, 45-degree flexion posterior–anterior weight-bearing view (Rosenberg view), lateral view, and axial view. The lateral view provides useful information

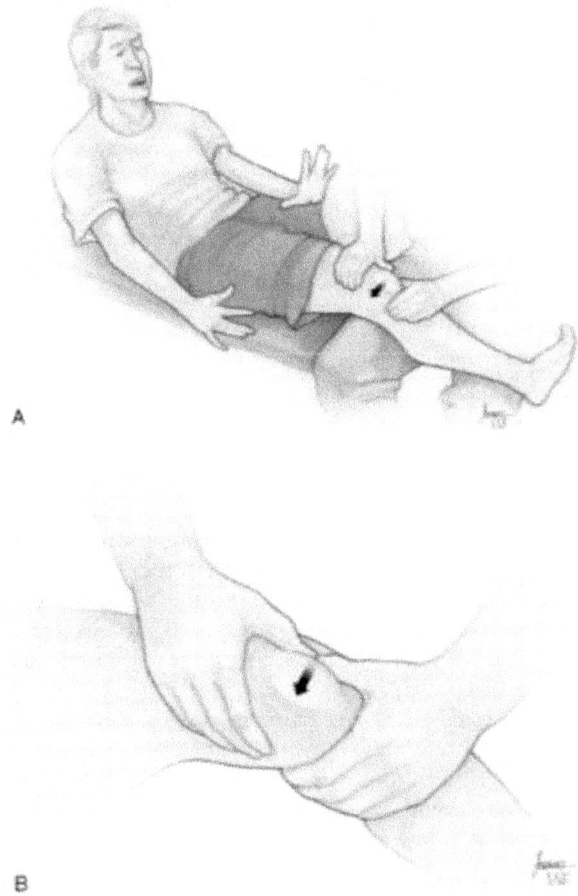

Figure 3.
Patellar apprehension test. The physician applies a lateral force to the medial border of the patella with the knee in 20 to 30 degrees of flexion. The patient experiences a sensation of the patella subluxating or dislocating in an outward (lateral) direction. Adapted from Steiner and Parker [30]. Reprinted with permission of The Cleveland Center for Medical Art & Photography © 2008. All Rights Reserved.

about the patellar height, trochlear depth, and patellar tilt. Patella alta is a known risk factor for patellar dislocation and can be determined on the lateral radiograph by numerous methods. These methods include the Insall-Salvati ratio [32], the modified Insall-Salvati ratio [33], the Blackburne-Peel ratio [34], and the Caton-Deschamps ratio [35]. A brief description of the above-mentioned radiographic measurements is provided under the heading – Assessment of Patellar Height – in Section 3 of this book chapter.

The Blackburne-Peel ratio, which is based on consistent bony landmarks, is the most reproducible and has the most moderate results for classification into patella alta and patella baja. The trochlear depth and patellar tilt can also be determined from the lateral radiograph of the knee. It is worth emphasizing that the lateral view of the knee must be a "true" lateral with the posterior borders of the femoral condyles overlapping for accurate interpretation and analysis of the trochlear depth and patellar tilt. The axial views as described by Merchant and colleagues [36] and Laurin and colleagues [37, 38] are commonly used. The axial view of the patellofemoral joint provides valuable information about any persistent subluxation or dislocation of the patella. In addition to the lateral patellar overhang, the sulcus angle can be determined on the axial view.

MRI has become the imaging modality of choice in the evaluation of patients with acute dislocations of the patella. Various pathologies such as, VMO edema, bone contusion, chondral and osteochondral injury, loose body, medial patellar retinacular injury, MPFL injury, and associated ligamentous and/or meniscal injury can be well visualized on a high-quality MRI study. The MPFL is almost universally disrupted in patients with acute lateral dislocation of the patella. The aforementioned MRI findings following acute dislocation of the patella are useful for the treating physician and allows him/her to formulate a sound treatment plan. Presence of a large osteochondral fragment, loose body, a complete tear of the MPFL, and associated ligamentous or meniscal injury may point the surgeon toward operative intervention [30].

2.7 Nonoperative treatment

Currently, there exists a debate in the orthopedic literature regarding nonoperative versus operative treatment of acute patellar dislocations. Most physicians recommend a more conservative, i.e. nonoperative approach, whereas some recommend immediate repair of the injured medial structures.

Maenpaa and Lehto [39] have reported a long-term study on nonoperative treatment of acute patellar dislocations. In their study, 100 patients were treated nonoperatively for primary acute patellar dislocations, either by plaster cast (N = 60); by posterior splint (N = 17); or by patellar bandage or brace (N = 23) for 2 to 4 weeks, followed by rehabilitation. Follow-up examinations were performed at an average of 13 years (range, 6 to 26 years) after the initial injury. The recurrence rate was 44% overall, yielding 0.17 redislocations per follow-up year; an additional 19% without recurrence had continued symptoms of pain and instability, and required surgery. The mean Kujala score at follow-up was 80, with significantly lower scores in those older than 30 years of age.

In the management of acute patellar dislocations, prospective, randomized controlled studies have shown higher Kujala scores (higher scores indicate better knee function) [40–42] and reduced rate of recurrent patellar dislocation [40–43] after surgical stabilization as compared with nonoperative treatment.

Despite above-mentioned studies, majority of patients with acute lateral dislocation of the patella are initially treated by nonoperative management. Nonoperative treatment is indicated for patients with acute, first-time dislocation of the patella without associated osteochondral fracture or loose bodies. The nonoperative treatment consists of immobilization in a plaster cast or a brace for about 4–6 weeks followed by a period of well-planed, supervised rehabilitation. Immobilization allows for healing of the injured soft tissues on the medial aspect of the knee. Some surgeons recommend early rehabilitation of the knee without immobilization to avoid harmful effects of immobilization (such as quadriceps weakness and wasting, knee stiffness, and chondrolysis). Whether immobilized or not, patients with acute patellar dislocation should expect a prolonged rehabilitation period before return to sport.

2.8 Operative treatment

Operative treatment is indicated for patients who have persistent pain, recurrent instability and diminished knee function, and who have failed a trial of nonoperative management. In our experience, the indications for initial operative treatment include presence of an osteochondral fragment, loose body, a complete tear or avulsion of the MPFL, palpable defects in the vastus medialis insertion, obvious tear in the medial patellar retinaculum, associated ligamentous or meniscal injury, and persistent asymmetric subluxation of the patella.

The surgical procedures include arthroscopy, lateral release, medial retinacular repair, MPFL repair with or without augmentation, realignment procedure, or combination of these surgical techniques. Repair and reconstruction should be undertaken to address identifiable, injured soft tissues on the medial aspect of the knee, whereas release or lengthening of the lateral patellar retinaculum should be performed to restore soft tissue balance of the patellofemoral joint. Realignment procedure is indicated for patients who have a clear underlying anatomic malalignment.

2.8.1 Arthroscopy

Arthroscopy helps to identify and treat the associated intra-articular pathologies, such as chondral and osteochondral injuries; meniscal tears; and ligamentous injuries. Arthroscopy can be performed alone or in combination with open procedures. Minor or small chondral or osteochondral fragments can be excised, and medium-sized or large chondral or osteochondral fragments can be fixed with the use of modern arthroscopic surgical technique, instrumentation, and implants.

2.8.2 Lateral release

We are extremely cautious in advocating an isolated lateral patellar retinaculum release procedure for the treatment of acute lateral dislocation of the patella. In our opinion, arthroscopic lateral release is strictly indicated for patients who have a documented patellar tilt without subluxation. Using a biomechanical cadaveric model, Desio et al. [8] have shown that the intact lateral patellar retinaculum actually prevents lateral displacement of the patella, contributing 10% of the restraining force. Several authors [44–46] have reported recurrent lateral dislocations of the patella, almost exclusively in groups of patients treated by lateral release. Moreover, iatrogenic medial subluxation and dislocation of the patella following lateral release have been reported by several authors [47, 48]. Fithian et al. [49] conducted a scientific survey of the International Patellofemoral Study Group to determine current views regarding lateral patellar release. The survey response rate was 60%. Isolated lateral release was estimated to account for only 1 to 5 surgical cases per respondent per year, or 2% of cases performed annually. The results of the survey showed that only 7% of respondents would consider a lateral release in a first-time lateral patellar dislocation with a tight lateral retinaculum, and 37% would consider a history of lateral patellar dislocation as a contraindication to lateral release procedure. The authors concluded that even among experienced knee surgeons with a special interest in disorders of the patellofemoral joint, isolated lateral release is rarely performed. Strong consensus was found that isolated lateral release should not be undertaken without previous planning in the form of objective clinical indications and preoperative informed consent. Therefore, in view of the above-mentioned findings, we emphasize that lateral release procedure should be used with caution in patients with acute lateral dislocation of the patella.

2.8.3 Medial retinacular repair

Disruption or stretching of the medial patellar retinaculum and MPFL almost always accompanies lateral dislocation of the patella. Hence, the mainstay of early surgical treatment in the acute, first-time patellar dislocation is repair or reefing of the injured medial soft tissue structures, often accompanied by a lateral release procedure.

2.8.4 Medial patellofemoral ligament repair and augmentation

Repair or reefing of the medial retinaculum often does not completely address the medial-sided pathology after acute lateral dislocation of the patella [30]. As mentioned previously, the MPFL is injured in about 90% of patients who sustain acute lateral dislocation of the patella. Therefore, it is logical that patellar stability may be restored by undertaking direct repair of the MPFL with or without augmentation (using a strip of fascia, slip of the medial patellar retinaculum, distal adductor magnus tendon, etc.). However, there is a limited clinical evidence showing the efficacy of such techniques. Going forward, high-quality, prospective randomized clinical studies utilizing a larger population are needed to firmly establish the role of MPFL repair and augmentation in patients with acute lateral dislocation of the patella. In contrast, MPFL reconstruction is a fairly well-established surgical technique and is usually reserved for cases of recurrent patellofemoral instability. A detailed discussion on MPFL reconstruction is provided in Section II of this chapter.

2.9 Rehabilitation

Traditionally and historically, nonoperative treatment has been the mainstay of therapy for patients with acute patellar dislocation. A comprehensive, well-planned supervised rehabilitation program is vital for a successful outcome. The initial goals of rehabilitation are to decrease joint effusion, regain both active and passive range of motion, and advance the weight-bearing status of the extremity. In the next phase, closed kinetic chain exercises, quadriceps strengthening, and proprioceptive exercises are begun. In the last phase of rehabilitation, emphasis is placed on proprioceptive feedback, and functional and sport-specific training [30]. Isokinetic, eccentric, and high-torque exercises can cause high articular cartilage pressures and should be avoided [50]. Core strengthening is emphasized. In addition, gluteal muscle strengthening should be undertaken to improve the external rotators of the hip, thus externally rotating the femur and decreasing the Q-angle. The ultimate goal of rehabilitation is to obtain a pain-free, mobile, stable and functional knee.

The patient is allowed to return to play when the following criteria have been met: Subjectively, there should be no pain, swelling, or sensation of giving-way/instability. Objectively, there should be no joint effusion, no tenderness, a negative patellar apprehension test, and a full, pain-free range of motion in the knee [30]. Quadriceps strength in the affected lower extremity should be at least 80% as compared with the contralateral side. The role and usefulness of patellar bracing and taping in the management of acute patellar dislocation is unclear. Patellofemoral instability symptoms may be reduced in some patients with a patellar cutout brace or patellar taping. Although patellar taping was originally reported to have a high success rate, researchers have been unable to reproduce these results [51]. Patellar bracing and/or taping should be regarded as adjuvants to physical therapy. Patient should be counseled regarding expectations and clinical outcomes of the nonoperative and operative treatment.

2.10 Summary

- There are two distinct groups of patellar dislocations; one group of patients with normal anatomy and a traumatic event, and the other group with predisposing anatomical factors and a history of patellar subluxation or dislocation without a traumatic event [30].

- The MPFL is the main restraint to lateral patellar subluxation/dislocation.
- The MPFL is injured in about 90% of patients who sustain acute lateral dislocation of the patella.
- Lateral patellar dislocation can occur following an indirect mechanism (noncontact injury) wherein the body rotates on a valgus, flexed knee relative to a planted foot, or as a result of a direct blow (contact injury) to the knee.
- A thorough history and a detailed physical examination, supplemented by plain radiographs and MRI, are vital for early, accurate diagnosis.
- The majority of first-time, acute traumatic lateral dislocations of the patella are treated nonoperatively, and this mode of treatment is supported by high-level evidence.
- Surgery is indicated for patients in following situations:

    1. Presence of an osteochondral fracture or major chondral injury.
    2. Substantial disruption of the medial soft tissue patellar stabilizers (medial retinaculum and MPFL).
    3. A persistent laterally subluxed patella.
    4. Recurrent, symptomatic lateral patellar subluxation or dislocation.
    5. Failure of a trial of nonoperative management.

- An organized, supervised rehabilitation program is crucial for optimal recovery and successful clinical outcome.
- Acute patellar dislocations can result in pain, recurrent instability, impairment of knee function, decreased level of sporting activity, and patellofemoral arthritis.
- Patients should be educated and counseled regarding expectations and clinical outcomes of nonoperative and operative treatment.

3. Patellofemoral instability: recurrent dislocation of the patella

Patellar instability by definition is a disorder where the patella pathologically subluxates or dislocates out of the trochlear groove. This most often involves multiple factors, such as acute trauma, chronic ligamentous laxity, connective tissue disorder, anatomical abnormality, or osseous malalignment [50]. Over a period of time, patients with patellar instability can have debilitating pain, limitations in knee function, loss of time from work and/or sports, and long-term arthritis.

Although medial, superior, and intra-articular dislocations of the patellae have been reported, most patellar dislocations are lateral. In clinical practice, lateral patellar subluxations or dislocations are far more common than medial subluxations or dislocations. Medial subluxation of the patella is usually iatrogenic. Medial subluxation may occur as a complication of an extensive lateral release, a lateral release performed for an incorrect indication, overtightening of the medial structures, or blunt or surgical trauma resulting in scarring and inferomedial tethering of the patella [50].

Two mechanisms of acute lateral patellar dislocation have been described: an indirect (noncontact) injury and a direct blow (contact injury) (**Figure 2**). The indirect mechanism is more common and involves the combination of a strong quadriceps contraction, a flexed and valgus knee position, and an internally rotated femur on an externally rotated tibia with the foot planted to the ground [50]. Patients with dislocations due to an indirect mechanism frequently have one or more predisposing anatomical risk factors. These risk factors include genu valgum, increased Q-angle, increased femoral anterversion (internal femoral torsion), external tibial torsion, patella alta, generalized ligamentous laxity, weakening or hypoplasia of the VMO, and trochlear dysplasia or hypoplasia (**Table 1**). Generalized ligamentous laxity is seen in various orthopedic disorders, such as Down syndrome, Ehlers Danlos syndrome, Marfan syndrome, osteogenesis imperfecta, and Morquio-Brailsford syndrome.

3.1 Clinical presentation

A thorough history should be obtained, focusing on the mechanism of injury, the onset and duration of symptoms, any previous history of patellar symptoms, and prior nonoperative or operative treatment. Patients should be asked whether the previous treatment modalities relieved their symptoms. Patients with patellofemoral instability usually present with a history of peripatellar pain, recurrent swelling, crepitus, giving-way or instability, and weakness in the affected extremity. The knee pain may get worse while going down the stair or up the stairs, and during squatting and kneeling. In few cases, the patient may complain of mechanical catching or locking in the knee, and this indicates presence of a loose body (chondral or osteochondral fragment) in the joint. The patient may report that "my kneecap slides, slips, shifts, pops or jumps out of place" or "my kneecap pops or jumps back into place" with certain positions of the knee. Symptoms may occasionally be preceded by a history of traumatic episode but more commonly, the clinical symptoms are insidious in onset.

3.2 Physical examination

A meticulous comprehensive physical examination of the affected extremity as well as the opposite extremity should be performed. The patient should be examined in standing, sitting, and supine positions, while barefoot and dressed in shorts [30]. Gait pattern, obesity, posture and body habitus should be documented [30]. Patients with significant knee pain may demonstrate antalgic gait. A quadriceps avoidance gait (typically seen in patients with anterior cruciate deficiency) with reduced knee flexion in stance phase may be observed in some patients with patellofemoral instability. A Trendelenburg gait with a drop in the contralateral pelvis during stance phase indicates gluteus medius weakness. This change in pelvic obliquity tightens the ipsilateral iliotibial band, causing pain over the lateral aspect of the knee [30].

The skin of the involved extremity should be examined for presence of traumatic scars or surgical incision(s), or evidence of vasomotor dysfunction (such as, alterations in sweating, skin color, and temperature) and trophic changes in the skin, hair, or nails. Any muscle asymmetry of the thigh or calf should be recorded using a measuring tape, by taking circumferential measurements at a standard distance proximal and distal to the knee.

The patient should be evaluated for any physical signs that may serve as prognosticators of patellar instability (**Table 1**). Generalized ligamentous hyperlaxity should be noted by examining finger metacarpophalangeal joint hyperextension, thumb-to-forearm apposition, knee hyperextension, and elbow hyperextension. Abnormalities in femoral anteversion should be measured by observing maximal prone internal and external hip rotation as well as rotation of the leg at the position of maximal prominence of the greater trochanter [52]. Similarly, transmalleolar axis and thigh-foot angle should be used to confirm excessive tibial torsion.

The range of motion and strength in the hip joint should be assessed as some patients with hip disorders may present with a referred knee pain. Examination of the foot should be performed. Some patients with lateral patellar dislocation may have pronation of the foot and hindfoot valgus. A complete neurovascular examination of the limb should be performed.

3.2.1 Sitting examination

The patient should next be examined in the sitting position, with the knees flexed at 90 degrees over the edge of the examination table. The position of the tibial tuberosity should be observed in relation to the center of the patella. Patella alta or baja can be easily observed from the side. The Q-angle (the angle between the quadriceps tendon and the patellar tendon) should be measured with the knee in flexion. Measurements of the Q-angle in full extension may be falsely low in patients with patellar subluxation. The angle is recorded by drawing one line from the anterior superior iliac spine to the center of the patella and another line from the center of the patella to the center of the tibial tuberosity. The mean Q-angle is about 10 degrees in men and 15 degrees in women [50].

Patellofemoral tracking is assessed as the patient sits on the edge of the examination table. The patient is asked to take the knee from flexion into full extension. The term *J sign* refers to an abnormal tracking pattern in which the patella sits lateral to the femoral sulcus in full extension; the movement of the patella appears in the shape of an upside-down *J* as the knee goes from flexion into full extension [30]. Conversely, the patella starts laterally with the knee in extension and makes an abrupt shift medially as it enters the femoral trochlea at about 20 to 30 degrees of knee flexion. The exact cause of the *J sign* is not known; however, factors such as VMO deficiency, underlying osseous morphology and soft tissue imbalance are postulated as causative factors for the occurrence of *J sign.*

3.2.2 Supine examination

The next stage of the patellofemoral examination consists of evaluation of the patella and related structures. Presence of joint effusion should be noted. The peripatellar soft tissues are carefully palpated. Tenderness over the medial femoral epicondyle region (Bassett's sign) may represent an injury to the MPFL in patients with acute or recurrent dislocations of the patella [53]. Tenderness on palpation of the inferior pole of the patella is often diagnostic of patellar tendinitis, whereas tenderness over the proximal pole of the patella may indicate quadriceps tendinitis. Tenderness within the substance of the distal quadriceps tendon or the proximal patellar tendon is suggestive of diffuse tendinosis. Tenderness along the medial border of the patella may represent injury to the medial patellar retinaculum and the MPFL. The MPFL should be palpated along its entire course from the femoral origin to the patellar insertion. The insertion of VMO should be palpated for tenderness or defect. Tenderness on the lateral border of the patella is often found in patients with excessive lateral pressure syndrome. Tenderness over the lateral femoral condyle is indicative of osteochondral fracture. In patients who have undergone previous surgery, the surgical incision area should be examined for the presence of neuroma. A diagnostic lidocaine injection is helpful to confirm a clinically suspected diagnosis of neuroma. Retinacular tenderness, hypersensitivity to palpation, and decreased patellar mobility are suggestive of Complex Regional Pain Syndrome Type I (previously known as Reflex Sympathetic Dystrophy). Active and passive range of motion in the affected knee should be evaluated and any deficit or asymmetry (as compared with the opposite, normal knee) should be recorded. A resisted straight-leg raise test is performed to rule out disruption of the extensor mechanism (i.e. quadriceps tendon and patellar tendon). The neurological and vascular status of the extremity should be assessed.

3.2.3 Patellar tilt test

Patellar tilt test is used to determine the tightness or integrity of the medial and lateral soft tissue restraints. The test is performed with the knee extended and the quadriceps relaxed. The examiner attempts to raise the patient's lateral patellar facet away from the lateral femoral trochlea. An inability to raise the lateral facet to the horizontal is indicative of lateral retinacular tightness and tethering of the lateral patella.

3.2.4 Patellar glide test

Patellar glide test is performed to assess the integrity of the medial and lateral patellar restraints. Patellar mobility is assessed by attempting to displace the patella medially and laterally. Throughout this portion of the examination, the knee is placed in full extension, with the quadriceps relaxed. The number of quadrants of medial and lateral glide is recorded as lateral and medial patellar pressure are applied. The amount of patellar glide on the affected side should be compared with that on the opposite, asymptomatic side. In a normal knee, the patella cannot be displaced more than half its width in either direction [50].

3.2.5 Patellar apprehension test

The patient lies supine on the examination table. The examiner passively translates the patella laterally with the knee flexed 20 to 30 degrees and the quadriceps relaxed. In a positive test, the patient experiences a feeling of impending subluxation or dislocation of the patella and this is called apprehension [54, 55]. (**Figure 3**). Some patients even make an attempt to hold the examiner's hand to prevent the patella from subluxating or dislocating laterally. Pain usually accompanies the apprehension; however, the latter is considered the major component of a positive test.

3.2.6 Patellar compression test

The patella should be palpated for retropatellar tenderness and crepitus which may suggest an injury to the articular cartilage. Compression of the patella during full range of motion of the knee may reproduce the associated pain. The location of the chondral injury may be estimated on the basis of the knee-flexion angle in which pain is experienced. The patellofemoral contact area moves proximally on the patella as the knee flexion increases. Articular lesions on the distal patella are painful during early knee flexion, whereas proximal patellar lesions are manifested with further knee flexion. Clinically suspected chondral lesions should be confirmed by MRI assessment to help in preoperative planning.

The flexibility of the lower extremity should be evaluated, especially in reference to hamstrings tightness. Excessive tightness of the hamstrings requires greater quadriceps force for knee extension, leading to increased transmission of contact pressure across the patellofemoral joint. Hamstring flexibility is best assessed by measuring the popliteal angle. Gastrocnemius and soleus tightness should also be evaluated. The flexibility of both muscles can be judged by ankle dorsiflexion with the knee extended. With the knee flexed, the gastrocnemius is relaxed, and the soleus is isolated. In both positions, the ankle should dorsiflex 15 to 20 degrees past neutral. Limitation of ankle dorsiflexion causes a compensatory increase in subtalar pronation, thereby increasing internal tibial rotation during gait [30]. The lower extremity should also be examined for iliotibial band tightness and the examination finding should be compared with that in the opposite limb. Iliotibial band tightness is assessed by performing the time-honored Ober's test [56]. With the patient in the lateral decubitus (with the affected extremity on top), the hip and knees are flexed to 90 degrees initially. The examiner then places one hand on the pelvis to stabilize and monitor for movement. The ipsilateral leg is abducted, brought into full extension at the hip and the knee, and then adducted toward the table. Tightness or pain may be elicited. The test is considered positive if the patient's leg does not lower beyond neutral as the examiner lowers it from an abducted and slightly extended position, suggesting shortness of the tensor fascia lata and iliotibial band. A negative test results in the leg returning normally toward the examination table.

3.2.7 Tests for associated meniscal injury

The medial and lateral joint lines should be examined for areas of tenderness. Medial joint line tenderness is suggestive of meniscal tear, arthrosis, or tear of the patellomeniscal ligament along its course to insertion on the anterior horn of the medial meniscus [30]. McMurray's test and Thessaly test are performed to rule out meniscal tear. The Thessaly test [57] is performed as follows: The patient stands on one leg while holding the examiner's hand for support. The examiner instructs the patient to rotate the body and leg internally and externally 3 times with the knee bent at 5 degrees and then at 20 degrees. The test should be first performed on the unaffected side so that the patient can properly perform movement as a practice run before testing the affected knee. The test is considered positive when pain or clicking occurs at the joint line. A locking or catching sensation is also suggestive of meniscal injury.

3.2.8 Tests for associated cruciate and collateral ligament injury

Patellar symptoms may be masked due to presence of concomitant anterior cruciate ligament deficiency; therefore, the Lachman and pivot shift tests should be performed. Posterior cruciate ligament insufficiency has been reported to be associated with patellofemoral arthrosis. Hence, the posterior drawer test is also an essential part of a complete physical examination. Valgus testing to determine the integrity of the medial collateral ligament is important in patients with a patellar dislocation because simultaneous medial collateral ligament and MPFL injuries can occur.

After completion of the physical examination, aspiration of an intra-articular effusion can be done to determine the diagnosis. A hemarthrosis implies a traumatic injury, whereas serosanguinous fluid may indicate an articular cartilage lesion. In patients with acute dislocations of the patella, it is important to examine the aspirate for the presence of fat droplets, which indicate the presence of an associated osteochondral fracture [50].

3.3 Radiographic studies

The radiographic investigations include plain radiographic series, stress radiography (less popular), Computed Tomography (CT) scan, and MRI examination. Recently, dynamic magnetic resonance imaging and 4-dimensional computed tomography have been introduced for better kinematic assessment of the patellofemoral maltracking during extension-flexion motion [58].

3.3.1 Plain radiographs

In all patients with recurrent dislocation of the patella, a complete plain radiographic series, consisting of standing anterior–posterior view, 45-degree flexion posterior–anterior weight-bearing view (Rosenberg view), lateral view, and axial view should be obtained. In patients with clinically diagnosed malalignment of the extremity, an additional full-length, standing alignment radiograph should also be obtained. Plain radiographs are a useful screening tool to rule out gross malalignment and fractures. However, they underestimate the presence of articular surface lesions.

3.3.2 The anteroposterior radiograph

The anteroposterior radiographs of the knee are useful to diagnose malalignment, patellar fracture, bipartite patella, and arthritis. Although patella alta and baja (infera) can be visualized on antero-posterior radiograph, they are best quantified on a 30-degree lateral radiographic view of the knee.

3.3.3 The lateral radiograph

A true lateral radiograph of the knee should be obtained, showing overlap of the distal and posterior cortices of the medial and lateral femoral condyles. The lateral view allows determination of the patellar height and depth of the femoral trochlea. Several measurements have been described to measure patella alta. Controversy exists as to which radiographic measurement is most accurate. When the patella does not engage in the trochlea by 15 to 20 degrees of knee flexion, patella alta may be present.

3.3.4 Assessment of patellar height

The Insall-Salvati [32], modified Insall-Salvati [33], Blackburne-Peel [34], and Caton-Deschamps [35] ratios are commonly used to measure the patellar height. A detailed description of these ratios has been published in standard orthopedic textbooks. The Insall-Salvati [32] index is based on the ratio of the length of the patellar tendon divided by the greatest length of the patella. The normal ratio defined by the authors is 1.0. A ratio of >1.2 indicates patella alta whereas, a ratio of <0.8 denotes patella baja. However, difficulty in determining the exact insertion site of the patellar tendon and abnormal morphology (such as elongated inferior pole of the patella) of the non-articular portion of the patella may falsely alter this ratio. Furthermore, the patellar tendon length varies between sexes in the normal population [59]. In order to eliminate these variables, Grelsamer and Meadows [33] proposed a modified Insall-Salvati ratio. This modified ratio is defined as the distance from the inferior point of the articular surface of the patella to the patellar tendon insertion into the tibial tuberosity, divided by the length of the articular surface of the patella. Using this method, patella alta is defined as a ratio greater than 2.0, a point at which only 3% of controls would be falsely identified as patella alta [33]. Blackburne and Peel [34] reported a ratio that is independent of the length of the patellar tendon. Their index is defined as the ratio of the length of the perpendicular line from the lower end of the articular surface of the patella to the tibial plateau line, divided by the length of the articular surface of the patella. Based on their study, a ratio of 0.8 is considered normal, a ratio of >1.0 indicates patella alta, whereas a ratio of <0.5 denotes patella baja [34]. Caton and Deschamps [35] have also described a ratio to address the difficulty in measuring the length of the patellar tendon. Their ratio is defined as the ratio of the distance from the inferior articular surface of the patella to the anterosuperior border of the tibia, divided by the length of the articular surface of the patella. Based on the Caton-Deschamp index, a ratio of >1.2 indicates patella alta and < 0.6 indicates patella baja. Seil et al. [60] recommended the Blackburne and Peel ratio to measure the patellar height because it showed the most intermediate classification results and the lowest interobserver variability.

3.3.5 Assessment of trochlear morphology

The morphology of the trochlea should be carefully assessed on a true lateral view of the knee as trochlear dysplasia is a known risk factor for recurrent patellar instability. On the true lateral radiograph, three anterior lines are visualized: the most anterior line is a projection of the medial femoral condyle, the middle line is a projection of the lateral femoral condyle, and the remaining line is a projection of the floor of the trochlea. Dejour et al. [61] have evaluated trochlear morphology and reported two separate measures in a radiographic study of the factors of patellar instability; First measure is the trochlear bump and the second is trochlear depth. The trochlear bump is defined as the distance between the projection of the anterior femoral cortex and the projection of the trochlea, which can be anterior positive or posterior negative. The trochlear bump was greater than +3 mm in 85% of patients with objective patellar instability [61]. The trochlear depth is defined as the depth of the trochlea along a line 15 degrees from the perpendicular to the tangent of the posterior femoral cortex. A depth of less than 4 mm was found in 85% of patients with objective patellar instability and in only 3% of controls [61].

One should also look for supratrochlear spur, crossing sign and double contour sign on the lateral radiograph of the knee. The supratrochlear spur is a global prominence of the trochlea. The crossing sign represents an abnormally elevated floor of the trochlear groove rising above the top of the wall of one of the femoral condyles. On the lateral radiograph of the knee, trochlear dysplasia is defined by the crossing sign [62] which refers to the crossing over of the trochlear floor condensation with the condensation of the most prominent aspect of the lateral trochlea and is found in 96% of the population with a history of true dislocation but in only 3% of healthy controls [61, 63]. The double contour sign is a radiographic line that represents the hypoplastic medial facet on the lateral view [64, 65].

Radiographically, trochlear dysplasia is defined by a sulcus angle of greater than 145 degrees as seen on axial radiographic views of the patellofemoral joint [66, 67]. Dejour and colleagues [67, 68] have classified trochlear dysplasia into 4 types as shown in **Figure 4**.

- In type A dysplasia, there is a crossing sign on the lateral radiographs and the trochlear groove is symmetric but shallower than normal, with a sulcus angle greater than 145° on axial images.

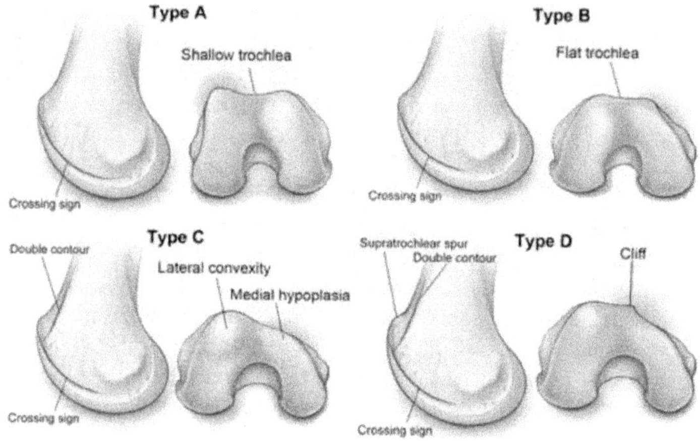

Figure 4.
Dejour classifications of trochlear dysplasia. Type A: Crossing sign, trochlear morphology preserved (fairly shallow trochlea, >145°). Type B: Crossing sign, supratrochlear spur, flat or convex trochlea. Type C: Crossing sign, double contour (projection on the lateral view of the hypoplastic medial facet). Type D: Crossing sign, supratrochlear spur, double contour, asymmetry of trochlear facets, vertical link between the medial and the lateral facet (cliff pattern). Reprinted with permission from: Onor et al. [69].

- In Type B dysplasia, there is a crossing sign as well as a supratrochlear spur on lateral radiographs, with a flat or convex trochlea on axial images.
- In Type C dysplasia, there is a crossing sign and a double contour sign on lateral radiographs, with lateral facet convexity and medial facet hypoplasia on axial images.
- In Type D dysplasia, there is a crossing sign, supratrochlear spur, and a double contour sign on lateral radiographs. There is asymmetry of the trochlear facets with medial facet hypoplasia. There is a vertical slope demonstrating the so-called "cliff pattern" on axial images because of asymmetry of the lateral and medial trochlear facets.

The Dejour classification is widely referred to in the literature and currently considered the gold standard for the description of trochlear dysplasia.

3.3.6 The Axial Radiograph

The axial views as described by Merchant and colleagues [36] and Laurin and colleagues [37, 38] are commonly used for the evaluation of the patellofemoral joint. The axial view is helpful for diagnosing lateral patellar tilt and also provides valuable information about any persistent subluxation or dislocation of the patella. The sulcus angle can be measured on the axial view. Tangential osteochondral fracture of the medial facet of the patella or osteochondral fracture of the lateral femoral condyle may be visualized on an axial radiograph.

3.3.7 Stress Radiographs

Stress radiography is widely practiced in Europe and less commonly utilized in USA. Stress radiographs are helpful in identifying patients with patellofemoral instability. Measurements on stress radiographs are more reliable predictors of lateral, medial, and multidirectional patellar instability than measurements made on static radiographs [50]. Moreover, they can provide useful objective information when evaluating the results of different treatment regimens. Patients who are unable to relax the extensor mechanism due to pain or who have bilateral symptoms are not candidates for stress radiography [50].

3.3.8 Computed Tomography

Computed tomography (CT) has been shown to be more accurate in detecting patellar malalignment than conventional axial radiography [70]. Among the advantages of CT over plain radiography are that there is no image overlap or distortion and that there are precise reference points for reliable measurements [50]. The conventional axial radiographs cannot assess the patellofemoral joint with the knee in full extension, whereas the cross-sectional nature of the CT scan allows the patellofemoral joint to be evaluated in such position and enhances detection of early lateral subluxation of the patella (within 0 to 30 degrees of knee flexion). Examination of the knee in extension is crucial because most patellar instability occur in the first 30 degrees of knee flexion, before the patella is constrained by the trochlea [30]. Measurements of congruence angle, lateral patellofemoral angle, patellar tilt, TT-TG distance, and rotational abnormalities of the femur and tibia have been studied extensively using a CT scan.

3.3.9 Tibial Tuberosity-Trochlear Groove (TT-TG) Distance

Computed Tomography scan can help in identifying lateralization of the tibial tuberosity, as measured by the TT-TG distance. An axial CT image demonstrating the femoral trochlear groove is superimposed on an axial image of the tibial tuberosity. A line is drawn on this superimposed image along the posterior margins of the femoral condyles. Two lines are then drawn perpendicular to this line, one bisecting the femoral trochlear groove and the other bisecting the anterior aspect of the tibial tuberosity. The distance between these two lines determines the extent of lateralization of the tibial tuberosity. A normal TT-TG distance is around 9 mm. A TT-TG distance >20 mm is considered abnormal. Values greater than 9 mm have been shown to identify patients with patellofemoral malalignment with a sensitivity of 85% and specificity of 95% [71].

3.3.10 Magnetic resonance imaging

Magnetic resonance imaging (MRI) combines the accuracy of osseous measurements made on CT scan with the ability to visualize the soft tissues. Furthermore, MR imaging can detect pathologies such as, articular cartilage lesion of the patella and/or the femoral condyle. Advantages of the MRI include ability to obtain images in multiple planes, better soft tissue resolution, and no risk of exposure to radiation. Sallay et al. [72] have reported the pathoanatomic features of patellar dislocations using MRI. The location of the injury was confirmed by surgical exploration. In their study, MRI revealed effusion in all 23 patients (100%), tears of the femoral attachment of the MPFL in 20 patients (87%), increased signal intensity and retraction of the vastus medialis muscle in 18 patients (78%), a bone bruise in the lateral femoral condyle in 20 (87%), and a bone bruise in the medial patella in 7 (30%). Arthroscopic examination revealed osteochondral lesions involving the patella and the lateral femoral condyle in 68% of cases. Open surgical exploration revealed tears of the MPFL off the femur in 15 of 16 patients (94%). Sallay et al. [72] also noted that the location of the bone bruise on the lateral femoral condyle was slightly anterior and superior to the typical bone bruise seen after an acute anterior cruciate

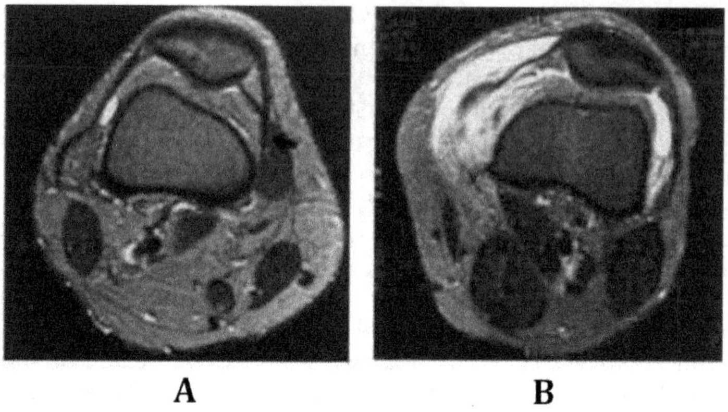

Figure 5.
(A). Axial MR image of the knee showing a normal MPFL. (B). Axial MR image of the knee demonstrating an avulsion of the MPFL from its femoral attachment. Reprinted with permission from Boden et al. [50].

ligament injury. An axial MRI image of the knee showing an avulsion of the MPFL from its femoral attachment is shown in **Figure 5**.

Injury to the VMO, which lies superficial to the MPFL, frequently presents as edema, hemorrhage, and/or elevation of the muscle away from the medial femoral condyle [73, 74]. Approximately 50–80% of injured MPFLs are disrupted at their femoral origin [73–75].

4. Principles of treatment of patellofemoral instability

4.1 Nonoperative treatment

Based on our extensive clinical experience (level V evidence), we have found that nonoperative treatment of chronic patellar dislocations (treated initially by a period of brief immobilization followed by rehabilitation) has produced less satisfactory or even dismal results, with nearly half of patients having recurrent dislocations or continued knee symptoms. Steiner and Parker [30] have also reported less satisfactory clinical outcomes following nonoperative treatment of patients with chronic patellofemoral instability. We believe that immobilization for patients with recurrent episodes of patellar dislocation may be used in the short-term for patient comfort; however, it is of little benefit in the long-term. A trial of rehabilitation may be offered to a patient who experiences only occasional dislocation and displays no obvious predisposing anatomic or radiographic abnormalities [30]. Rehabilitation may be augmented by the use of a patellar brace or orthosis if tolerated by the patient. On the other hand, patients who have predisposing anatomical risk factors (**Table 1**) or those who experience recurrent patellar dislocation with activities of daily living will likely require operative treatment.

4.2 Operative treatment

Operative treatment for patients with recurrent patellar instability should be directed at the underlying causative pathoanatomy that can be determined by careful history-taking, meticulous physical examination, and pertinent radiographic studies. We emphasize an individualized treatment approach rather "one-size-fits-all" approach. Surgical intervention should be based on clear understanding of the underlying pathoanatomic risk factor(s) and radiographic abnormality as shown below:

1. Reconstruction of the MPFL is indicated for patients with recurrent instability, with or without trochlear dysplasia, who have a normal TT-TG distance and a normal patellar height.

2. Distal realignment procedures should be performed for patients who have an increased TT-TG distance (>20 mm) or patella alta.

3. A standard medialization of the tibial tuberosity can be performed if there is a normal patellar height and trochlear anatomy, and an increased TT-TG distance (>20 mm). Distalization of the tuberosity can be added if there is concomitant patella alta, and anteromedialization of the tuberosity is performed if there is lateral and/or distal patellar facet chondrosis.

4. Patients with moderate-to-severe trochlear dyslpasia can be treated by trochleoplasty.

5. Corrective derotation osteotomy may be required for patients with rotational (torsional) abnormality of the femur or tibia.

Patients with recurrent patellofemoral instability often have multiple anatomical and/or radiographic risk factors. In such a scenario, a combination of abovementioned surgical procedures is necessary to restore patellar stability.

4.2.1 Arthroscopic assessment

A thorough arthroscopic evaluation of the knee joint should be performed. The articular surfaces of the patella and femoral trochlea should be assessed. The extent and type of chondral lesion are determined by probing the articular surface. Large, unstable chondral lesions should be fixed, whereas the small fragments are excised. The superomedial portal is particularly useful in evaluating patellar tracking and patellar tilt [76]. The lateral facet should align with the trochlea by 20 to 25 degrees of knee flexion and the mid-patellar ridge should align with the trochlea by 35 to 40 degrees of knee flexion. Any lateral overhang of the patella should be documented while the patella is engaging the femoral trochlea. Evidence of patellar tilt should be noted.

4.2.2 Lateral retinacular release

In our opinion, isolated lateral release has a very limited role in the management of patellofemoral instability. This procedure may be combined (when indicated) with other procedures such as MPFL reconstruction or distal realignment. Lateral release is effective in reducing patellar tilt. It is important to keep in mind that excessive or unindicated lateral release procedure can result in iatrogenic medial subluxation or dislocation of the patella.

4.2.3 Proximal realignment procedures

The goal of proximal realignment surgery is to reestablish a dynamic balance of forces around the patella. In 1979, Insall and associates described the "tube" realignment procedure for the treatment of chondromalacia patellae [77]. The procedure consists of release of the medial and lateral retinacular tissue, which are sewn together over the quadriceps proximal to the patella. Since then, modifications of this procedure involving a lateral release, with a lateral and 1-cm distal advancement of the vastus medialis, have been described in the treatment of patellar dislocation.

4.2.4 Distal realignment procedures

Historically numerous surgical procedures (such as Roux-Goldthwait procedure, Hauser procedure, Elmslie-Trillat procedure – to name a few) for restoring patellofemoral stability have been described. Few of these reconstructive techniques are still popular in some parts of the word. The Hauser technique has fallen out of favor because of high incidence of patellofemoral arthritis at long-term follow-up. The Elmslie-Trillat procedure allows medialization without posterior transfer of the tibial tuberosity in combination with lateral release and medial capsular reefing. Carney and associates [78] have reported the long-term outcome of the Roux-Elmslie-Trillat procedure for patellar instability. In their study, 18 patients who underwent the Roux-Elmslie-Trillat procedure for dislocation or subluxation of the patella were identified from a group previously evaluated at a mean follow-up of 3 years. The prevalence of recurrent subluxation or dislocation in patients with patellofemoral malalignment who underwent the Roux-Elmslie-Trillat procedure was similar (7%) at 3 and 26 years' of follow-up. Fifty-four percent of the patients rated their affected knee as good or excellent at 26 years' of follow-up. The long-term functional status of the affected knee in patients who underwent the Roux-Elmslie-Trillat procedure declined.

Anteromedial tibial tuberosity transfer has been described by Fulkerson [79, 80]. In this procedure, an osteotomy of variable obliquity is made. Such an osteotomy allows the degree of anterior and medial transfer of the tibial tuberosity that can be independently adjusted to address the patient's individual pathology. The Fulkerson procedure (anteromedial tibial tuberosity transfer) corrects the Q-angle with medialization of the tibial tuberosity and unloads the patellofemoral joint with anteriorization of the tibial tuberosity. A hinge of bone is maintained intact at the distal aspect of the tuberosity to facilitate healing. After the tibial tuberosity has been transferred anteriorly and medially, the bone pedicle is locked into position with two cortical screws. Molina and associates [81] have showed that the most predictable way of increasing contact area and decreasing patellofemoral stress is transfer of the tibial tuberosity 1 cm anteriorly and 0.5 to 1 cm medially.

The indications for anteromedial tibial tuberosity transfer are:

1. Patients with recurrent patellar instability who have an increased TT-TG distance (>20 mm).

2. Patients with patellofemoral malalignment who have degenerative changes in the distal and lateral articular surface of the patella.

The contraindications for anteromedial tibial tuberosity transfer are:

1. Patients who have a normal TT-TG distance.

2. Presence of significant chondrosis affecting the proximal and/or medial facet of the patella.

3. Skeletally immature patients with patellar subluxation or dislocation.

4. Relative contraindications include smoking and severe osteoporosis.

The tibial tuberosity transfer procedure should not be performed in skeletally immature patients (who have open growth plates) with recurrent patellar instability due to the risk of premature closure of the physis and subsequent development of genu recurvatum.

Complications of anteromedial tibial tuberosity transfer include skin slough, hematoma, wound infection, compartment syndrome, knee stiffness, persistent knee pain, delayed union or non-union at the osteotomy site, symptomatic hardware, hardware failure (loosening, migration or breakage of the hardware), risk of proximal tibial facture, and progressive chondral deterioration.

Fracture of the proximal part of the tibia or of the tibial tuberosity after anteromedial tibial tuberosity transfer has been reported by several authors [82–84]. In order to prevent the occurrence of such a complication, various preventive measures have been suggested; these strategies include avoidance of step cuts [82], an osteotomy of at least 5 cm in length and 0.75 cm in thickness to avoid fracture of the tibial tuberosity [82], protected weight-bearing for six to eight weeks in a hinged knee brace, and advancement to full weight-bearing only when the osteotomy site has fully healed radiographically [83–85].

Stetson et al. [83] reviewed the records of 234 patients who underwent anteromedialization of the tibial tubercle with oblique osteotomy. In their series, six patients (2.6%) had fractures of the proximal tibia postoperatively, within 13 weeks of the Fulkerson osteotomy. All fractures occurred after a change in the postoperative physical therapy regimen from partial weight-bearing to immediate full weight-bearing. Given this increase in fracture incidence, a more conservative postoperative physical therapy regimen was recommended. The authors concluded that patients should be non-weight-bearing initially, advanced gradually to partial weight-bearing, and allowed full weight-bearing only after the osteotomy site shows radiographic evidence of complete healing.

Cosgarea et al. [85], in their biomechanical study, performed oblique and flat osteotomies on 13 pairs of fresh-frozen cadaveric knees. The knees were then tested to failure on a materials testing system by exerting a load through the quadriceps tendon at a rate of 1000 N/sec to simulate a stumble injury. The authors found that the failure mechanism for flat osteotomies was more likely to be a tubercle "shingle" fracture, while oblique osteotomies more frequently failed through a tibial fracture or fixation failure in the posterior tibial cortex. These authors recommended flat osteotomy for patients with isolated recurrent patellar instability and an oblique osteotomy in patients who have concomitant patellofemoral pain or degenerative changes in the articular cartilage. In cases where an oblique osteotomy is used, the authors recommended postoperative brace protection and restricted weight-bearing until the osteotomy site heals.

4.2.5 Trochleoplasty

Different surgical techniques have been developed to correct the pathologic trochlear morphology seen in patients with recurrent patellofemoral instability. These techniques include deepening of a shallow or flat trochlear groove (trochleoplasty), elevation of the anterior portion of the femoral condyles (trochlear osteotomy), and/or removal of a prominent trochlear bump. Numerous variations in these techniques and retrospective case series of their results have been reported. However, there are no prospective, randomized controlled studies in the literature that support the use of these techniques [30]. Trochleoplasty is more popular in Europe. There are concerns about possible irreversible damage to the articular cartilage and subchondral bone of the femoral trochlea, and these concerns have limited the use of trochleoplasty in the United States.

Trochleoplasty is a complex, challenging and technically demanding surgical procedure. Several authors have reported their experience with the use of trochleoplasty in the management of trochlear dysplasia in patients with patellofemoral instability [67, 68, 86–95]. Indications for a sulcus-deepening trochleoplasty include abnormal patellar tracking with a *J-sign*, usually manifested by a TT-TG distance of greater than 10 to 20 mm, and/or a dome-shaped trochlea noted on a perfect lateral radiograph of the knee with overlap of the posterior femoral condyles, and radiographic evidence of trochlear dysplasia in a patient with recurrent patellofemoral instability [89]. In a trochleoplasty procedure, a strip of cortical bone around the edge of the trochlea is elevated and the cancellous bone of the trochlea is exposed. The new trochlear sulcus is then created, proximal and about 3 to 6 degrees lateral to the previous sulcus, by removing the cancellous bone. Next, the trochlear bone shell is impacted into the new sulcus and fixed with two small staples. Alternatively, the bone shell can be secured using resorbable sutures [87, 90]. Early postoperative complications include arthrofibrosis and bothersome patellofemoral crepitus. Meticulous surgical technique in combination with postoperative continuous passive motion (CPM) are vital for maintaining range of motion of the knee and to ensure optimal clinical outcome.

Von Knoch et al. [90] reported the clinical and radiological outcome of trochleoplasty for recurrent patellar dislocation in association with trochlear dysplasia. Thirty-eight consecutive patients (45 knees) were treated by trochleoplasty, medial reefing, with or without reconstruction of the MPFL. The patients were reviewed at a mean follow-up of 8.3 years (range, 4 to 14 years). A total of 33 knees were available for radiological assessment. None of the patients had recurrence of dislocation after trochleoplasty. Preoperatively, patellofemoral pain was present in 35 knees. Postoperatively, 15 (43%) of 35 knees had worsening of the patellofemoral pain. The most recent Kujala score averaged 95 points (range, 80 to 100 points). The depth of the trochlea increased and the trochlear boss height was reduced. Although trochleoplasty was effective in preventing future patellar dislocations, it did not halt the progression of patellofemoral arthritis. At latest follow-up, ten (30%) of the 33 knees had osteoarthritic changes in the patellofemoral compartment.

Rouanet et al. [95] reported the long-term results of sulcus deepening trochleoplasty for patellofemoral instability. In their study, 34 cases were reviewed after a mean follow-up of 15 years (range, 12 to 19 years). No recurrent objective instability was observed. Seven knees had additional surgery after a mean follow-up of 7 years. Furthermore, 7 cases required conversion to total knee arthroplasty because of progression of osteoarthritis. Overall, there was an improvement in the knee function postoperatively. Patients were satisfied in 65% of the cases. At the time of the final follow-up, osteoarthritis was present in 33/34 cases. The authors concluded that the sulcus deepening trochleoplasty corrects patellofemoral instability in patients with severe trochlear dysplasia and the long-term functional outcome is better in this group. However, it does not prevent patellofemoral osteoarthritis. The sulcus deepening trochleoplasty procedure should be limited to patients who have severe trochlear dysplasia in conjunction with supratrochlear spurs, and this procedure should be combined with other surgical techniques to realign the extensor mechanism of the knee.

In conclusion, we believe that trochleoplasty has a limited but important role in the management of patients with recurrent patellofemoral instability with concurrent moderate-to-severe trochlear dysplasia. In such cases, trochleoplasty should be undertaken in combination with other surgical procedures, such as MPFL reconstruction or distal realignment procedure.

4.2.6 Medial Patellofemoral Ligament (MPFL) Reconstruction

Various authors have reported that the MPFL is universally disrupted in patients with lateral patellar dislocation and that its integrity is of primary importance to maintain stability of the patella [6, 8, 9, 72, 75, 96]. Hence, it is important to undertake reconstruction of MPFL (when indicated) in patients with recurrent patellofemoral instability to restore the patellofemoral biomechanics and kinematics. Medial patellofemoral ligament reconstruction has become one of the most common and widely used procedures to regain stability in patients with recurrent lateral dislocation of the patella. Recent studies have demonstrated low recurrence rates, improved patient-reported outcome measures, and a high rate of return to sports. Reconstruction of the MPFL is typically indicated for patients with recurrent patellofemoral instability, with or without trochlear dysplasia, who have a normal TT-TG distance and a normal patellar height. The procedure may be performed with concomitant procedures, such as distalization of the tibial tuberosity in a patient with patella alta, or trochleoplasty in a patient with high-grade trochlear dysplasia.

Numerous surgical techniques have been reported for reconstruction of the MPFL. A detailed description of all available techniques is beyond the scope of this chapter. The MPFL reconstruction can be performed using various sources of graft material, such as the medial retinaculum [97], adductor magnus tendon [98–102], patellar tendon [103, 104], quadriceps tendon [105–115], and most commonly, hamstring tendon (gracilis or semitendinosus tendon) [116–136]. In general, about 80–96% good to excellent results following isolated MPFL reconstruction have been reported.

Over the years, various methods of fixation of the tendon graft have been reported; these methods of fixation include staples, spiked washers, sutures, bone tunnels, interference screws, and bone anchors [30]. It is worth noting that variation in the location and length of the graft can greatly alter the compressive forces at the medial aspect of the patellofemoral joint [30].

4.3 At What Knee Flexion Angle the Graft Should be Fixed?

There is still no clear consensus of opinion regarding the ideal knee flexion angle at which the tendon graft should be fixed during MPFL reconstruction. Most authors prefer to fix the graft with the knee at 30 to 60 degrees of flexion. Patel et al. [137] conducted a systematic review to determine the effect of knee flexion angle during graft fixation on outcomes and complications following MPFL reconstruction. Of the 3399 studies, 17 studies satisfied the inclusion criteria. A total of 556 patients with a mean age of 24 years underwent MPFL reconstructions, with 458 patients in the 0° to 30° fixation group and 98 in the 45° to 90° fixation group. The authors concluded that the knee flexion angle during MPFL graft fixation ranges from 20° to 90°. Graft fixation at both low and high knee flexion angles during MPFL reconstruction showed excellent patient-reported outcomes and low patellar redislocation rates overall, with no clear differences between the 2 groups based on the available data.

4.4 Use of Autograft versus Allograft for MPFL Reconstruction

Kumar et al. [138] completed a retrospective chart review on patients younger than 18 years of age who underwent MPFL reconstruction for recurrent instability after failed nonoperative management. The patients were divided into autograft or allograft hamstring cohorts for comparison. Primary outcome measures were return to normal activity, incidence of redislocation/subluxation, pain, stiffness, Kujala scores, and other complications. After criteria were applied, there were 59 adolescents (38 girls and 21 boys; mean ± SD age of 15.2 ± 1.7 years). Allograft was used in 36 patients and the autograft in 23. The patients were reviewed at a mean follow-up of 4.1 ± 1.9 years (allograft, 3.3 ± 1.1 years; autograft, 5.7 ± 2.1 years;

$P \leq 0.001$). The authors identified no significant differences in return to activity, pain score changes, and incidences of failure between patients undergoing MPFL reconstruction with allograft versus autograft. Although teenagers with surviving autograft MPFL reconstruction reported statistically higher Kujala scores, the mean score difference of 5 points was not clinically significant. It appears that using allograft tendon instead of autograft tissue for MPFL reconstruction in this teenage population does not adversely affect the long-term outcomes.

The choice of autograft or allograft for MPFL reconstruction is based on surgeon and/or patient preference. A thorough preoperative counseling should be undertaken, and advantages and disadvantages of each graft source should be discussed with the patient before choosing the tendon graft for MPFL reconstruction.

4.5 Single-Bundle or Double-Bundle MPFL Reconstruction?

Singhal et al. [139] carried out a meta-analysis of studies reporting outcomes of MPFL reconstruction using hamstring tendon autograft in a double-bundle configuration and patellar fixation via mediolateral patellar tunnels. The primary outcome examined was the postoperative Kujala score. The authors identified 320 MPFL reconstructions in nine relevant articles. The combined mean postoperative Kujala score was 92 using a fixed effects model and 89 using random effect modeling. The reported rate of complications with MPFL reconstruction was 12.5% (40 of 320), with stiffness of the knee being the most common. The authors concluded that high-quality evidence in assessing double-bundle MPFL reconstruction is lacking. The current literature consists of a mixture of prospective and retrospective case series. High-quality, prospective randomized controlled trials are needed before definitive conclusions can be drawn regarding the superiority of one form of surgical technique over the other.

Kang et al. [140] performed a systematic review of the single-bundle (SB) and double-bundle (DB) MPFL reconstruction procedures using the hamstring tendon autografts, and compared the clinical outcomes including the Kujala score, postoperative apprehension, recurrent subluxation or dislocation, and complications. Thirty-one articles were included, involving 1063 patients (1116 knees). Two hundred and forty-four patients (254 knees) underwent SB reconstruction, whereas 819 patients (862 knees) underwent DB reconstruction. The pooled mean values of Kujala score improvement were similar in both groups. The SB group had a significantly greater rate of postoperative apprehension (8%) than the DB group (4%). There were no significant differences between the SB and DB groups in the rates of recurrent subluxation or dislocation and complications. The authors concluded that the DB procedure for isolated MPFL reconstruction demonstrates similar outcomes as compared to the SB technique regarding improvement of knee function, recurrent subluxation or dislocation, and complications. The SB technique may have a greater risk of postoperative apprehension, whereas the DB technique may cause more stiffness.

4.6 Outcomes of MPFL Reconstruction in Skeletally Immature Patients

Shamrock et al. [141] performed a systematic review and meta-analysis of the literature to evaluate the outcomes and complications of MPFL reconstruction in skeletally immature patients. Seven studies that entailed 132 MPFL reconstructions (126 patients) met the inclusion criteria. There were 73 females (58% of the cohort) and the mean age was 13 years (range, 6 to 17 years). Mean postoperative follow-up was 4.8 years (range, 1.4 to 10 years). Autograft was used for all reconstructions, with gracilis tendon (61%) being the most common. Methods of femoral fixation included interference screw (39%), suture anchor (39%), and soft tissue pulley around the medial collateral ligament or adductor tendon (22%). Pooled Kujala scores improved from 59 to 85 after MPFL reconstruction. The total reported complication rate was 25% and included 5 redislocations (4%) and 15 subluxation events (11%). No cases of premature physeal closure were noted. Neither autograft choice nor the method of femoral fixation influenced recurrent instability or overall complication rates. These findings suggest that MPFL reconstruction in skeletally immature patients is a viable and reasonable treatment option, with significant improvement in patient-reported outcomes and redislocation event rates of less than 5% at nearly 5-year follow-up. Further high-quality research should be undertaken to determine optimal surgical technique and graft options.

4.7 Return to Play

Few studies have reported on return to play after patellar stabilization in patients with patellofemoral instability [142–145].

Schneider and associates [142] performed a systematic review and meta-analysis to evaluate the outcomes of isolated MPFL reconstruction for the treatment of recurrent patellofemoral instability. Fourteen articles met the inclusion criteria and were included in this review. The mean age of the patients was 24 years. The mean postoperative Tegner score was 5.7 and the pooled estimated mean postoperative Kujala score was 86. Eighty-four per cent of the patients returned to sports after surgery. The pooled total risk of recurrent instability after surgery was 1%, with a positive apprehension sign risk of 4% and a reoperation risk of 3%. The authors concluded that a high percentage of young patients return to sports after isolated MPFL reconstruction for chronic patellar instability, with short-term results demonstrating a low incidence of recurrent instability, postoperative apprehension, and reoperations.

Sherman and colleagues [143] evaluated the existing literature regarding return to play (RTP) and return to prior performance (RPP) following patellar stabilization surgery. These authors found that there is a lack of validation and universal adoption of standardized RTP guidelines. The best available studies to date would suggest high RTP rates (84–100%), average RPP rates (33–77%), and a highly variable timeframe (3 to 12 months) for return to sport. Sherman et al. [143] concluded that the best available data on RTP and RPP following patellofemoral instability is based on lower quality of evidence studies, expert opinion, and published societal guidelines.

Manjunath et al. [144] performed a systematic review to determine both the rate and timing of return to play after MPFL reconstruction, and the rate of further patellar instability. Their review found 27 studies including 1278 patients meeting the inclusion criteria. The majority of patients were women (58%), and the total group had a mean age of 22 years. The mean follow-up was 39 months. The overall rate of return to play was 85% (with 68% returning to the same level of play). The average time to return to play was 7 months postoperatively. The rate of recurrent instability events following reconstruction was 5%.

Platt et al. [145] undertook a systematic review and meta-analysis to evaluate return to sport after MPFL reconstruction for patellar instability. Twenty-three articles met the inclusion criteria after full-text review. A total of 930 patients were analyzed, including 786 athletes. The overall mean age of the patients was 21 years. Women represented 61% of all patients. The mean follow-up was 3 years (range, 0.8 to 8.5 years). The return to sport rate was 93%. Patients returned to or surpassed their preoperative level of activity in 71% of cases. An osteotomy was performed in 11% of the athletes. Return to sport did not differ significantly in patients undergoing MPFL reconstruction without osteotomy versus those receiving additional osteotomy. Patients returned to sport at a mean of 6.7 months (range, 3 to 6 months) postoperatively. The overall complication rate was 9%. The most common complication was recurrence of instability.

We emphasize that the treating surgeon should counsel their patients preoperatively regarding their expectations and outcomes of treatment. Based on abovementioned studies, a high rate of return to sport after MPFL reconstruction surgery is expected. In our experience, most athletes return to play around 6 to 8 months after undergoing MPFL reconstruction.

4.8 Complications of MPFL Reconstruction

Postoperative complications following MPFL reconstruction include subcutaneous hematoma, wound infection, dehiscence, seroma after graft harvest, persistent pain, knee stiffness, flexion contracture, recurrent instability, patellar fracture, and deep vein thrombosis. The cause of recurrent patellar instability may be technically inadequate MPFL reconstruction or failure to address other concomitant pathology. Persistent pain may be caused by the over-constrained MPFL, unaddressed chondral defect in the patellofemoral compartment, or patellar fracture.

Shah and associates [146] performed a systematic review to determine the rate of complications associated with MPFL reconstruction. A total of 164 complications occurred in 629 knees (26%). These complications included wound infection, knee pain, restriction of knee flexion, recurrent patellar instability, and patellar fracture. Twenty-six patients returned to the operating room for additional procedures.

Parikh and colleagues [147] have reported the early complications (<3 years) of MPFL reconstruction in young patients. A total of 179 knees underwent MPFL reconstruction during the study period. There were 38 complications (16%) in 29 knees. The major complications included recurrent lateral patellar instability, knee motion stiffness with flexion deficits, patellar fractures, and patellofemoral arthrosis/pain. In their series, 18 of 38 (47%) complications were secondary to technical factors and were considered preventable. Female gender and bilateral MPFL reconstructions were risk factors associated with postoperative complications. Patients should be counseled preoperatively on the risk of potential complications that may occur after MPFL reconstruction.

Common fixation techniques for MPFL reconstruction at the patella include transosseous bone tunnels [148, 149], suture anchors [122, 150, 151], and interference screws [152–154]. It has been reported that the patellar tunnel techniques present a higher risk of postoperative patellar fractures, particularly for those that pass completely through the patella [146, 147, 155–159]. In view of the high risk of patellar fracture with the use of transosseous tunnel technique, the suture anchor fixation was introduced [154, 160]. Suture anchors provide a stable fixation and are gaining increasing popularity. Good to excellent results have been reported with the use of suture anchors for fixation of the tendon graft in MPFL reconstruction [122, 150].

4.9 Authors' Preferred Treatment of MPFL Reconstruction

In order to eliminate the risk of patellar fracture (that may occur using the patellar tunnel technique), the senior author of this paper (AJS), prefer to use suture anchors to fix the tendon graft to the medial border of the patella. Kurowicki et al. [130] have reported the Patella Footprint Technique of MPFL reconstruction. In our opinion, this surgical technique provides a safe, reliable and reproducible method of restoring patellofemoral stability. The Patella Footprint Technique minimizes the stress risers in the patella by using suture anchor fixation that creates a ligamentous footprint instead of tendon healing into a bony socket in the patella.

4.10 The Authors' Operative Technique of Medial Patellofemoral Ligament Reconstruction using the Patella Footprint Technique

4.10.1 Step 1: Patient Preparation and Diagnostic Arthroscopy

The patient is placed in the supine position. Using a surgical marking pen, the skin incisions and anatomical landmarks (i.e. the medial two-thirds of the patellar border, the pes anserinus, adductor tubercle, and medial femoral epicondyle) are marked as shown in **Figure 6**. After the induction of general anesthesia, the patient is examined for range of motion and the presence of 4-quadrant translation of the patella with minimal force applied. After performing the examination under anesthesia, the patient is prepped and draped in a sterile fashion. Using standard anterolateral and anteromedial portals, diagnostic arthroscopy of the affected knee is undertaken. Arthroscopic chondroplasty is performed if the patient has significant chondromalacia of the patellofemoral joint.

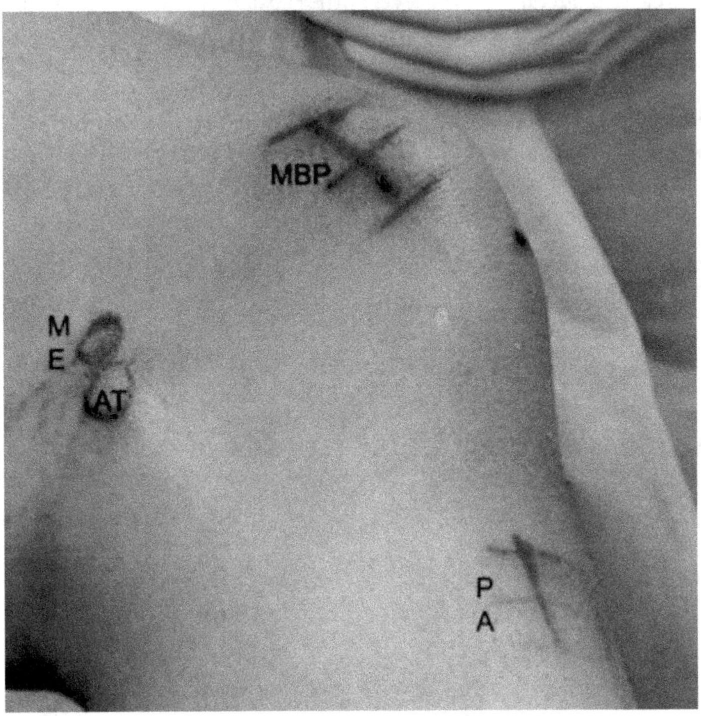

Figure 6.
Patient is placed in the supine position with the left knee in 45° of flexion providing an anteromedial view of the knee. Using a surgical marking pen, the anatomical landmarks are drawn. First, the medial border of the patella (MBP) is palpated and the proximal two-thirds is marked. The pes anserinus (PA) is marked at the anteromedial border of the proximal tibia. On the medial aspect of the knee, the adductor tubercle (AT) can be palpated just distal to the medial femoral epicondyle (ME). Proper identification of these anatomical landmarks is essential to performing this MPFL reconstruction with relative ease. Reproduced with permission from: Kurowicki et al. [130].

4.10.2 Step 2: Graft Harvesting and Preparation

A longitudinal incision is made over the pes anserinus, and dissection carried out down to the level of the sartorial fascia. The sartorial fascia is identified and incised proximal to and in line with the gracilis tendon. The gracilis tendon is bluntly dissected off of the sartorial fascia, and brought out of the wound using a hemostat (**Figure 7A** and **B**).

The open hamstring stripping device (Stryker Orthopedics, Mahwah, NJ) is used to harvest a gracilis tendon autograft, maintaining the distal attachment during the harvesting process. Once harvested, the gracilis tendon is detached sharply at its insertion taking care to avoid damage to the semitendinosus tendon. The muscle belly is removed from the gracilis tendon using a periosteal elevator. A whip stitch is applied to the distal end of the gracilis tendon using a No. 2 orthocord suture (DePuy Mitek, Warsaw, IN). The gracilis tendon graft is placed in a moist lap sponge while attention is now turned to the placement of suture anchors in the medial border of the patella.

4.10.3 Step 3: Medial Patellar Dissection With Suture Anchor Placement and Bone Debridement

Next, a longitudinal incision is made over the medial border of the patella, and dissection is carried out down to the level of the capsule. A longitudinal arthrotomy is performed just medial to the patellar tendon. The proximal-third of the medial aspect of the patella is debrided with a rongeur down to a base of bleeding bone, creating a footprint for insertion of the gracilis tendon graft. Two GRYPHON suture anchors (DePuy Mitek) are placed in the medial aspect of the patella: the first suture anchor at the junction of the proximal-third and middle-third of the medial border of the patella, and the second suture anchor, 5 mm to 10 mm proximal to the first (**Figure 8**).

4.10.4 Step 4: Soft Tissue Tunneling

Using the adductor tubercle and the medial femoral epicondyle as anatomical reference points, a blunt instrument is used to develop an intra-articular, extrasynovial plane, tunneling toward the anatomic insertion of the MPFL on the femur (**Figure 9**).

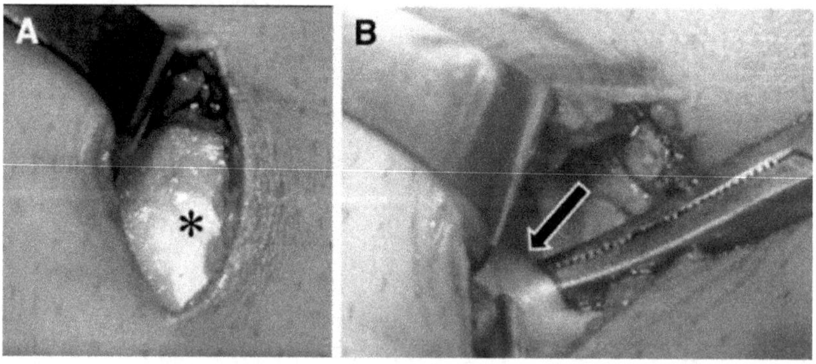

Figure 7.
With the patient in the supine position and the left knee flexed at 45°, a longitudinal incision is made over the pes anserinus and dissection is performed down to the level of the sartorial fascia, indicated by the asterisk (*) in Figure A. The sartorial fascia is then incised proximally and in line with the gracilis tendon (the arrow denotes the gracilis tendon in Figure B). Blunt dissection of the sartorial fascia off of the gracilis tendon is performed. Reproduced with permission from: Kurowicki et al. [130].

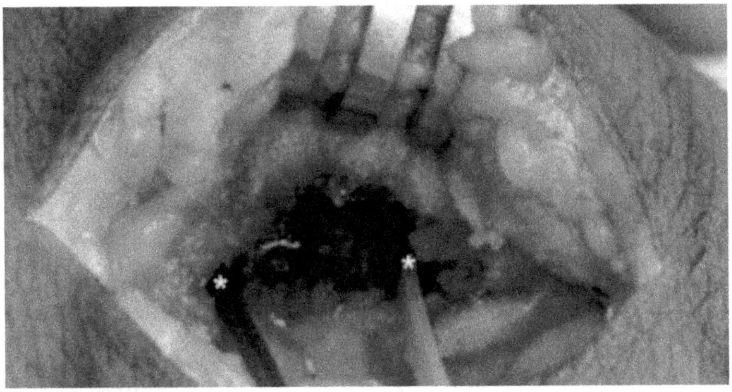

Figure 8.
With the patient in the supine position and the left knee flexed at 45°, a longitudinal incision is made over the medial aspect of the patella just medial to the border. Dissection is carried out down to the level of the capsule, and a longitudinal arthrotomy is performed just medial to the patellar border. The proximal-third of the medial aspect of the patella is debrided with a rongeur down to a base of bleeding bone, creating a footprint for graft insertion. The asterisks (*) indicate the placement of 2 GRYPHON suture anchors (DePuy Mitek) approximately 5 mm to 10 mm from each other. Reproduced with permission from: Kurowicki et al. [130].

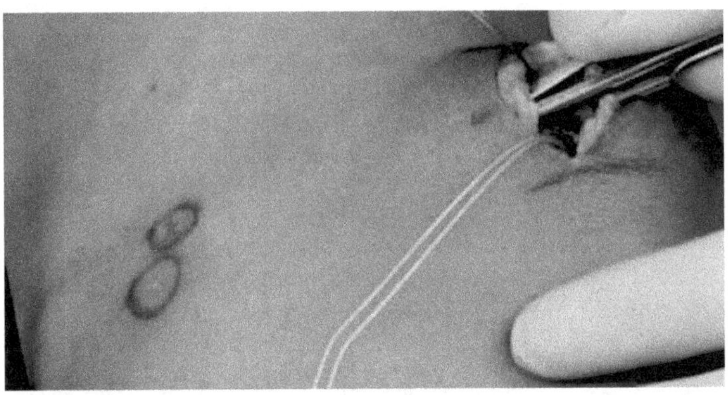

Figure 9.
Formation of an intra-articular, extrasynovial plane for tunneling toward the anatomic insertion of the MPFL on the femur using a blunt instrument with the patient positioned supine and the left knee flexed at 45°. The blue star represents the medial femoral epicondyle, and the green star represents the adductor tubercle. The anatomic origin of the MPFL on the femur can be found in the saddle area between the proximal-posterior to the medial epicondyle and distal-anterior to the adductor tubercle. Reproduced with permission from: Kurowicki et al. [130].

4.10.5 Step 5: Femoral Tunnel Formation, Graft Preparation, and Femoral Graft Fixation

An incision is made over the site of anatomic origin of the MPFL on the femur. A guidewire is placed to approximately 30 mm of depth at the anatomic attachment of the MPFL on the femur, which can be identified in the saddle area proximal-posterior to the medial epicondyle and distal-anterior to the adductor tubercle (Kruckeberg et al. 2018). The femur is drilled and the drill hole is tapped. One end of the whip stitch applied to the gracilis tendon autograft is loaded through a 7 mm × 23 mm MILAGRO interference screw (DePuy Mitek) with the assistance of the CHIA PERCPASSER suture passer (DePuy Mitek). The tendon graft is then pushed into the drill hole with a pickup or a freer, and the screw is advanced until flush with the cortex of the femur (**Figure 10A** and **B**). A free needle is used to sew

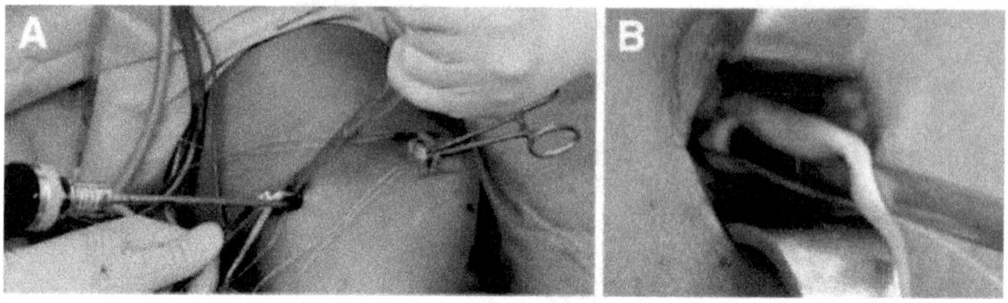

Figure 10.
(A) With the patient supine and the left knee in 45° of flexion, an incision is made over the saddle area proximal-posterior to the medial epicondyle and distal-anterior to the adductor tubercle on the femur. A guidewire is placed to approximately 30 mm of depth, the femur is drilled, and the drill hole is taped. One end of the whip stitch applied to the gracilis tendon autograft is loaded through a 7 mm × 23 mm interference screw (DePuy Mitek) and the tendon is dunked into the drill hole. (B) The screw is advanced until flush with the cortex of the femur. Reproduced with permission from: Kurowicki et al. [130].

the unused end of the suture through the graft, and it is tied to the end that was previously passed through the suture anchor.

4.10.6 Step 6: Deliver the Graft Through the Soft Tissue Tunnel and Tension the Graft

The gracilis tendon graft is now passed through the intra-articular, extrasynovial plane using a hemostat (**Figure 11**). With the knee held in 45° of flexion, the graft is marked where it aligns with the more distal suture anchor, and then from there the distance between the 2 suture anchors is marked off on the graft.

4.10.7 Step 7: Secure Distal and Then Proximal End of the Graft to the Patella

A free needle is used to whip stitch the graft to the appropriate suture anchor at each level. The unused end of the graft is pulled to take up the slack, bringing the

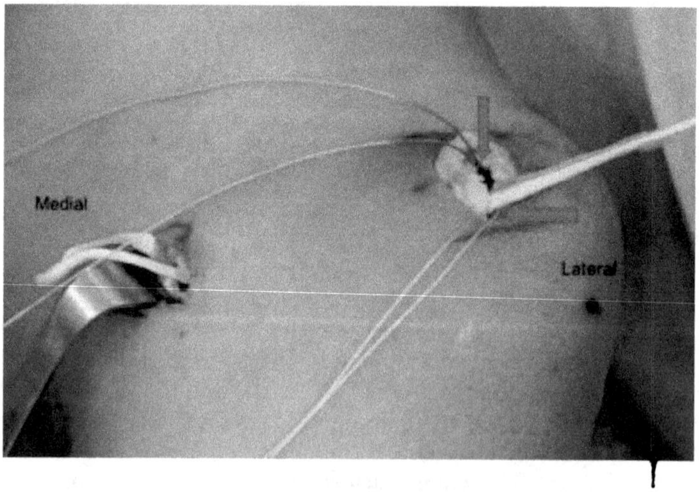

Figure 11.
The patient is in the supine position, the left knee flexed to 45°, when the gracilis tendon autograft is passed from the femoral fixed side through the intra-articular, extrasynovial plane using a hemostat and exiting out the opening at the medial border of the patella. Once the graft is passed, with the knee held in 45° of flexion, the graft is marked where it aligns with the more distal suture anchor, and then from there the distance between the 2 suture anchors is marked off on the graft. Arrows denote the location of 2 suture anchors. Reproduced with permission from: Kurowicki et al. [130].

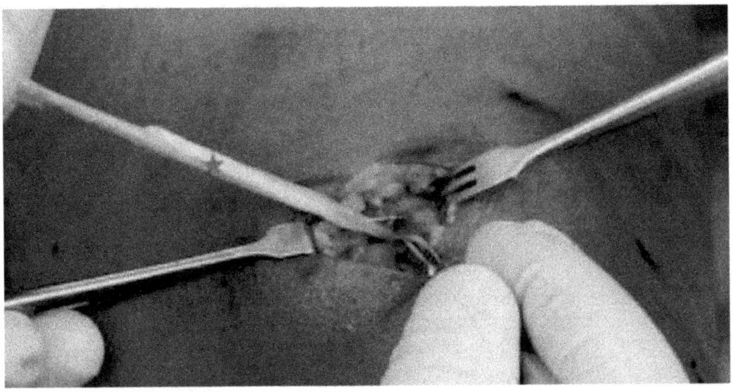

Figure 12.
The patient is supine with the knee in 45° of flexion and a free needle is used to whip stitch the graft to the appropriate suture anchor at each level. The unused end of the graft is pulled to take up the slack, bringing the graft down to the bone and suture anchor. The knots are subsequently tied, starting with the distal anchor and then the proximal anchor, and the excess graft is cut off. The blue star denotes excess graft. Reproduced with permission from: Kurowicki et al. [130].

graft down to the bone and anchor. The knots are subsequently tied, starting with the distal anchor and then the excess graft is cut off (**Figure 12**).

4.10.8 Step 8: Evaluate Graft Tensioning

The knee is taken through a range of motion to confirm that the graft is not overtensioned. Translation of the patella is confirmed to be less than 2 quadrants.

4.10.9 Step 9. Wound Closure

The capsule is repaired in a "pants-over-vest" fashion with a No. 2 orthocord suture (DePuy Mitek). The skin incision is closed with a subcuticular vicryl suture followed by a running monocryl.

4.11 Postoperative rehabilitation protocol

Postoperatively, the patient is weight bearing as tolerated with the brace in 0° to 30° of flexion for the first week, progressing to 60° of flexion by week 2 and 90° of flexion by week 4. With the assistance of a physical therapist, the patient

Pearls	Pitfalls
1. Proper tunnel and footprint position	1. Malposition leads to anisometric graft placement
2. Avoid graft overtensioning by marking in 45° of knee flexion	2. Postoperative pain and stiffness due to overtensioned graft
3. Address concomitant pathology when needed; consider tibial tuberosity transfer if the TT-TG[#] distance is >20 mm, or consider osteochondritis dissecans repair for a full-thickness chondral defect	3. Recurrence of dislocation due to unaddressed pathology or recurrent pain due to chondral defect in the patella

[#]TT-TG, tibial tuberosity-trochlear groove.
[*]Adapted from Kurowicki et al. [130].

Table 2.
Pearls and pitfalls of patellar footprint technique of MPFL reconstruction.[*]

Advantages
1. Anatomic interference femoral screw allows for proper graft isometry and promotes osseous ingrowth
2. Use of two bioresorbable suture anchors on the patella creates a ligamentous footprint to decrease the propagation of patellar stress risers
3. Gracilis tendon provides a stronger construct compared with the native MPFL while limiting hamstring morbidity
4. ensioning in 45° of knee flexion allows for some bony restraint by trochlea yet prevents overtensioning of the graft
5. L-configuration diminishes patellar rotation
Disadvantages
1. Interference screw fixation on the patellar side provides a biomechanically stronger fixation as compared with the suture anchor fixation [154]
Adapted from Kurowicki et al. [130].

Table 3.
*Advantages and disadvantages of patellar footprint technique of MPFL reconstruction.**

undertakes quadriceps strengthening (especially, the VMO) exercises for the first 6 weeks. At more than 6 weeks postoperatively, if patients have achieved a near-full range of motion and can maintain a strong quadriceps contraction, discontinuation of the brace is acceptable. **Table 2** highlights the pearls and pitfalls of the Patella Footprint Technique of MPFL reconstruction. **Table 3** outlines the advantages and disadvantages of our described operative technique. The surgical technique described in this chapter provides an easy to replicate anatomical MPFL reconstruction with suture anchor patellar fixation. However, future studies are warranted comparing the outcomes between different fixation options, as well as evaluating long-term clinical outcomes.

5. Discussion

Patellofemoral instability typically affects the young and athletically active patient population. Most physicians recommend an initial trial of nonoperative management for patients who present with first-time patellar dislocation, without intra-articular osteochondral fragments, severe injury to the medial patellar soft tissue stabilizers, and significant patellofemoral malalignment or dysplasia. One of the challenges around nonoperative management of patellar dislocation is the complexity of interventions offered and the various rehabilitation regimens that are practiced in different institutions. Numerous physical therapy protocols have been described. The goals of physical therapy are to decrease pain, restore the range of motion of the knee, strengthen the quadriceps musculature, address the deficiencies in the trunk, hip or foot biomechanics that may predispose to patellar instability, improve the joint function, enhance the quality of life, and increase patient satisfaction. Unfortunately, there are little data or validated, objective evidence to determine which nonoperative treatment regimen is best for the management of patients with acute patellar dislocation.

We are aware that some physicians recommend nonoperative management as the first-line treatment for patients with chronic, recurrent patellar instability. However, in our clinical experience (expanding over a period of 40 years), the nonoperative treatment of chronic patellar dislocations treated by an initial period of immobilization (using a cast or a brace) followed by rehabilitation has produced less satisfactory clinical outcomes; many of these patients have continued knee symptoms and recurrent patellar dislocations. There remains a paucity of scientific evidence on how to optimally manage patients with recurrent patellar dislocation (particularly, whether these patients should be given an initial trial of nonoperative treatment, how long the nonoperative treatment should be continued, and when surgical intervention should be recommended). This remains a subject of further clinical research. We believe many of the patients with chronic, symptomatic, recurrent patellar dislocations have predisposing anatomical risk factors (**Table 1**) and these patients invariably require operative treatment.

The natural history of acute patellar dislocation is that of a relatively high rate of recurrent instability, and long-term functional limitations and inability to return to baseline level of activity. Hence, surgery often plays an important role in the management of these patients. Prospective randomized trials comparing different surgical techniques are needed to determine which treatment options provide optimal clinical outcomes with restoration of knee function, low recurrence rate of patellar instability, and decreased risk of patellofemoral arthritis. The main goal of surgery is to restore the integrity of the MPFL and optimize the alignment of the lower extremity.

The MPFL acts as an important checkrein during the first 30 degrees of flexion (before the patella engages with the trochlea), thus allowing for a smooth knee motion. Rupture of the MPFL is often seen in patients with recurrent lateral patellar dislocation, leading to abnormal patellofemoral contact pressures, and resulting in pain, knee dysfunction, and early-onset arthritis. Hence, it is vital to undertake anatomic MPFL reconstruction to restore the kinetics and biomechanics of the patellofemoral joint.

Medial patellofemoral ligament reconstruction has become one of the most common and widely used surgical procedures to regain stability in patients with recurrent lateral dislocation of the patella. Recent studies have demonstrated low recurrence rates, improved patient-reported outcome measures, and a high rate of return to sports. No gold standard currently exists for MPFL reconstruction. Various surgical techniques of MPFL reconstruction have been reported employing different methods of graft fixation and tensioning. A detailed description of all available surgical techniques is beyond the scope of this chapter. Shah and associates [146] performed a systematic review to determine the rate of complications associated with MPFL reconstruction. In their study, a total of 164 complications occurred in 629 knees (26%). Therefore, efforts must be made to develop new operative techniques in order to minimize potentially devastating complications and optimize clinical outcomes.

Numerous graft sources, operative techniques, and fixation methods have been described with favorable clinical outcomes for reconstruction of the MPFL for patients with symptomatic patellofemoral instability. Several surgical techniques have been reported for fixation of the graft to the patella; these techniques include the use of suture anchors, interference screws, and transosseous tunnels. However, to date, no particular method has emerged as superior with regard to clinical outcome. Formation of a stress riser in the patella can result in a catastrophic complication after MPFL reconstruction. Large-diameter (4.5 mm), transverse, or long-oblique patellar bone tunnels have been associated with an increased risk of patellar fracture after MPFL reconstruction [147]. Schiphouwer et al. [159] reported a retrospective case series of 179 patients (192 knees) who underwent MPFL reconstruction, with or without additional bony realignment procedures. In their series, MPFL reconstruction was performed using two, transverse patellar bone tunnels. Seven patients (3.6%) sustained a patellar fracture without adequate trauma. This study highlights the associated, increased risk seen with the use of transverse patellar bone tunnel while performing MPFL reconstruction. Recently, Deasey et al. [161] have shown that the use of small-diameter (3.2-mm), oblique patellar bone tunnels was not associated with an increased risk of patellar fracture in comparison with the use of suture anchors for patellar fixation. Deasey et al. [161] concluded that the use of small (3.2-mm), short, oblique patellar tunnels can be a safe and reliable method of patellar graft fixation in MPFL reconstruction.

Russ and colleagues [154] have shown that the use of transpatellar bone tunnels with interference screw fixation offers a biomechanically stronger fixation as compared to the use of suture anchors. Despite being biomechanically weaker, Russ et al. [154] did find that suture anchor fixation nevertheless allows for a reconstruction that withstands greater mechanical loads before failure than the native MPFL. The use of suture anchors also minimizes the risk of violating the articular surface when reaming the tunnels and decreases the risk of patellar fracture. Song and colleagues [150] prospectively evaluated the clinical and radiographic outcomes following anatomic MPFL reconstruction using patellar suture anchor fixation for patients with recurrent patellar instability. Twenty patients (20 knees) were enrolled in this study. The median age of the patients was 21 years, and the median follow-up was 34.5 months (range, 24 to 50 months). Reconstruction was performed using a hamstring autograft fixed with two suture anchors at native patellar site of the MPFL. The preoperative Kujala scores were 52.6 ± 12.4 and the postoperative Kujala scores were 90.9 ± 4.5 ($p < 0.001$). The preoperative Lysholm scores were 49.2 ± 10.7 and the postoperative Lysholm scores were 90.9 ± 5.2 ($p < 0.001$). The Tegner score increased from 3.0 (range 1 to 4) preoperatively to 5.0 (range 4 to 7) postoperatively ($p < 0.001$). No patient experienced a patellar fracture or recurrent dislocation in their series. This study shows that anatomic MPFL reconstruction using two suture anchors is a reliable treatment option for management of patients with recurrent patellofemoral instability.

We have previously reported our surgical technique of MPFL reconstruction that uses two suture anchors along the patella for graft fixation to provide a biomechanically favorable construct [130]. In our clinical experience, anatomic MPFL reconstruction (utilizing the autogenous gracilis tendon and patella footprint technique) has produced satisfactory clinical and functional outcomes in majority of the patients. We emphasize that MPFL reconstruction requires precise graft placement at the anatomic origin and insertion points of the MPFL. Anatomic graft placement, appropriate graft length and tension are critical to prevent over-constraint of the patellofemoral joint while undertaking reconstruction of the MPFL. By utilizing two suture anchors in the patella, the MPFL footprint was secured in a single-bundle setting to restore the native MPFL anatomy and patellar stability [130]. Furthermore, we ensure a secure fixation by submerging the tail of the gracilis graft with the interference screw at the femoral footprint. We believe our Patellar Footprint Surgical Technique provides an easy to replicate anatomical MPFL reconstruction utilizing an autogenous gracilis tendon graft that is secured to the medial border of the patella using two suture anchors [130]. **Table 2** highlights the pearls and pitfalls of the Patella Footprint Technique of MPFL reconstruction. The advantages and disadvantages of our described surgical technique are outlined in **Table 3**. Future studies are warranted comparing the outcomes between different fixation options, as well as exploring the long-term clinical and functional outcomes.

Reconstruction of the MPFL is typically indicated for patients with recurrent patellofemoral instability, with or without trochlear dysplasia, who have a normal TT-TG distance and a normal patellar height. The procedure may be performed with concomitant procedures, such as distalization of the tibial tuberosity in a patient with patella alta, or trochleoplasty in a patient with high-grade trochlear dysplasia.

Distal patellofemoral realignment procedure (such as the anteromedial tibial tuberosity transfer) is indicated for patients with recurrent instability, who have an increased TT-TG distance, abnormally high Q-angle, patella alta, lateral and/or distal patellar chondrosis, and absence of trochlear chondrosis. The degree of anteriorization, distalization, and/or medialization of the tibial tuberosity depends on the presence of associated arthrosis of the lateral patellar facet and/or the presence of patella alta. It is worth noting that the distal realignment procedure is contraindicated in patients who have a normal TT-TG distance or in those patients who have associated proximal and/or medial patellar chondrosis.

Groove-deepening trochleoplasty is a complex and technically challenging surgical procedure. This procedure is indicated for patients with Dejour type-B and type-D trochlear dysplasia, whereas a lateral elevation or proximal recession trochleoplasty is indicated for patients with Dejour type-C dysplasia.

6. Conclusions

- Recurrent patellofemoral instability is a common cause of knee pain and functional disability in adolescent and young adult patients, resulting in loss of time from work and/or sports.

- There are numerous factors that contribute to recurrent patellofemoral instability; these factors include tear of the MPFL, weakening or hypoplasia of the VMO, trochlear dysplasia, increased TT-TG distance (>20 mm), valgus malalignment, increased Q-angle, malrotation secondary to internal femoral or external tibial torsion, patella alta, and generalized ligamentous laxity.

- A detailed history and a thorough physical examination are crucial to clinch an early, accurate diagnosis.

- Imaging studies play an important role to confirm the clinical diagnosis and also help to identify concomitant intra-articular pathologies. CT scans are useful for assessment of the trochlear morphology, TT-TG distance, patellar tilt, as well as femoral and tibial torsions. MRI scans are used to identify the soft tissue injury (especially, injury to the medial patellar retinaculum, MPFL and VMO). It also helps to detect the osteochondral fractures, loose bodies and bone bruises involving the medial patellar facet and lateral femoral condyle in acute cases.

- In general, nonoperative management of chronic patellar instability with immobilization followed by rehabilitation has produced unsatisfactory clinical results.

- A diligent attempt should be made to identify the underlying pathologic abnormality in each case and the surgical treatment should be customized to correct the offending anatomic and radiographic abnormality.

- An individualized case-by-case approach is recommended based on the underlying anatomical risk factors and radiographic abnormality.

- Careful preoperative patient selection is crucial to ensure optimal clinical outcome.

- Patients should be counseled preoperatively regarding expectations and outcomes of treatment.

- Most of the current surgical treatment options for chronic patellofemoral instability are based on Level-IV evidence. Multicenter, prospective randomized controlled studies are necessary to determine the optimal surgical treatment for patients with chronic, recurrent patellar instability.

- Isolated lateral release of the patella has not proven to be of long-term benefit for the treatment of patellofemoral instability. It may be performed (when indicated) as an adjunct procedure to MPFL reconstruction or to distal realignment of the extensor mechanism.

- Patients with recurrent instability, with or without trochlear dysplasia, who have a normal TT-TG distance and a normal patellar height, are candidates for surgical reconstruction of the MPFL, using either autograft or allograft (based on patient and/or surgeon preference).

- MPFL reconstruction requires precise graft placement at the anatomic origin and insertion points of the MPFL. Anatomic graft placement, appropriate graft length and tension are critical to prevent over-constraint of the patellofemoral joint while undertaking reconstruction of the MPFL.

- Distal patellofemoral realignment procedure (such as the anteromedial tibial tuberosity transfer) is indicated for patients with recurrent instability, who have an increased TT-TG distance, patella alta, lateral and/or distal patellar chondrosis, and absence of trochlear chondrosis. The degree of anteriorization, distalization, and/or medialization of the tibial tuberosity depends on the presence of associated arthrosis of the lateral patellar facet and/or the presence of patella alta.

- The distal realignment procedure is contraindicated in patients who have a normal TT-TG distance or in those with associated proximal and/or medial patellar chondrosis.

- Groove-deepening trochleoplasty is indicated for patients with Dejour type-B and type-D trochlear dysplasia, whereas a lateral elevation or proximal recession trochleoplasty is indicated for patients with Dejour type-C dysplasia.

- Associated injury to meniscus, cruciate ligament or collateral ligament should be recognized and appropriately treated.

- Pain, recurrent instability and patellofemoral arthrosis are likely complications of any surgical procedure that is performed for patients with patellofemoral instability.

Conflict of interest

AJS has received research support from ISO-biologics, is a paid consultant for Mitek, is a board or committee member of the American Academy of Orthopedic Surgery and the New Jersey Orthopedic Society, and has stock or stock options in Biomet, CONMED Linvatec, Johnson & Johnson, Pfizer, Smith & Nephew, and Stryker. The remaining authors declare no conflict of interest.

Author details

Deepak V. Patel*, Iciar M. Dávila Castrodad, Jennifer Kurowicki, Vincent K. McInerney and Anthony J. Scillia
St. Joseph's University Hospital and Regional Medical Center, Paterson, New Jersey, USA

*Address all correspondence to: bonepatel@yahoo.com

References

[1] Hawkins RJ, Bell RH, Anisette G. Acute patellar dislocations: The natural history. Am J Sports Med. 1986;14(2): 117-120.

[2] Casteleyn PP, Handelberg F. Arthroscopy in the diagnosis of occult dislocation of the patella. Acta Orthop Belg. 1989;55(3):381-383.

[3] Atkin DM, Fithian DC, Marangi KS, Stone ML, Dobson BE, Mendelsohn C. Characteristics of patients with primary acute lateral patellar dislocation and their recovery within the first 6 months of injury. Am J Sports Med. 2000;28(4): 472-479.

[4] Fithian DC, Paxton EW, Stone ML, Silva P, Davis DK, Elias DA, White LM. Epidemiology and natural history of acute patellar dislocation. Am J Sports Med. 2004;32(5):1114-1121.

[5] Warren LF, Marshall JL. The supporting structures and layers on the medial side of the knee: An anatomical analysis. J Bone Joint Surg Am. 1979;61(1):56-62.

[6] Conlan T, Garth WP Jr, Lemons JE. Evaluation of the medial soft-tissue restraints of the extensor mechanism of the knee. J Bone Joint Surg Am. 1993;75(5):682-693.

[7] Feller JA, Feagin JA Jr, Garrett WE Jr. The medial patellofemoral ligament revisited: An anatomical study. Knee Surg Sports Traumatol Arthrosc. 1993;1(3-4):184-186.

[8] Desio SM, Burks RT, Bachus KN. Soft tissue restraints to lateral patellar translation in the human knee. Am J Sports Med. 1998;26(1):59-65.

[9] Hautamaa PV, Fithian DC, Kaufman KR, Daniel DM, Pohlmeyer AM. Medial soft tissue restraints in lateral patellar instability and repair. Clin Orthop. 1998;349: 174-182.

[10] Nomura E, Horiuchi Y, Kihara M. Medial patellofemoral ligament restraint in lateral patellar translation and reconstruction. Knee. 2000;7(2): 121-127.

[11] Tuxoe JI, Teir M, Winge S, Nielsen PL. The medial patellofemoral ligament: A dissection study. Knee Surg Sports Traumatol Arthrosc. 2002;10(3):138-140.

[12] Smirk C, Morris H. The anatomy and reconstruction of the medial patellofemoral ligament. Knee. 2003; 10(3):221-227.

[13] Steensen RN, Dopirak RM, McDonald WG 3rd. The anatomy and isometry of the medial patellofemoral ligament: Implications for reconstruction. Am J Sports Med. 2004;32(6):1509-1513.

[14] Mochizuki T, Nimura A, Tateishi T, Yamaguchi K, Muneta T, Akita K. Anatomic study of the attachment of the medial patellofemoral ligament and its characteristic relationships to the vastus intermedius. Knee Surg Sports Traumatol Arthrosc. 2013;21(2):305-310.

[15] Fujino K, Tajima G, Yan J, Kamei Y, Maruyama M, Takeda S, Kikuchi S, Shimamura T. Morphology of the femoral insertion site of the medial patellofemoral ligament. Knee Surg Sports Traumatol Arthrosc. 2015; 23(4):998-1003.

[16] Shea KG, Polousky JD, Jacobs JC Jr, Ganley TJ, Aoki SK, Grimm NL, Parikh SN. The patellar insertion of the medial patellofemoral ligament in children: A cadaveric study. J Pediatr Orthop. 2015;35(4):e31-e35.

[17] Aframian A, Smith TO, Tennent TD, Cobb JP, Hing CB. Origin and insertion

of the medial patellofemoral ligament: A systematic review of anatomy. Knee Surg Sports Traumatol Arthrosc. 2017;25(12):3755-3772.

[18] Hinckel BB, Gobbi RG, Demange MK, Pereira CAM, Pécora JR, Natalino RJM, Miyahira L, Kubota BS, Camanho GL. Medial patellofemoral ligament, medial patellotibial ligament, and medial patellomeniscal ligament: Anatomic, histologic, radiographic, and biomechanical study. Arthroscopy. 2017;33(10):1862-1873.

[19] Kikuchi S, Tajima G, Yan J, Kamei Y, Maruyama M, Sugawara A, Fujino K, Takeda S, Doita M. Morphology of insertion sites on patellar side of medial patellofemoral ligament. Knee Surg Sports Traumatol Arthrosc. 2017;25(8):2488-2493.

[20] Ji G, Sun Y, Lu J, Niu Y, Wang F. Functional regions of the medial patellofemoral ligament. J Knee Surg. 2019;32(1):80-84.

[21] Tanaka MJ. Femoral origin anatomy of the medial patellofemoral complex: Implications for reconstruction. Arthroscopy. 2020;36(12):3010-3015.

[22] Schottle PB, Schmeling A, Rosenstiel N, Weiler A. Radiographic landmarks for femoral tunnel placement in medial patellofemoral ligament reconstruction. Am J Sports Med. 2007;35(5):801-804.

[23] Loeb AE, Tanaka MJ. The medial patellofemoral complex. Curr Rev Musculoskelet Med. 2018;11(2): 201- 208.

[24] Tanaka MJ, Voss A, Fulkerson JP. The anatomic midpoint of the attachment of the medial patellofemoral complex. J Bone Joint Surg Am. 2016;98(14):1199-1205.

[25] Tanaka MJ. The anatomy of the medial patellofemoral complex. Sports Med Arthrosc. 2017;25(2):e8-e11.

[26] Tanaka MJ. Variability in the patellar attachment of the medial patellofemoral ligament. Arthrosc - J Arthrosc Relat Surg. 2016;32(8):1667-1670.

[27] Fulkerson JP, Edgar C. Medial quadriceps tendon-femoral ligament: Surgical anatomy and reconstruction technique to prevent patella instability. Arthrosc Tech. 2013;2(2):e125–e128.

[28] Amis AA, Firer P, Mountney J, Senavongse W, Thomas NP. Anatomy and biomechanics of the medial patellofemoral ligament. Knee. 2003;10(3):215-220.

[29] Mountney J, Senavongse W, Amis AA, Thomas NP. Tensile strength of the medial patellofemoral ligament before and after repair or reconstruction. J Bone Joint Surg Br. 2005;87(1):36-40.

[30] Steiner T, Parker RD. Subluxation and Dislocation: Patellofemoral instability – Acute dislocation of the patella. In DeLee JC, Drez D Jr, Miller MD (eds): Orthopaedic Sports Medicine: Principles and Practice, 3rd Edition. Saunders, Elsevier. Philadelphia, PA, USA, 2010, pp 1534-1547.

[31] Stefancin JJ, Parker RD. First-time traumatic patellar dislocation: A systematic review. Clin Orthop. 2007;455:93-101.

[32] Insall J, Salvati E. Patella position in the normal knee joint. Radiology. 1971;101(1):101-104.

[33] Grelsamer RP, Meadows S. The modified Insall-Salvati ratio for assessment of patellar height. Clin Orthop. 1992;282:170-176.

[34] Blackburne JS, Peel TE. A new method of measuring patellar height. J Bone Joint Surg Br. 1977;59(2):241-242.

[35] Caton J, Deschamps G, Chambat P, Lerat JL, Dejour H. [Patella infera: Apropos of 128 cases]. [Article in

French]. Rev Chir Orthop Reparatrice Appar Mot. 1982;68(5):317-325.

[36] Merchant AC, Mercer RL, Jacobsen RH, Cool CR. Roentgenographic analysis of patellofemoral congruence. J Bone Joint Surg Am. 1974;56(7):1391-1396.

[37] Laurin CA, Lévesque HP, Dussault R, Labelle H, Peides JP. The abnormal lateral patellofemoral angle: A diagnostic roentgenographic sign of recurrent patellar subluxation. J Bone Joint Surg Am. 1978;60(1):55-60.

[38] Laurin CA, Dussault R, Levesque HP. The tangential x-ray investigation of the patellofemoral joint: X-ray technique, diagnostic criteria and their interpretation. Clin Orthop. 1979;144:16-26.

[39] Mäenpää H, Lehto MU. Patellar dislocation: The long-term results of nonoperative management in 100 patients. Am J Sports Med. 1997;25(2):213-217.

[40] Camanho GL, Viegas AC, Bitar AC, Demange MK, Hernandez AJ. Conservative versus surgical treatment for repair of the medial patellofemoral ligament in acute dislocations of the patella. Arthroscopy. 2009;25(6): 620-625.

[41] Bitar AC, Demange MK, D'Elia CO, Camanho GL. Traumatic patellar dislocation: Nonoperative treatment compared with MPFL reconstruction using patellar tendon. Am J Sports Med. 2012;40(1):114-122.

[42] Petri M, Liodakis E, Hofmeister M, Despang FJ, Maier M, Balcarek P, Voigt C, Haasper C, Zeichen J, Stengel D, Krettek C, Frosch KH, Lill H, Jagodzinski M. Operative vs conservative treatment of traumatic patellar dislocation: Results of a prospective randomized controlled clinical trial. Arch Orthop Trauma Surg. 2013;133(2);209-213.

[43] Sillanpää PJ, Mattila VM, Mäenpää H, Kiuru M, Visuri T, Pihlajamäki H. Treatment with and without initial stabilizing surgery for primary traumatic patellar dislocation: A prospective randomized study. J Bone Joint Surg Am. 2009;91(2):263-273.

[44] Jensen CM, Roosen JU. Acute traumatic dislocations of the patella. J Trauma. 1985;25(2):160-162.

[45] Dainer RD, Barrack RL, Buckley SL, Alexander AH. Arthroscopic treatment of acute patellar dislocations. Arthroscopy. 1988;4(4):267-271.

[46] Vainionpää S, Laasonen E, Silvennoinen T, Vasenius J, Rokkanen P. Acute dislocation of the patella: A prospective review of operative treatment. J Bone Joint Surg Br. 1990;72(3):366-369.

[47] Hughston JC, Deese M. Medial subluxation of the patella as a complication of lateral retinacular release. Am J Sports Med. 1988;16(4):383-388.

[48] Miller PR, Klein RM, Teitge RA. Medial dislocation of the patella. Skeletal Radiol. 1991;20(6):429-431.

[49] Fithian DC, Paxton EW, Post WR, Panni AS; International Patellofemoral Study Group. Lateral retinacular release: A survey of the International Patellofemoral Study Group. Arthroscopy. 2004;20(5): 463-468.

[50] Boden BP, Pearsall AW, Garrett WE Jr, Feagin JA Jr. Patellofemoral instability: Evaluation and management. J Am Acad Orthop Surg. 1997;5(1):47-57.

[51] Kowall MG, Kolk G, Nuber GW, Cassisi JE, Stern SH. Patellar taping in the treatment of patellofemoral pain:

A prospective randomized study. Am J Sports Med. 1996;24(1):61-66.

[52] Ruwe PA, Gage JR, Ozonoff MB, DeLuca PA. Clinical determination of femoral anteversion: A comparison with established techniques. J Bone Joint Surg Am. 1992;74(6):820-830.

[53] Bassett FH III. Acute dislocation of the patella, osteochondral fractures, and injuries to the extensor mechanism of the knee. Instr Course Lect. 1976;25: 40-49.

[54] Hughston JC. Subluxation of the patella. J Bone Joint Surg Am. 1968;50(5):1003-1026.

[55] Dimon JH 3rd. Apprehension test for subluxation of the patella. Clin Orthop. 1974;103:39.

[56] Ober FR. The role of the iliotibial band and fascia lata as a factor in the causation of low-back disabilities and sciatica. J Bone Joint Surg Am. 1936;18(1):105-110.

[57] Karachalios T, Hantes M, Zibis AH, Zachos V, Karantanas AH, Malizos KN. Diagnostic accuracy of a new clinical test (the Thessaly test) for early detection of meniscal tears. J Bone Joint Surg Am. 2005;87(5): 955-962.

[58] Haj-Mirzaian A, Thawait GK, Tanaka MJ, Demehri S. Diagnosis and characterization of patellofemoral instability: Review of available imaging modalities. Sports Med Arthrosc Rev. 2017;25(2):64-71.

[59] Marks KE, Bentley G. Patella alta and chondromalacia. J Bone Joint Surg Br. 1978;60(1):71-73.

[60] Seil R, Muller B, Georg T, Kohn D, Rupp S. Reliability and interobserver variability in radiological patellar height ratios. Knee Surg Sports Traumatol Arthrosc. 2000;8(4):231-236.

[61] Dejour H, Walch G, Nove-Josserand L, Guier C. Factors of patellar instability: An anatomic radiographic study. Knee Surg Sports Traumatol Arthrosc. 1994;2(1):19-26.

[62] Parikh SN, Rajdev N, Sun Q. The growth of trochlear dysplasia during adolescence. J Pediatr Orthop. 2018;38(6):e318-e324.

[63] Dejour H, Walch G, Neyret P, Adeleine P. [Dysplasia of the femoral trochlea]. [Article in French]. Rev Chir Orthop Reparatrice Appar Mot. 1990;76(1):45-54.

[64] Tavernier T, Dejour D. [Knee imaging: What is the best modality] [Article in French]. J Radiol. 2001;82(3) (pt 2):387-405, 407-408.

[65] Lippacher S, Dejour D, Elsharkawi M, Dornacher D, Ring C, Dreyhaupt J, Reichel H, Nelitz M. Observer agreement on the Dejour trochlear dysplasia classification: A comparison of true lateral radiographs and axial magnetic resonance images. Am J Sports Med. 2012;40(4):837-843.

[66] Malghem J, Maldague B. Depth insufficiency of the proximal trochlear groove on lateral radiographs of the knee: Relation to patellar dislocation. Radiology. 1989;170(2):507-510.

[67] Dejour D, Le Coultre B. Osteotomies in patello-femoral instabilities. Sports Med Arthrosc Rev. 2007;15(1):39-46.

[68] Dejour D, Saggin P. The sulcus deepening trochleoplasty - The Lyon's procedure. Int Orthop. 2010;34(2): 311-316.

[69] Onor GI Jr, Yalcin S, Kaar SG, Lee Pace J, Ferrua P, Farrow LD. The evaluation of trochlear osseous morphology: An epidemiologic study. Orthop. J Sports Med. 2021;9(4): 2325967121994548.

doi: 10.1177/2325967121994548. eCollection 2021 April.

[70] Inoue M, Shino K, Hirose H, Horibe S, Ono K. Subluxation of the patella: Computed tomography analysis of patellofemoral congruence. J Bone Joint Surg Am. 1988;70(9):1331-1337.

[71] Jones RB, Barlett EC, Vainright JR, Carroll RG. CT determination of tibial tubercle lateralization in patients presenting with anterior knee pain. Skeletal Radiol. 1995;24(7):505-509.

[72] Sallay PI, Poggi J, Speer KP, Garrett WE. Acute dislocation of the patella: A correlative pathoanatomic study. Am J Sports Med. 1996;24(1): 52-60.

[73] Sanders TG, Morrison WB, Singleton BA, Miller MD, Cornum KG. Medial patellofemoral ligament injury following acute transient dislocation of the patella: MR findings with surgical correlation in 14 patients. J Comput Assist Tomogr. 2001;25(6):957-962.

[74] Elias DA, White LM, Fithian DC. Acute lateral patellar dislocation at MR imaging: Injury patterns of medial patellar soft-tissue restraints and osteochondral injuries of the inferomedial patella. Radiology. 2002;225(3):736-743.

[75] Nomura E, Horiuchi Y, Inoue M. Correlation of MR imaging findings and open exploration of medial patellofemoral ligament injuries in acute patellar dislocations. Knee. 2002;9(2):139-143.

[76] Schreiber SN. Proximal superomedial portal in arthroscopy of the knee. Arthroscopy 1991;7(2): 246-251.

[77] Insall J, Bullough PG, Burstein AH. Proximal "tube" realignment of the patella for chondromalacia patellae. Clin Orthop Relat Res. 1979;144:63-69.

[78] Carney JR, Mologne TS, Muldoon M, Cox JS. Long-term evaluation of the Roux-Elmslie-Trillat procedure for patellar instability: A 26-year follow-up. Am J Sports Med. 2005;33(8):1220-1223.

[79] Fulkerson JP. Anteromedialization of thc tibial tuberosity for patellofemoral malalignment. Clin Orthop. 1983;177:176-181.

[80] Fulkerson JP, Becker GJ, Meaney JA, Miranda M, Folcik MA. Anteromedial tibial tubercle transfer without bone graft. Am J Sports Med. 1990;18(5): 490-497.

[81] Molina A, Ballester J, Martin C, Munoz I, Vazquez J, Torres J. Biomechanical effects of different surgical procedures on the extensor mechanism of the patellofemoral joint. Clin Orthop. 1995;320:168-175.

[82] Koeter S, Diks MJF, Anderson PG, Wymenga AB. A modified tibial tubercle osteotomy for patellar maltracking: Results at two years. J Bone Joint Surg Br. 2007;89(2):180-185.

[83] Stetson WB, Friedman MJ, Fulkerson JP, Cheng M, Buuck D. Fracture of the proximal tibia with immediate weightbearing after a Fulkerson osteotomy. Am J Sports Med. 1997;25(4):570-574.

[84] Bellemans J, Cauwenberghs F, Brys P, Victor J, Fabry G. Fracture of the proximal tibia after Fulkerson anteromedial tibial tubercle transfer: A report of four cases. Am J Sports Med. 1998;26(2):300-302.

[85] Cosgarea AJ, Schatzke MD, Seth AK, Litsky AS. Biomechanical analysis of flat and oblique tibial tubercle osteotomy for recurrent patellar instability. Am J Sports Med. 1999;27(4):507-512.

[86] Bereiter H, Gautier E. The trochleaplasty as a surgical therapy of

recurrent dislocation of the patella in dysplastic trochlea of the femur. Arthroskopie. 1994;7:281-286.

[87] Schottle PB, Fucentese SF, Pfirrmann C, Bereiter H, Romero J. Trochleaplasty for patellar instability due to trochlear dysplasia: a minimum 2-year clinical and radiological follow-up of 19 knees. Acta Orthop. 2005;76(5):693-698.

[88] Verdonk R, Jansegers E, Stuyts B. Trochleoplasty in dysplastic knee trochlea. Knee Surg Sports Traumatol Arthrosc. 2005;13(7):529-533.

[89] Donell ST, Joseph G, Hing CB, Marshall TJ. Modified Dejour trochleoplasty for severe dysplasia: Operative technique and early clinical results. Knee. 2006;13(4):266-273.

[90] von Knoch F, Bohm T, Burgi ML, von Knoch M, Bereiter H. Trochleaplasty for recurrent patellar dislocation in association with trochlear dysplasia: A 4- to 14-year follow-up study. J Bone Joint Surg Br. 2006;88(10):1331-1335.

[91] Koeter S, Pakvis D, van Loon CJM, van Kampen A. Trochlear osteotomy for patellar instability: Satisfactory minimum 2-year results in patients with dysplasia of the trochlea. Knee Surg Sports Traumatol Arthrosc. 2007;15(3): 228-232.

[92] Utting MR, Mulford JS, Eldridge JDJ. A prospective evaluation of trochleoplasty for the treatment of patellofemoral dislocation and instability. J Bone Joint Surg Br. 2008;90(2):180-185.

[93] Faruqui S, Bollier M, Wolf B, Amendola N. Outcomes after trochleoplasty. Iowa Orthop J. 2012;32:196-206.

[94] Banke IJ, Kohn LM, Meidinger G, Otto A, Hensler D, Beitzel K, Imhoff AB, Schottle PB. Combined trochleoplasty and MPFL reconstruction for treatment of chronic patellofemoral instability: A prospective minimum 2-year follow-up study. Knee Surg Sports Traumatol Arthrosc. 2014;22(11):2591-2598.

[95] Rouanet T, Gougeon F, Fayard JM, Remy F, Migaud H, Pasquier G. Sulcus deepening trochleoplasty for patellofemoral instability: A series of 34 cases after 15 years postoperative follow-up. Orthop Traumatol Surg Res. 2015;101(4):443-447.

[96] Vainionpaa S, Laasonen E, Patiala H, Rusanen M, Rokkannen P. Acute dislocation of the patella: Clinical, radiographic and operative findings in 64 consecutive cases. Acta Orthop Scand. 1986;57(4):331-333.

[97] Cossey AJ, Paterson R. A new technique for reconstructing the medial patellofemoral ligament. Knee. 2005;12(2):93-98.

[98] Avikainen VJ, Nikku RK, Seppanen-Lehmonen TK. Adductor magnus tenodesis for patellar dislocation: Technique and preliminary results. Clin Orthop. 1993;297:12-16.

[99] Sillanpää P, Mattila VM, Visuri T, Mäenpää H, Pihlajamäki H. Ligament reconstruction versus distal realignment for patellar dislocation. Clin Orthop. 2008;466(6):1475-1484.

[100] Sillanpää PJ, Mäenpää HM, Mattila VM, Visuri T, Pihlajamäki H. A mini-invasive adductor magnus tendon transfer technique for medial patellofemoral ligament reconstruction: A technical note. Knee Surg Sports Traumatol Arthrosc. 2009;17(5): 508-512.

[101] Jacobi M, Reischl N, Bergmann M, Bouaicha S, Djonov V, Magnussen RA. Reconstruction of the medial patellofemoral ligament using the

adductor magnus tendon: An anatomic study. Arthroscopy. 2012;28(1):105-109.

[102] Malecki K, Fabis J, Flont P, Niedzielski KR. The results of adductor magnus tenodesis in adolescents with recurrent patellar dislocation. Biomed Res Int. 2015;2015:456858. doi: 10.1155/2015/456858. Epub 2015 Feb 16.

[103] Camanho GL, Bitar AC, Hernandez AJ, Olivi R. Medial patellofemoral ligament reconstruction: A novel technique using the patellar ligament. Arthroscopy. 2007;23(1): 108.e1-4.

[104] Bitar AC, Demange MK, D'Elia CO, Camanho GL. Traumatic patellar dislocation: Nonoperative treatment compared with MPFL reconstruction using patellar tendon. Am J Sports Med. 2012;40(1):114-122.

[105] Teitge RA, Torga-Spak R. Medial patellofemoral ligament reconstruction. Orthopedics. 2004;27(10):1037-1040.

[106] Noyes FR, Albright JC. Reconstruction of the medial patellofemoral ligament with autologous quadriceps tendon. Arthroscopy. 2006;22(8):904.e1-7.

[107] Steiner TM, Torga-Spak R, Teitge RA. Medial patellofemoral ligament reconstruction in patients with lateral patellar instability and trochlear dysplasia. Am J Sports Med. 2006;34(8):1254-1261.

[108] Goyal D. Medial patellofemoral ligament reconstruction: The superficial quad technique. Am J Sports Med. 2013;41(5):1022-1029.

[109] Fink C, Veselko M, Herbort M, Hoser C. MPFL reconstruction using a quadriceps tendon graft: Part 2: Operative technique and short term clinical results. Knee. 2014;21(6): 1175-1179.

[110] Nelitz M, Williams SR. Anatomic reconstruction of the medial patellofemoral ligament in children and adolescents using a pedicled quadriceps tendon graft. Arthrosc Tech. 2014;3(2):e303-308.

[111] Vavalle G, Capozzi M. Isolated reconstruction of the medial patellofemoral ligament with autologous quadriceps tendon. J Orthop Traumatol. 2016;17(2):155-162.

[112] Nelitz M, Dreyhaupt J, Williams SRM. Anatomic reconstruction of the medial patellofemoral ligament in children and adolescents using a pedicled quadriceps tendon graft shows favourable results at a minimum of 2-year follow-up. Knee Surg Sports Traumatol Arthrosc. 2018;26(4):1210-1215.

[113] Peter G, Hoser C, Runer A, Abermann E, Wierer G, Fink C. Medial patellofemoral ligament (MPFL) reconstruction using quadriceps tendon autograft provides good clinical, functional and patient-reported outcome measurements (PROM): A 2-year prospective study. Knee Surg Sports Traumatol Arthrosc. 2019;27(8):2426-2432.

[114] Fisher M, Singh S, Samora WP 3rd, Beran MC, Klingele KE. Outcomes of MPFL reconstruction utilizing a quadriceps turndown technique in the adolescent/pediatric population. J Pediatr Orthop. 2021;Apr 23. doi: 10.1097/BPO.0000000000001836. Online ahead of print.

[115] Olotu O, Siddiqui A, Peterson D, de D. The superficial "swing-down" quadriceps tendon autograft is a viable option for medial patellofemoral ligament reconstruction: A systematic review. Arthroscopy. 2021; May 4:S0749-8063(21)00440-0. doi: 10.1016/j.arthro.2021.04.048. Online ahead of print.

[116] Drez D Jr, Edwards TB, Williams CS. Results of medial patellofemoral ligament reconstruction in the treatment of patellar dislocation. Arthroscopy. 2001;17(3):298-306.

[117] Deie M, Ochi M, Sumen Y, Yasumoto M, Kobayashi K, Kimura H. Reconstruction of the medial patellofemoral ligament for the treatment of habitual or recurrent dislocation of the patella in children. J Bone Joint Surg Br. 2003;85(6):887-890.

[118] Ellera Gomes JL, Stigler Marczyk LR, Cesar de Cesar P, Jungblut CF. Medial patellofemoral ligament reconstruction with semitendinosus autograft for chronic patellar instability: A follow-up study. Arthroscopy. 2004;20(2):147-151.

[119] Deie M, Ochi M, Sumen Y, Adachi N, Kobayashi K, Yasumoto M. A long-term follow-up study after medial patellofemoral ligament reconstruction using the transferred semitendinosus tendon for patellar dislocation. Knee Surg Sports Traumatol Arthrosc. 2005;13(7):522-528.

[120] Fernandez E, Sala D, Castejon M. Reconstruction of the medial patellofemoral ligament for patellar instability using a semitendinosus autograft. Acta Orthop Belg. 2005;71(3):303-308.

[121] Schöttle PB, Fucentese SF, Romero J. Clinical and radiological outcome of medial patellofemoral ligament reconstruction with a semitendinosus autograft for patella instability. Knee Surg Sports Traumatol Arthrosc. 2005;13(7):516-521.

[122] Mikashima Y, Kimura M, Kobayashi Y, Miyawaki M, Tomatsu T. Clinical results of isolated reconstruction of the medial patellofemoral ligament for recurrent dislocation and subluxation of the patella. Acta Orthop Belg. 2006;72(1):65-71.

[123] Nomura E, Inoue M. Hybrid medial patellofemoral ligament reconstruction using the semitendinosus tendon for recurrent patellar dislocation: Minimum 3 years' follow-up. Arthroscopy. 2006;22(7):787-793.

[124] Han H, Xia Y, Yun X, Wu M. Anatomical transverse patella double tunnel reconstruction of medial patellofemoral ligament with a hamstring tendon autograft for recurrent patellar dislocation. Arch Orthop Trauma Surg. 2011;131(3):343-351.

[125] Ladenhauf HN, Berkes MB, Green DW. Medial patellofemoral ligament reconstruction using hamstring autograft in children and adolescents. Arthrosc Tech. 2013;2(2):e151-154.

[126] Wang HD, Dong JT, Gao SJ. Medial patellofemoral ligament reconstruction using a bone groove and a suture anchor at patellar: a safe and firm fixation technique and 3-year follow-up study. J Orthop Surg Res. 2016;11(1):138.

[127] Monllau JC, Erquicia JI, Ibañez M, Gelber PE, Ibañez F, Masferrer-Pino A, Pelfort X. Reconstruction of the medial patellofemoral ligament. Arthrosc Tech. 2017;6(5):e1471-e1476.

[128] Niu J, Qi Q, Fu K, Duan G, Liu C, Wang F. Medial patellofemoral ligament reconstruction with semi-patellar tunnel fixation: Surgical technique and mid-term follow-up. Med Sci Monit. 2017;23:5870-5875.

[129] Vasso M, Corona K, Toro G, Rossini M, Schiavone Panni A. Anatomic double-bundle medial patellofemoral ligament reconstruction with autologous semitendinosus: Aperture fixation both at the femur and the patella. Joints. 2017;5(4):256-260.

[130] Kurowicki J, Mease SJ, Palacios S, Festa A, McInerney VK, Scillia AJ. Patella footprint technique - A surgical method for medial patellofemoral ligament reconstruction. Arthrosc Tech. 2018;7(6):e595-e600.

[131] Sim JA, Lim JK, Lee BH. Anatomic double-bundle medial patellofemoral ligament reconstruction with aperture fixation using an adjustable-length loop device: A 2-year follow-up study. BMC Musculoskelet Disord. 2018;19(1):346. doi: 10.1186/s12891-018-2261-x. PMID: 30253770; PMCID: PMC6156865.

[132] Devgan A, Yadav U, Sharma P, Rohilla R, Devgan R, Mudgil P, Verma A, Dhupper V. Implantless patellar fixation in medial patellofemoral ligament reconstruction. Chin J Traumatol. 2019;22(5):281-285.

[133] Mochizuki Y, Kaneko T, Kawahara K, Toyoda S, Ikegami H, Musha Y. A 2-year follow-up of isolated medial patellofemoral ligament reconstruction by using soft suture anchor and adjustable cortical fixation system. J Orthop. 2019;16(4):356-360.

[134] Gao G, Liu P, Xu Y. Treatment of patellar dislocation with arthroscopic medial patellofemoral ligament reconstruction using gracilis tendon autograft and modified double-patellar tunnel technique: Minimum 5-year patient-reported outcomes. J Orthop Surg Res. 2020;15(1):25.

[135] Ye M, Zhang H, Liang Q. Clinical outcomes after medial patellofemoral ligament reconstruction using transosseous sutures versus suture anchors: A prospective nonrandomized controlled trial. Orthop J Sports Med. 2020 May 4;8(5):2325967120917112. doi: 10.1177/2325967120917112. PMID: 32490023; PMCID: PMC7238809.

[136] Zhang H, Ye M, Liang Q. Clinical outcomes after medial patellofemoral ligament reconstruction with suture fixation of the gracilis tendon via transosseous tunnels. Orthop J Sports Med. 2020;8(2):2325967119900373. doi: 10.1177/2325967119900373. PMID: 32095487; PMCID: PMC7011329.

[137] Patel NK, de Sa D, Vaswani R, Kay J, Musahl V, Lesniak BP. Knee flexion angle during graft fixation for medial patellofemoral ligament reconstruction: A systematic review of outcomes and complications. Arthroscopy. 2019;35(6):1893-1904.

[138] Kumar N, Bastrom TP, Dennis MM, Pennock AT, Edmonds EW. Adolescent medial patellofemoral ligament reconstruction: A comparison of the use of autograft versus allograft hamstring. Orthop J Sports Med. 2018 May 24;6(5):2325967118774272. doi: 10.1177/2325967118774272. eCollection 2018 May.

[139] Singhal R, Rogers S, Charalambous CP. Double-bundle medial patellofemoral ligament reconstruction with hamstring tendon autograft and mediolateral patellar tunnel fixation: A meta-analysis of outcomes and complications. Bone Joint J. 2013;95-B(7):900-905.

[140] Kang H, Zheng R, Dai Y, Lu J, Wang F. Single- and double-bundle medial patellofemoral ligament reconstruction procedures result in similar recurrent dislocation rates and improvements in knee function: A systematic review. Knee Surg Sports Traumatol Arthrosc. 2019;27(3): 827-836.

[141] Shamrock AG, Day MA, Duchman KR, Glass N, Westermann RW. Medial patellofemoral ligament reconstruction in skeletally immature patients: A systematic review and meta-analysis. Orthop J Sports Med. 2019 Jul 29;7(7):2325967119855023. doi: 10.1177/2325967119855023. PMID: 31384615; PMCID: PMC6664654.

[142] Schneider DK, Grawe B, Magnussen RA, Ceasar A, Parikh SN, Wall EJ, Colosimo AJ, Kaeding CC, Myer GD. Outcomes after isolated medial patellofemoral ligament reconstruction for the treatment of recurrent lateral patellar dislocations: A systematic review and meta-analysis. Am J Sports Med. 2016;44(11): 2993-3005.

[143] Sherman SL, Deasis DP, Garrone AJ, Voss EE, Oliver HA. Return to play after patellar stabilization. Curr Rev Musculoskelet Med. 2018;11(2): 280-284.

[144] Manjunath AK, Hurley ET, Jazrawi LM, Strauss EJ. Return to play after medial patellofemoral ligament reconstruction: A systematic review. Am J Sports Med. 2021;49(4):1094-1100.

[145] Platt BN, Bowers LC, Magnuson JA, Marx SM, Liu JN, Farr J, Stone AV. Return to sport after medial patellofemoral ligament reconstruction: A systematic review and meta-analysis. Am J Sports Med. 2021 Mar 15:363546521990004. doi: 10.1177/0363546521990004. Online ahead of print. PMID: 33720789.

[146] Shah JN, Howard JS, Flanigan DC, Brophy RH, Carey JL, Lattermann C. A systematic review of complications and failures associated with medial patellofemoral ligament reconstruction for recurrent patellar dislocation. Am J Sports Med. 2012;40(8):1916-1923.

[147] Parikh SN, Nathan ST, Wall EJ, Eismann EA. Complications of medial patellofemoral ligament reconstruction in young patients. Am J Sports Med. 2013;41(5):1030-1038.

[148] Christiansen SE, Jacobsen BW, Lund B, Lind M. Reconstruction of the medial patellofemoral ligament with gracilis tendon autograft in transverse patellar drill holes. Arthroscopy. 2008;24(1):82-87.

[149] Matthews JJ, Schranz P. Reconstruction of the medial patellofemoral ligament using a longitudinal patellar tunnel technique. Int Orthop. 2010;34(8):1321-1325.

[150] Song SY, Kim IS, Chang HG, Shin JH, Kim HJ, Seo YJ. Anatomic medial patellofemoral ligament reconstruction using patellar suture anchor fixation for recurrent patellar instability. Knee Surg Sports Traumatol Arthrosc. 2014;22(10):2431-2437.

[151] Calanna F, Pulici L, Carimati G, Quaglia A, Volpi P. Medial patello-femoral ligament (MPFL) reconstruction using suture anchors fixation: Preliminary results. Muscles Ligaments Tendons J. 2016;6(1):64-70.

[152] Schöttle PB, Hensler D, Imhoff AB. Anatomical double-bundle MPFL reconstruction with an aperture fixation. Knee Surg Sports Traumatol Arthrosc. 2010;18(2):147-151.

[153] Hapa O, Akşahin E, Özden R, Pepe M, Yanat AN, Doğramacı Y, Bozdağ E, Sünbüloğlu E. Aperture fixation instead of transverse tunnels at the patella for medial patellofemoral ligament reconstruction. Knee Surg Sports Traumatol Arthrosc. 2012;20(2): 322-326.

[154] Russ SD, Tompkins M, Nuckley D, Macalena J. Biomechanical comparison of patellar fixation techniques in medial patellofemoral ligament reconstruction. Am J Sports Med. 2015;43(1):195-199.

[155] Thaunat M, Erasmus PJ. Recurrent patellar dislocation after medial patellofemoral ligament reconstruction. Knee Surg Sports Traumatol Arthrosc. 2008;16(1):40-43.

[156] Lippacher S, Reichel H, Nelitz M. [Patellar fracture after patellar stabilization] [Article in German]. Orthopade. 2010;39(5):516-518.

[157] Parikh SN, Wall EJ. Patellar fracture after medial patellofemoral ligament surgery: A report of five cases. J Bone Joint Surg Am. 2011;93(17): e97(1-8).

[158] Sanchis-Alfonso V, Montesinos-Berry E, Ramirez-Fuentes C, Leal-Blanquet J, Gelber PE, Monllau JC. Failed medial patellofemoral ligament reconstruction: Causes and surgical strategies. World J Orthop. 2017;8(2): 115-129.

[159] Schiphouwer L, Rood A, Tigchelaar S, Koeter S. Complications of medial patellofemoral ligament reconstruction using two transverse patellar tunnels. Knee Surg Sports Traumatol Arthrosc 2017;25(1):245-250.

[160] Lenschow S, Schliemann B, Gestring J, Herbort M, Schulze M, Kösters C. Medial patellofemoral ligament reconstruction: Fixation strength of 5 different techniques for graft fixation at the patella. Arthroscopy. 2013;29(4):766-773.

[161] Deasey MJ, Moran TE, Lesevic M, Burnett ZR, Diduch DR. Small, short, oblique patellar tunnels for patellar fixation do not increase fracture risk or complications in MPFL reconstruction: A retrospective cohort study. Orthop J Sports Med. 2020;8(10):2325967120 954430. doi: 10.1177/23259671209 54430. eCollection 2020 Oct. PMID: 33062759.

Chapter 5

The Meniscus Deficient Knee: Options for Repair and Reconstruction

Matthew Brown

Abstract

The preservation of the structure of the meniscus despite a tear has been widely discussed in the literature. However, meniscectomy continues to be the most-performed meniscus surgery. In a percentage of patients, knee pain and swelling, as well as tibial plateau bony edema, follow meniscus resection; this panoply of symptoms is known as "post-meniscectomy syndrome". The management of this condition requires meniscus transplant in case of total meniscectomy or a meniscus scaffold in the case of a partial resection. This chapter aims to discuss the indication, surgical technique, and outcomes of collagen meniscus implants (CMI) for partial resections and meniscus transplants for full resections.

Keywords: meniscus transplant, collagen meniscus implant, post-meniscectomy syndrome, meniscus scaffold, osteoarthritis

1. Introduction

It is essential to understand the anatomy and biomechanics of the knee joint before performing a sub-total or total meniscectomy due to the possible catastrophic consequences at a long-term follow-up. Moreover, the medial and the lateral compartment of the knee have different kinematic properties and the clinician must take into account the different degree of mobility, bony structure, and load distribution between these two compartments. Biomechanical studies have demonstrated the essential role of the menisci on load transfer, in that a total meniscectomy can increase the contact area by 33 to 50 percent in a fully extended knee [1].

Walker et al. demonstrated that the lateral compartment is much more dependent on meniscal function than the medial one. The lateral meniscus carries a higher percentage of load transfer than the medial meniscus. This is due to a higher load being transferred directly by the exposed cartilage surface of the medial compartment [1]. The different bony morphology of the tibiofemoral compartments also play a part in this. In the sagittal plane, the medial convexity of the femoral condyle and the concavity of the tibial plateau provide a degree of congruity, even after a meniscectomy. While, on the lateral side, both the convexity of the femoral condyle and the lateral tibial plateau make this compartment much more prone to an increase in peak contact pressures after meniscectomy [2].

Clinically, the differences between the medial and lateral meniscus have been confirmed by worse results reported after lateral meniscectomy compared to medial meniscectomy at a long-term follow-up [3, 4]. These findings are even more stark if the meniscectomy is performed during adolescence: in a prospective 30 years of follow-up study, about 80% of patients after medial meniscectomy maintained good or excellent clinical results; in comparison to less than 50% for lateral meniscectomy [5].

The causal relationship of knee arthritis with meniscectomy led to the investigation of meniscal allograft transplantation for the post-meniscectomy patient experiencing pain and demonstrating arthritic changes [6]. Basic science studies have shown that although meniscal allografts cannot fully replicate the function of the native meniscus, the grafts are able to significantly improve joint contact area and decrease contact pressures [7, 8]. Also, early clinical series demonstrated isolated meniscal allograft transplantation to be a feasible procedure [9, 10]. However, the initial studies had variable outcomes due to significant differences in indications, surgical techniques, and tissue processing methods.

As experience was gained, the variables became more defined and the results improved. Numerous short and midterm studies have shown that meniscal allografts are able to provide pain relief and increase function with high rates of graft survivorship [11, 12]. More recently, a long-term study has been published demonstrating >50% graft survival at 20 years [13].

However, if a subtotal meniscectomy has previously been performed, a meniscal scaffold may be a more appropriate procedure, despite the relative lack of relevant articles with extended follow-up. There are two different scaffold types available on the market: the collagen meniscus implant (CMI) derived from a bovine collagen and the Actifit, a polyurethane scaffold [14, 15]. 3D printed scaffolds have been recently proposed as an experimental treatment and only a few case reports are available, while CMI and Actifit have been widely studied.

2. Biomechanics

After a meniscal tear, the effectiveness of meniscal repair strictly relies on the tissue quality and defect location with respect to the vascular supply. Tears in the vascularized "red" peripheral zone are more likely to heal, while the more common lesions in the avascular "white" zone have poor healing potential [16, 17]. When the majority of the meniscus is not salvageable, a meniscectomy is usually performed. It has been well documented that meniscectomy increases the risk of degenerative joint disease of the knee. For example, Persson et al. demonstrated that in almost 2,500 patients followed for more than 20 years, the risk of developing arthritis after a partial meniscectomy was almost 6 times higher than the standard population, with a 17% absolute risk [18].

Structurally, it has been demonstrated that meniscal allografts should be frozen, not sterilized using chemicals or radiation. It the first published series of isolated meniscal allografts, Milakowski et al. found that graft processing methods were vital to the success of the procedure [19]. He reported that lyophilized grafts lead to inferior results compared to fresh frozen grafts. While clinical series have not shown benefit of cryopreserved over fresh frozen, basic science studies have shown slightly better mechanic properties with cryopreserved, with a higher elastic modulus and point of rupture [20].

While meniscus allograft transplantation appropriately addresses a prior total or subtotal meniscectomy, an allograft is not a solution for the treatment of a partial meniscus defect. The Collagen Meniscus Implant (Ivy Sports Medicine, Germany) is a porous biologic scaffold. It consists of 97% type I collagen purified from bovine Achilles tendon while the remaining portion is composed of glycosaminoglycan (GAG). The specific size of the scaffold's micropores are controlled to increase the fibrocartilage maturation while avoiding pseudo-capsule formation and foreign body reaction [21].

The second scaffold type consists of a synthetic polyurethane-based material composed of flexible segments made from polycaprolactone 80% and stiff segments made from urethane 20% (Actifit; Orteq Sports Medicine, London, UK). The scaffold slowly biodegrades, with an estimated decomposition time of 4 to 6 years. The implant itself is also highly porous to allow for sufficient ingrowth [22]. Both the Actifit and the CMI implants come in separate configurations for medial or lateral meniscus defects.

3. Surgical technique

The indications for both meniscus allograft and scaffold vary by surgeon, but in general, the patient should have previously undergone a total or partial meniscectomy, respectively, and present with discomfort only in the compartment previously operated upon. Maximal osteoarthritis allowed is grade III and a minimum 2 mm joint space. Also, if the knee is clinically unstable, it should be stabilized at the time of the procedure with respect to the anterior cruciate ligament. If operative knee alignment is more than 3–5 degrees different concerning the involved compartment compared to the contralateral knee, an osteotomy should be performed to unload the affected compartment.

For meniscus allograft transplant, the traditional methodology denotes the use of medial side double bone plugs, and a press-fit bone bridge (keyhole) method on the lateral side (**Figure 1**). On the medial side bone plugs are used due to graft size and anterior attachment variability, while on the lateral side bone bridges are used due to horn proximity [13]. In the case of a concomitant ACL and lateral meniscus, the femoral and tibial ACL tunnels are drilled initially and then the lateral meniscus trough is made. The femoral side of the ACL is then secured, followed by placement of the lateral meniscal allograft, and finally the tibial side of the ACL is secured. While a number of papers have investigated all-soft tissue constructs, several basic science studies have demonstrated improved biomechanical function with bony meniscal attachments [23, 24].

For meniscus scaffolds, surgical technique is similar for both devices. This begins with arthroscopic resection of the surrounding damaged tissue and subsequent implantation of a custom-sized scaffold. The sized scaffold is then sutured to the meniscal rim and capsule using standard techniques (**Figure 2**).

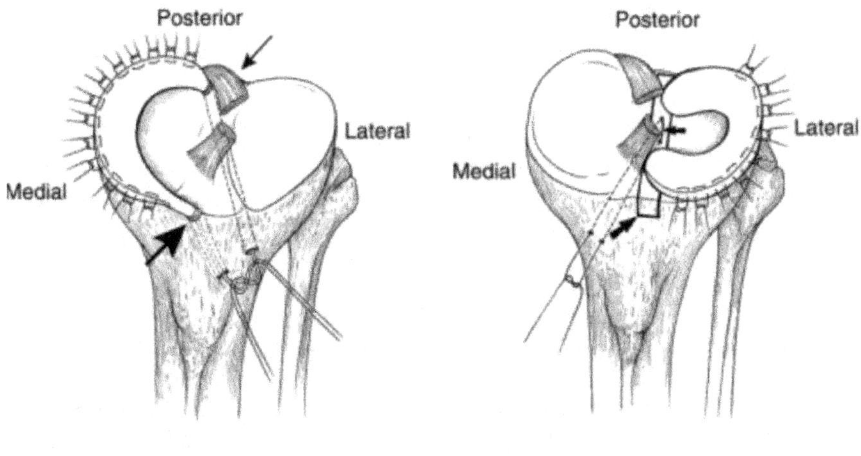

Figure 1.
Lateral keyhole technique with suture fixation and medial bone plug technique with suture fixation.

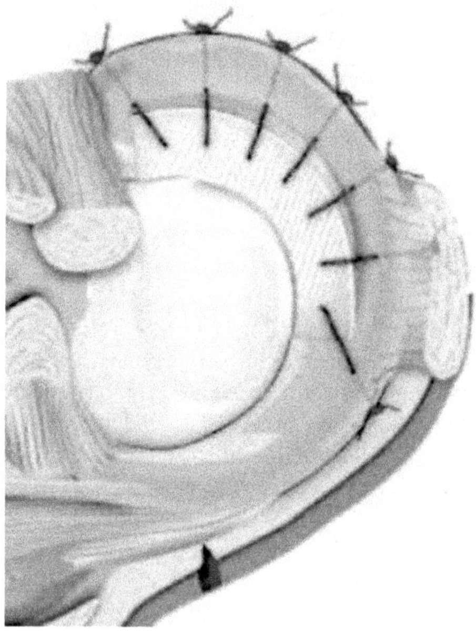

Figure 2.
Custom meniscal scaffold sizing and fixation.

Initially, a partial meniscectomy is performed, with surgical debridement back to the vascularized zone of the damaged portion of the native meniscus. It is particularly important that the meniscal rim be continuous, especially at the popliteal hiatus of the lateral meniscus. If there is complete loss of the tissue in front of the popliteus tendon, it should be considered a total loss and thus a contraindication for a meniscus scaffold. After debridement, the resulting void is sized along the peripheral edge using the meniscal ruler supplied with the scaffold. The scaffold is then cut to fit, placed into the knee, and finally sutured to the native meniscus. The surgeon can use an all-inside, inside-out, or outside-in suture technique depending on the area to be sutured and their experience and preference [25].

4. Clinical outcomes

Early results showed meniscus transplant could be a viable procedure; however, the initial results were mixed and raised concerns of long-term durability. It the first series of isolated meniscal allografts, Milakowski et al. demonstrated that graft processing methods were vital to the success of the procedure [9]. He reported the use of lyophilized grafts lead to inferior results compared to fresh frozen grafts. In the first American published series, Garrett et al. reported success in 35 of 43 patients (81%) at 2 to 7-year follow-up [26]. However, 6 of the 11 patients with grade IV chondromalacia failed, leading to the conclusion that while beneficial, grafts should not be placed in knees with advanced arthritis.

In the early experience of Noyes et al. they reported a high failure rate [27]. They evaluated 38 patients with 40 grafts, with a follow-up at an average of 40 months (24–62 months). While clinically the patients did significantly better, on MRI 30% of grafts demonstrated "altered characteristics" with another 28% demonstrating gross failure. Patients with no pre-operative arthritis demonstrated 10 abnormal MRIs out of 22, while the arthritic group showed abnormalities in 13 of 18, again demonstrating the folly of allograft implantation in arthritic knees.

Over time, graft processing methods, patient selection parameters, and surgical techniques were refined. With these improvements, meniscus allograft transplant ceased being seen as experimental (**Table 1**) [28].

Numerous short and mid-term studies reported that the vast majority of the grafts did not require reoperation, and a significant number of patients had decreased pain and improved function [29–32]. In a large series, Verdonk et al. reported a survivorship of 79% in the first 100 patients at a mean of 7.2 years [33].

Kim et al. published the most optimistic longer-term data on meniscal allograft transplantation, with 2 failures in 49 knees after a minimum follow-up of 8 years. The 10-year survival rate was 98.0% and the 15-year survival rate was 93.3% according to their Kaplan–Meier analysis [34].

Carter et al. demonstrated 10-year results in 40 of his original 46 patients [35]. Thirty-two (80%) stated they had improvement in symptoms from the preoperative level. The 10 year mean IKDC score improved from the pre-op mean 50.6 (range 32.2–68.9) to 70.1 (range 39.1–93.1). Seven patients required partial meniscectomies, for a 10-year graft survivorship of 83%. Of thirty-four patients with plain radiographs available at the time of implantation and at 10 years for comparison, fourteen had no change, 15 had mild osteoarthritis, and 5 moderate to advanced progression.

Noyes et al. in his later series, 58/72 patients had follow-up at a mean of 11.9 years ± 3.2 years [36]. Twenty-six underwent reoperation for a total graft survival rate of 55.2%. While demonstrating lower survivorship, their study group had greater chondral abnormalities and malalignment at baseline. Twenty patients underwent OATS procedures, and fourteen underwent an osteotomy in conjunction with the meniscal allograft at the time of implantation.

Van der Wal et al. reported on 63 meniscal allografts transplanted in 57 patients evaluated at 13.8 ± 2.8 years. Nineteen patients had grade IV chondromalacia at baseline, and their grafts were not secured with bone [37]. Their failure rate was 29% (18 grafts) and twelve patients (21%) were converted to a TKR at a mean follow-up of 10.8 years (range 4.3–13.7). They acknowledged that the degree of chondromalacia, ACL deficiency, and graft fixation contributed to failures, with these results confirming that strict patient selection is vital for long term success.

Case studies	**Year**	**Follow-up (y)**	**Survivorship (%)**
Garrett	1993	2+	81
Noyes	2004	2+	72
Verdonk	2006	5+	79
Kim	2017	8+	98
Carter	2012	10+	83
Noyes	2016	8+	55
Van der Waal	2009	11+	71
Carter	2020	20+	56
Systematic reviews			
Novaretti		10	73.5
		15	60
Bin	Medial	10+	53
	Lateral	10+	57

Table 1.
Selected meniscal transplant studies survivorship rates.

Systematic reviews have emerged providing data with compiled results at ten-plus years after meniscal transplant implantation. Novaretti et al. combined 11 studies with 688 meniscal allograft transplants and found a 10-year survivorship of 73.5%, and a 15-year survivorship of 60.3% [18]. Bin et al. evaluated the long-term survivorship of medial versus lateral meniscal transplants at greater than ten years in a meta-analysis of 9 studies totaling 694 grafts, and found that 52.6% of medial and 56.6% of lateral grafts were intact [19].

The one study to discuss 20-year follow-up was Carter et al. where 48/56 (86.7%) of patients were able to be contacted, and of those, had 21 required surgical treatment of the graft. Thirteen patients had an isolated partial meniscectomy. Eight patients had knee arthroplasty with 1 having prior partial graft removal and one also had a high tibial osteotomy (HTO). The average time to arthroplasty was 12.7 years. The graft survivorship was therefore 56.2% [13].

The take-away points from the usage of meniscal transplants involve proper patient selection, use of a properly prepared graft, and implantation in an appropriate knee. When an average-weight patient without varus or valgus knee abnormalities has a fresh meniscal allograft placed in a stable knee without moderate or severe arthritis or chondral loss, the graft survival can potentially be greater than twenty years.

The data supporting meniscal scaffold implantation does not go back nearly as long as meniscal transplant but is also robust. Clinical studies report outcomes for CMI ranging up to 12 years, while the longest study on Actifit reports up to 8 years, both demonstrating improvements in all knee clinical outcome scales (**Table 2**).

For the CMI implant, Monllau et al. demonstrated 83% good and excellent results at 10-year follow-up for 22 patients [38]. In a randomized trial comparing the long-term results of patients with ACL rupture and partial medial meniscus defects treated with ACL reconstruction and partial medial meniscectomy versus medial CMI implant, Bulgheroni et al. demonstrated significant improvement of all clinical scores at an average of 9.6 years [39]. Also, Zaffagnini et al. showed prospective study results between medial CMI implantation and partial medial meniscectomy [40]. The CMI group showed significantly lower VAS for pain, higher objective IKDC, and Tegner scores at 10-year follow-up.

The Actifit results are similarly impressive. Schuttler et al. demonstrated significant improvement in VAS from 5 preoperatively to 1 at 4 years of follow-up in a group of 18 Actifit patients [41]. Leroy et al. also showed, with a minimal follow-up of 5 years, 15 patients improved from 5.3 and 50 preoperative VAS and subjective IKDC scores respectively to 2.9 and 79 [42]. Finally, a meta-analysis of 613 Actifit patients demonstrated both VAS and Tegner scores improving significantly remaining higher up to 72 months [43]. Overall, there has been degeneration of the

Case studies (CMI)	Year	Follow-up (y)	Survivorship (%)
Monllau	2011	10+	83
Bulgheroni	2015	6+	not listed
Zaffagnini	2011	10+	88
Leroy	2017	5+	77
(Actifit)			
Schuttler	2016	2+	100
Systematic reviews			
Filardo	2015	CMI/Actifit 2+	94

Table 2.
Selected meniscal scaffold studies survivorship rates.

scaffold over time with some resulting increase in osteoarthritis, with a reported rate of 9.9% at a mean follow-up of 40 months and 6.7% at a mean follow-up of 44 months, for the Actifit and CMI patients, respectively [43].

The vast majority of meniscal scaffold literature has been published on medial implants, with a recent systematic review including 396 CMI with only 10% of them were implanted in the lateral compartment [44]. Zaffagnini et al. investigated 43 patients at 24± 1.9 months after lateral CMI implant. Their Lysholm score improved from 64.3 ± 18.4 preoperatively to 93.2 ± 7.2 at final follow-up, with pain experienced during strenuous activity and at rest was significantly reduced. At 2 years of follow-up, roughly 60% of patients reported activity levels similar to their preinjury values with a satisfaction rate of 95%. The presence of a higher BMI, the need for concomitant procedures, and a chronic injury pattern resulted in reduced outcomes [45].

Finally, Hirschmann et al. demonstrated the results of a series of 67 patients undergoing medial or lateral CMI implantation associated with ACL reconstruction (45%), high tibial osteotomy (7.5%) or microfracture (4.5%). At one year the cohort demonstrated a marked decrease in pain with a subsequent improvement in the Tegner, IKDC and Lysholm scores, with comparable results of the medial and the lateral groups [46].

And so, for the meniscal scaffolds, the useage and survivorship appear to be similar to those of the transplants; however, these implants are placed into patients with contained meniscal defects as opposed to the full meniscal loss which necessitates the use of a meniscus transplant. When an average-weight patient without varus or valgus knee abnormalities has a meniscal scaffold placed in a partially debreided meniscus in an otherwise stable knee without moderate or severe arthritis or chondral loss, the graft survival can potentially be greater than ten years based on current data.

5. Conclusions

For the patient with "post-meniscectomy syndrome" with either a partially or entirely deficient meniscus, surgical treatment options exist which have demonstrated both short, medium, and in the case of meniscus allograft, long term success. Allografts have demonstrated greater than 50% survivorship at 20-year follow-up, while scaffolds have demonstrated the progressive reabsorption with substitution with a meniscus-like tissue with a potential chondroprotective effect in shorter-term studies. For both allografts and scaffolds, patient selection and the treatment of concomitant knee pathology is mandatory in order to achieve both short and long-term clinical improvement.

Author details

Matthew Brown
University of Arizona, Phoenix, AZ, USA

*Address all correspondence to: mjb9rc@mail.missouri.edu

References

[1] Walker PS, Hajek JV. The load-bearing area in the knee joint. J Biomech. 1972;5(6):581-589.

[2] McDermott ID, Amis AA. The consequences of meniscectomy. J Bone Joint Surg Br. 2006;88(12):1549-1556.

[3] Jørgensen U, Sonne-Holm S, Lauridsen F, et al. Long-term follow-up of meniscectomy in athletes. A prospective longitudinal study. J Bone Joint Surg Br. 1987;69(1):80-83.

[4] Hede A, Larsen E, Sandberg H. The long term outcome of open total and partial meniscectomy related to the quantity and site of the meniscus removed. Int Orthop. 1992;16(2): 122-125.

[5] McNicholas MJ, Rowley DI, McGurty D, et al. Total meniscectomy in adolescence. A thirty year follow-up. J Bone Joint Surg Br. 2000;82(2):217-221.

[6] Allen PR, Denham RA, Swan AV. Late degenerative changes after meniscectomy: Factors affecting the knee after operation. J Bone Joint Surg Br 1984;66:666-671.

[7] Wang H, Chen T, Gee AO, et al. Altered regional loading patterns on articular cartilage following meniscectomy are not fully restored by autograft meniscal transplantation. Osteoarthritis Cartilage 2015;23: 462-468.

[8] Spang JT, Dang AB, Mazzocca A, et al. The effect of medial meniscectomy and meniscal allograft transplantation on knee and anterior cruciate ligament biomechanics. Arthroscopy 2010;26: 192-201

[9] Milachowski KA, Weismeier K, Wirth CJ. Homologous meniscus transplantation. Experimental and clinical results. Int Orthop 1989;13:1-11.

[10] Garrett JC, Steensen RN. Meniscal transplantation in the human knee: A preliminary report. Arthroscopy 1991;7:57-62.

[11] McCormick F, Harris JD, Abrams GD, et al. Survival and reoperation rates after meniscal allograft transplantation: Analysis of failures for 172 consecutive transplants at a minimum 2-year follow-up. Am J Sports Med 2014;42:892-897.

[12] Zaffagnini S, Grassi A, Marcheggiani Muccioli GM, et al. Is sport activity possible after arthroscopic meniscal allograft transplantation? Midterm results in active patients. Am J Sport Med 2016;44:625-632.

[13] Carter TR, Brown MJ. Meniscal allograft survivorship and outcomes 20 years after implantation. Arthroscopy. 2020 Aug;36(8):2268-2274.

[14] Filardo G, Petretta M, Cavallo C, et al. Patient-specific meniscus prototype based on 3D bioprinting of human cell-laden scaffold. Bone Jt Res. 2019;8(2):101-106.

[15] Ghodbane SA, Brzezinski A, Patel JM, et al. Partial meniscus replacement with a collagen-hyaluronan infused three-dimensional printed polymeric scaffold. Tissue Eng Part A. 2019;25(5-6):379-389.

[16] Longo UG, Campi S, Romeo G, et al. Biological strategies to enhance healing of the avascular area of the meniscus. Stem Cells Int 2012;2012:528359.

[17] Goodwillie AD, Myers K, Sgaglione NA. Current strategies and approaches to meniscal repair. J Knee Surg 2014;27(6):423-434.

[18] Persson F, Turkiewicz A, Bergkvist D, Neuman P, Englund M. The risk of symptomatic knee osteoarthritis

after arthroscopic meniscus repair vs partial meniscectomy vs the general population. Osteoarthritis Cartilage. 2018;26:195-201.

[19] Milachowski KA, Weismeier K, Wirth CJ. Homologous meniscus transplantation. Experimental and clinical results. Int Orthop 1989;13:1-11.

[20] Ahmad S, Singh VA, Hussein SI. Cryopreservation versus fresh frozen meniscal allograft: A biomechanical comparative analysis. J Ortho Surg 2017;25:1-7

[21] Klompmaker J, Jansen HW, Veth RP, et al. Porous implants for knee joint meniscus reconstruction: A preliminary study on the role of pore sizes in ingrowth and differentiation of fibrocartilage. Clin Mater. 1993;14(1):1-11.

[22] Filardo G, Andriolo L, Kon E, et al. Meniscal scaffolds: Results and indications. A systematic literature review. Int Orthop 2015;39(1):35-46.

[23] Jauregui JJ, Wu ZD, Meredith S, Griffith C, Packer JD, Henn RF 3rd. How should we secure our transplanted meniscus? A meta-analysis. Am J Sports Med 2018;46:2285-2290.

[24] Seitz AM, Dürselen L. Biomechanical considerations are crucial for the success of tendon and meniscus allograft integration—A systematic review. Knee Surg Sports Traumatol Arthrosc 2019;27:1708-1716.

[25] de Caro F, Perdisa F, Dhollander A, et al. Meniscus scaffolds for partial meniscus defects. Clin Sports Med. 2020 Jan;39(1):83-92.

[26] Garrett JC. Meniscal transplantation: A review of 43 cases with 2- to 7- year follow-up. Sports Med Arthroscopy Rev 1993:1;164-157.

[27] Noyes FR, Barber-Westin SD, Rankin M. Meniscal transplantation in symptomatic patients less than fifty years old. J Bone Joint Surg Am 2004 Jul;86:1392-1404.

[28] Getgood A, LaPrade RF, Verdonk P, et al. International meniscus reconstruction experts forum (IMREF) 2015 consensus statement on the practice of meniscal allograft transplantation. Am J Sports Med 2017;45:1195-1205.

[29] Myers P, Tudor F. Meniscal allograft transplantation: How should we be doing it? A systematic review. Arthroscopy 2015 31:911-925.

[30] Novaretti JV, Patel NK, Lian J, et al. Long-term survival analysis and outcomes of meniscal allograft transplantation with minimum 10-year follow-up: A systematic review. Arthroscopy 2019;35:659-667.

[31] Bin SI, Nha KW, Cheong JY, Shin YS. Midterm and long-term results of medial versus lateral meniscal allograft transplantation: A meta-analysis. Am J Sports Med 2018; 46:1243-1250.

[32] Lee BS, Kim HJ, Lee CR, et al. Clinical outcomes of meniscal allograft transplantation with or without other procedures: A systematic review and meta-analysis. Am J Sports Med 2018;46:3047-3056

[33] Verdonk PC, Demurie A, Almqvist KF, Veys EM, Verbruggen G, Verdonk R. Transplantation of viable meniscal allograft. Journal Bone Joint Am 2006;88:109-118.

[34] Kim JM, Bin SI, Lee BS et al. Long-term survival analysis of meniscal allograft transplantation with bone fixation. Arthroscopy 2017;33:387-393.

[35] Carter TR, Rabago MA: Meniscal allograft transplantation: 10 year follow-up. Arthroscopy 2012;28 suppl 1;e17-18.

[36] Noyes FR and Barber-Westin SD. Long-term survivorship and function of meniscus transplantation. Am J Sports Med 2016;44:2330-2338.

[37] van der Wal RJ, Thomassen BJ, van Arkel ER. Long-term clinical outcome of open meniscal allograft transplantation. Am J Sports Med 2009;3:2134-2139.

[38] Monllau JC, Gelber PE, Abat F, et al. Outcome after partial medial meniscus substitution with the collagen meniscal implant at a minimum of 10 years' follow-up. Arthroscopy 2011;27(7): 933-943.

[39] Bulgheroni E, Grassi A, Bulgheroni P, et al. Long-term outcomes of medial CMI implant versus partial medial meniscectomy in patients with concomitant ACL reconstruction. Knee Surg Sports Traumatol Arthrosc 2015;23:3221-3227.

[40] Zaffagnini S, Marcheggiani Muccioli GM, Lopomo N, et al. Prospective long-term outcomes of the medial collagen meniscus implant versus partial medial meniscectomy. A minimum 10-year follow-up study. Am J Sports Med 2011;39(5).

[41] Schuttler KF, Haberhauer F, Gesslein M, et al. Midterm follow-up after implantation of a polyurethane meniscal scaffold for segmental medial meniscus loss: Maintenance of good clinical and MRI outcome. Knee Surg Sports Traumatol Arthrosc 2016;24(5): 1478-1484.

[42] Leroy A, Beaufils P, Faivre B, et al. Actifit polyurethane meniscal scaffold: MRI and functional outcomes after a minimum follow-up of 5 years. Orthop Traumatol Surg Res 2017;103(4): 609-614.

[43] Filardo G, Andriolo L, Kon E, et al. Meniscal scaffolds: Results and indications. A systematic literature review. Int Orthop 2015;39(1):35-46.

[44] Grassi A, Zaffagnini S, Marcheggiani Muccioli GM, et al. Clinical outcomes and complications of a collagen meniscus implant: A systematic review. Int Orthop. 2014;38(9):1945-1953.

[45] Zaffagnini S, Marcheggiani Muccioli GM, Bulgheroni P, et al. Arthroscopic collagen meniscus implantation for partial lateral meniscal defects: A 2-year minimum follow-up study. Am J Sports Med. 2012;40(10): 2281-2288.

[46] Hirschmann MT, Keller L, Hirschmann A, et al. One-year clinical and MR imaging outcome after partial meniscal replacement in stabilized knees using a collagen meniscus implant. Knee Surg Sports Traumatol Arthrosc Off J ESSKA. 2013;21(3): 740-747.

Section 2

Wrist

Chapter 6

Wrist Arthroscopy

Uldis Krustins and Jānis Krustins

Abstract

This article is dedicated to our special interest in hand surgery - arthroscopy. We are the initiators of the wrist arthroscopy in our clinic as well as in country. In this chapter we can only sketch some aspects of this fascinating, intriguing and specific direction of hand surgery. Indications for arthroscopic surgery and application in different wrist conditions including novel techniques. There is a short historical review at the beginning - names and contribution of the pioneers of the wrist arthroscopy, development of instruments and surgical possibilities. This is followed by arthroscopic anatomy of the portals and structures accessible via these portals. The most common arthroscopic procedures in our practice are listed and described, such as arthroscopic treatment of ganglions and bone cysts, intercarpal ligament or TFCC tears, application of the arthroscopy in treatment of the articular distal radius fractures, scaphoid fractures and nonunions The text is supplemented with photos of our patients.

Keywords: wrist, arthroscopy, carpal injuries, distal radius fracture, TFCC

1. Introduction

Since wrist arthroscopies for diagnostical purposes were first reported and described in 1979, it has become an important diagnostic and therapeutic tool in the hands of trained specialists during the last decades. Nowadays it is widely used in the treatment of acute wrist injuries as well as different chronic conditions and degenerative diseases. Arthroscopy has assumed an important place in wrist surgery. The wide list of indications for wrist arthroscopy is continuously growing and requires specific operative skills and specialized training before entering the operating room for real surgery. At this point it's necessary to highlight the huge investment of International Wrist Arthroscopy Society (IWAS) and Asia Pacific Wrist Association (APWA) in training programs, courses and workshops all around the world. Today arthroscopic methods are proposed in the treatment of almost all soft tissue and osseous problems of the wrist. They include synovitis, fibrosis, stiffness, triangular fibrocartilage complex (TFCC) problems, ganglion cysts, scapholunate- (SLIL) and lunotriquetral ligament (LTIL) tears, intra-articular distal radius fracture (DRF) and nonunion treatment, arthroscopic arthrolysis, treatment of scaphoid fractures and nonunions, arthroscopic treatment of Kienböck's disease, arthroscopically assisted partial wrist fusions, etc. We can be grateful to the industry, that they have been able to listen to our wishes and create the tools needed for our surgeries. Since authors have been limited in the size of the manuscript as well as many well illustrated books on this topic have already been published, we will address only the most frequent problems of wrist arthroscopy in our practice.

2. History of the wrist arthroscopy

Early arthroscopic explorations mostly focused on a knee joint, but M. Burman in the early thirties experimented with a use of arthroscopy in other joints, including the wrist joint. In 1970, the 1.7 mm No. 24 arthroscope was developed, allowing a wide angle of vision and clear focus utilizing a small diameter. M. Watanabe, who started to use arthroscopy in 1950s and developed the famous No. 21, used this scope to examine 21 wrists in 1970–1972. He developed dorsal approaches on the ulnar side of the extensor pollicis longus tendon to access the radiocarpal joint. Watanabe reported on 67 wrist arthroscopies, including visualization of the distal radioulnar joint. He also included 39 arthroscopies of the thumb carpometacarpal joint and metacarpophalangeal joints as well as 9 interphalangeal joint arthroscopies [1]. Y.C. Chen was an another enthusiast and pioneer of the wrist arthroscopy in 1970s. In 1979 he published an article about 90 arthroscopies of the wrist and finger joints in 34 clinical cases and 2 amputed arms with No.24 arthroscope. Eighty-four wrist and finger joints of four cadavers and two amputated arms were also dissected for macroscopic observation. This article was also illustrated with some color photographies taken with arthroscope [2].

In 1986 Terry Whipple published paper on wrist artrhroscopy technics and described the safe wrist artrhroscopy portals which are still used today [3]. The first wrist arthroscopy course was organized by Terry Whipple, Gary Poehling and James Roth in Winston-Salem, North Carolina, USA in 1986. The first textbook dedicated to the wrist arthroscopy was published in 1992 by T. Whipple. During the next decades the popularity of the wrist arthroscopy has grown, new indications and techniques have been developed. In 1997 P.C.Ho organized the 1st Hong Kong Wrist Arthroscopy course. With growing international interest in wrist arthroscopy, Christophe Mathoulin founded the European Wrist Arthroscopy Society (EWAS) in 2005 and the first EWAS cadaveric wrist arthroscopy course was organized in Strasbourg. In

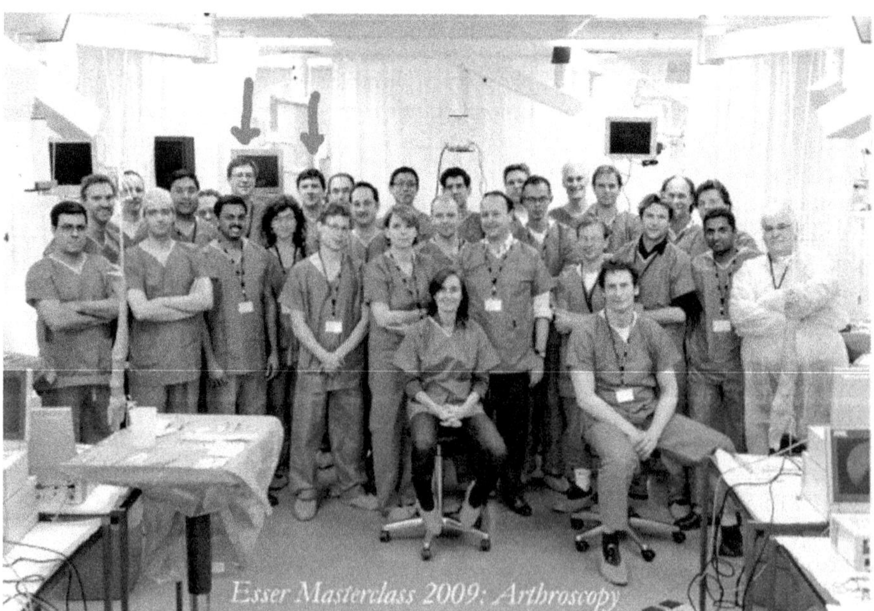

Figure 1.
Authors attending their first wrist arthroscopy course in Rotterdam in 2009 – Uldis Krustins (left), Janis Krustins (right).

2015 P.C. Ho and G. Bein developed the Asian Pacific Wrist Association (APWA). Both of them are wrist-specific international educational organizations with world-wide network of wrist arthroscopy courses and workshops (**Figure 1**). In 2019, EWAS evolved into the IWAS – International Wrist Arthroscopy Society.

3. Setup and equipment

Wrist arthroscopy requires standard arhroscopic equipment – arthroscopy column with monitor, video camera, video and photo recordingdevice, light source with fiber optic cable which nowadays can be integrated in one small box motorized shavers, radiofrequency ablators and X-Ray C arm and traction system. The patient is positioned supine on the operation table with the affected arm on a hand table. The arm is abducted 90° and the elbow flexed 90° allowing a vertical position of the forearm, wrist and hand. In this position the wrist is kept in neutral prono-supination. The surgeon is positioned at the head of the patient with the assistant beside or facing the surgeon. The arthroscopy column may be on the other side of the patient facing the surgeon (**Figure 1**). X-ray C arm is used when necessary and is not in the way of the staff all the time (**Figures 2** and **3**).

Arthroscopic wrist procedures usually are performed under the regional block anesthesia with a pneumatic tourniquet placed on the upper arm, but there are surgeons who propose to do wrist arthroscopies under portal site local anesthesia (PSLA) without tourniquet [4]. Traditionally wrist arthroscopies were performed using irrigation, but it can be easily inspected and treated also in "dry technique" [5]. However, dry arthroscopy also has its limits. For example when radiofrequency ablators are used, water is necessary as milieu conductor and to prevent temperature peaks and possible joint damage. Also when using a burr the aspiration may be blocked by small cartilage and bone fragments and water facilitates the aspiration [6].

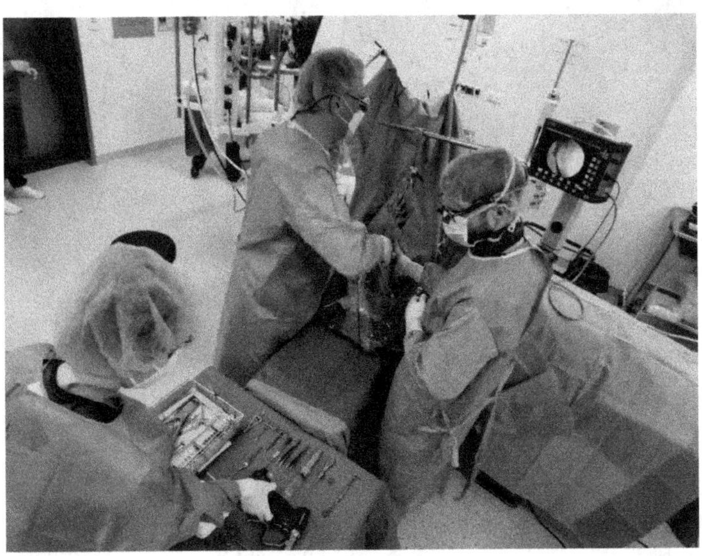

Figure 2.
Standard setup and position of the staff during the wrist arthroscopy.

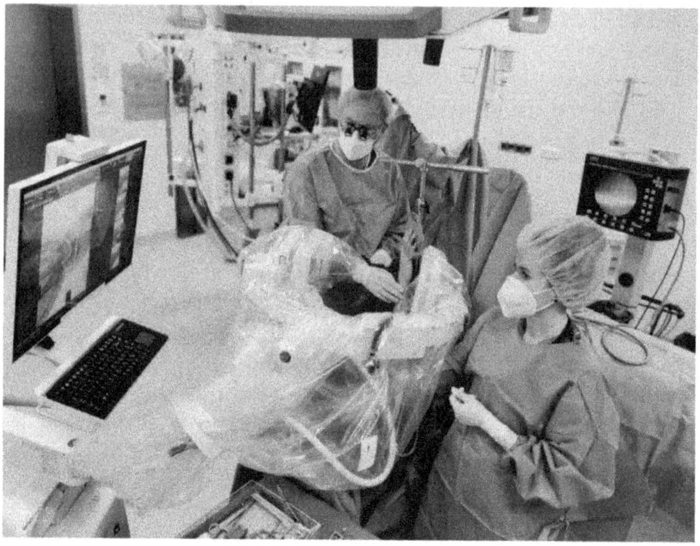

Figure 3.
Use of C arm during the surgery.

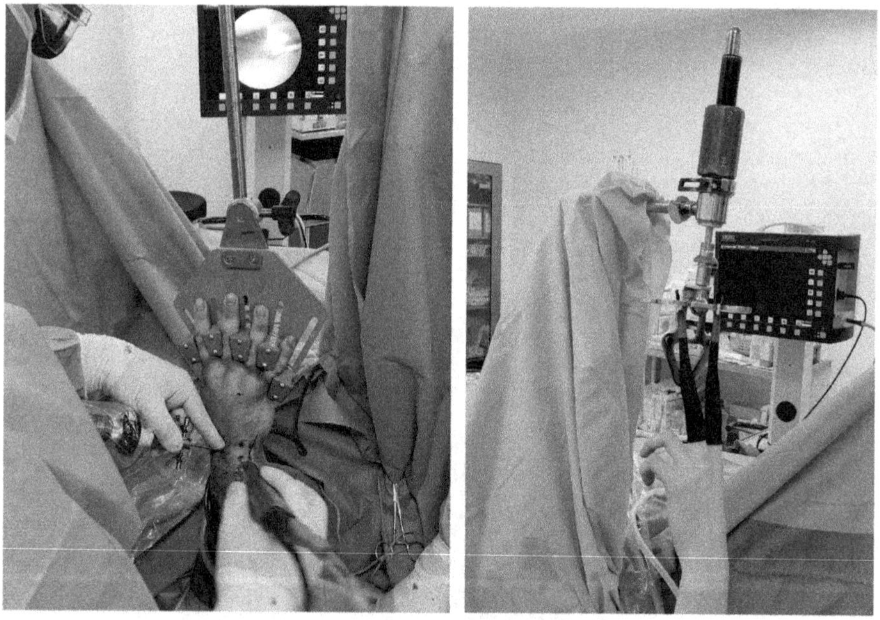

(a) (b)

Figure 4.
Different finger traps and traction devices (4a - K.L.Martin; 4b -Smith & Nephew).

Arthroscopic manipulations in wrist require vertical traction to separate bones and create space for instruments and scope. The traction applied is usually 3.5 to 7 kg for wrist joint and 2 to 3 kg for the thumb [6, 7]. There are different types of wrist vertical traction towers – with Chinese finger traps or special traction hands for all fingers. Authors use K.L.Martin and Smith & Nephew wrist traction towers (**Figure 4a, b**).

4. Instruments

The most important instrument, of course, is the scope. In wrist small arthroscopes, between 1.9 mm and 2.7 mm, with camera angulated at 30°, are usually used Arthroscopes are shorter (60 to 80 mm), too. The second most important tool is a probe which helps to explore the joint and serves as an extension of the surgeon's finger [8]. A variety of differently angled punches, baskets with or without the option of incorporating a suction mechanism and grasping forceps in various sizes are useful for specific manipulations (**Figure 5**). A motor is fitted with abrasive instruments, such as shavers or burrs of appropriate sizes: 2 to 3 mm in diameter and 6 to 8 cm long. Basic instruments also include a shaver for synovial resection and a burr for bony resection. A special electric bipolar diathermy machine is used for efficient tissue resection by vaporization. An irrigation system is used for joint cleaning. The equipment can be completed by different instruments or kits for specific arthroscopic procedures.

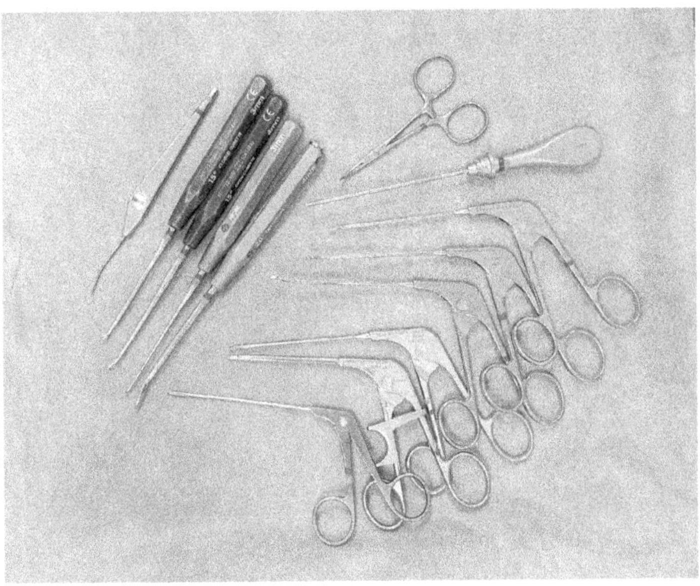

Figure 5.
Set of manual instruments for wrist arthroscopy.

5. Wrist arthroscopy portals

The map of safe wrist arthroscopy portals was first designed by Terry L. Whipple and co-authors in 1986 after anatomical studies of fresh cadaveric wrists which were arthroscoped an then tediously dissected to determine the relationship of each portal to the closest neurovascular and tendinous structures [3]. Seven dorsal wrist portals were identified - five portals for radio-carpal joint with relation to the six extensor compartments (1-2; 3-4; 4-5; 6R and 6 U), one for midcarpal joint – distally from the 3-4 portal and the seventh portal for DRUJ. Anatomical studies proved that 1-2,6 U and 6R portals are the most perilous due the proximity of the radial artery and dorsal radial and ulnar sensory nerve branches. The midcarpal, 3-4,4-5 and DRUJ portals are relatively safe, since neurovascular structures are usually remote [9]. Later additional portals for midcarpal and radio-carpal joint, DRUJ as well as portals and techniques for small joint arthroscopy were described [9–14].

Localization of portals first has to be checked by palpation with fingertip, then standard intramuscular injection needle can be inserted to determine the exact orientation of the portal. Small and shallow horizontal incisions using no. 15 blade are recommended. Then skin, subcutaneous tissues and join capsule can be dissected using mosquito clip to push away any important structures without injuring them. It's suggested to use a curved mosquito clip which can easily slip over the curve of the dorsal rim of the radius or proximal carpal bones.

The normal inclination of the dorsal radius and lunate must be taken into consideration when entering the joints with trocar and never use sharp trocars. The insertion angle usually is about 10° proximally to parallel of the dorsal joint axis, to match the distal articular curves of the bones (**Figure 6**).

Volar portals can be used for visualization of the dorsal capsular structures like dorsal radiocarpal ligament (DRCL), palmar aspects of the carpal ligaments or as occasional accessory portals in arthroscopic assisted surgeries of the distal radius fractures or carpal injuries [13–15].

Localization, function of radiocarpal portals and structures at risk are presented in **Table 1** and for midcarpal portals in **Table 2**.

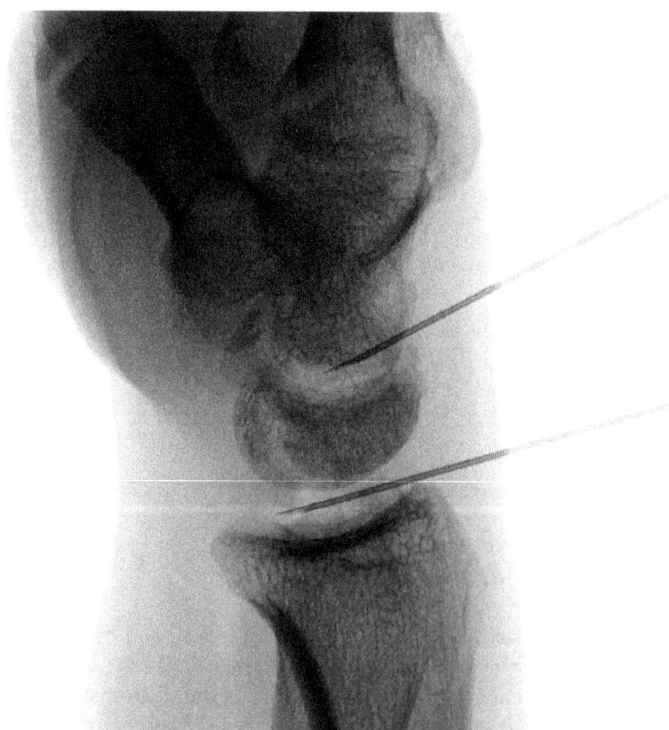

Figure 6.
Insertion angle of the instruments.

Portal	Localization and function	Structures at risk
1-2	Between APL and ECRB tendons at the dorsal aspect of the anatomical snuffbox. Used rarely, mostly to reach the radial styloid process and radial part of the joint, as well as for removal of the volar ganglion cysts or washout of the joint.	Radial artery, superficial sensory branch of the radial nerve
3-4	1 cm distally from the Lister`s tubercle, between the EPL and EDC tendons. Always used as a primary portal for visualization of the joint. Almost a complete panoramic view of the volar radiocarpal joint.	EPL and EDC tendons
4-5	Axis of the 4th metacarpal, between the EDC and EDM tendons. Portal for instrumentation and visualization of the TFCC.	EDC and EDM tendons
6R	At the radial aspect of the ECU tendon. Additional portal for instrumentation or visualization or reconstruction of the TFCC	Dorsal branch of the ulnar nerve
6U	At the ulnar aspect of the ECU tendon. Additional portal for instrumentation, visualization of the reposition of DRF fragments or for reconstruction of the ulnar part of the TFCC	Dorsal branch of the ulnar nerve
VR	2 cm long incision parallel to FCR tendon. Used for evaluation of the DRCL and volar part of the SLIL or fixation of the DRF fragments	Palmar cutaneous branch of the radial nerve, radial artery and volar cutaneous branch of the median nerve
VU	2 cm long incision parallel to ulnar margin of the flexor tendons. Used for the evaluation of the volar part of the LTIL and dorsal ulnar capsule.	Ulnar artery, ulnar nerve and distal palmar branch of the ulnar nerve

APL – m. abductor pollicis longus, *DRCL* – dorsal radio-carpal ligament, *ECRB* – m. extensor carpi radialis, *ECRL* – m. extensor carpi radialis longus, *ECU* – m. extensor carpi ulnaris, *EDC* – m. extensor digitorum communis, *EDM* – m. extensor digiti minimi, *EPL* – m. extensor pollicis longus, *FCR* – m. flexor carpi radialis, *DRF – distal radius fracture, LTIL – luno-triquetral interosseus ligament, SLIL - scapho-lunate interosseus ligament, TFCC – triangular fibrocartilage complex, VR – volar radial portal, VU – volar ulnar portal.*

Table 1.
Radiocarpal portals.

Portals	Localization and function	Structures at risk
MCR	Localized 1 cm distally from the 3-4 portal, between ECRB and EDC tendons. Visualization of the scapho-lunate, scapho-capitate and scapho-trapezium-trapezoideum joints.	ECRB and EDC tendons
MCU	Localized 1 cm distally from the 4-5 portal, on the axis of the 4th metacarpal bone, between EDC and EDM tendons. Visualization of the luno-triquetral, luno-capitate and. triquetro-hamate joints	EDC and EDM tendons
STT	Localized on the axis of the 2nd metacarpal bone, ulnary from the EPL tendon, at the level of the scapho-trapezio-trapezoidal joint. Used for instrumentation and resection of the distal scaphoid in STT arthritis	Radial artery, EPL, ECRB and ECRL tendons, terminal branches of the sensory branch of the radial nerve
STT-R	Localized radially to APL tendon at the same level as STT portal. Used for resection of the distal pole of the scaphoid	APL tendon, terminal branches of the sensory branch of the radial nerve

APL – m. abductor pollicis longus, *ECRB* – m. extensor carpi radialis, *ECRL* – m. extensor carpi radialis longus, *EDC* - m. extensor digitorum communis, *EDM* – m. extensor digiti minimi, *EPL* – m. extensor pollicis longus, *MCR – midcarpal radial portal, MCU – midcarpal ulnar portal, STT - scapho-trapezio-trapezoidal portal, STT-R - scapho-trapezio-trapezoidal radial portal.*

Table 2.
Midcarpal portals.

6. Structures which can be identified via dorsal radiocarpal portals

The images below (**Figures 7–18**) illustrate the anatomical structures of the wrist that can be identified from different standard portals.

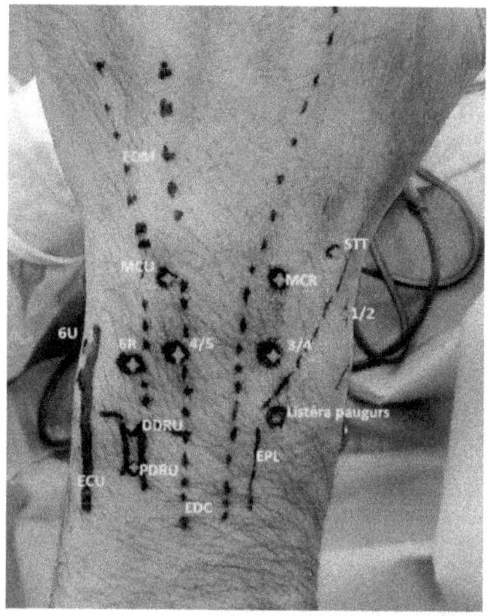

Figure 7.
Standard dorsal portals of the wrist. MCR – midcarpal radial portal, MCU – midcarpal ulnar portal, STT - scapho-trapezio-trapezoidal portal, DDRU – dorsal distal radioulnar joint portal, PDRU – proximal distal radioulnar joint portal, ECU – m. extensor carpi ulnaris, *EDC –* m. extensor digitorum communis, *EDM –* m. extensor digiti minimi, *EPL –* m. extensor pollicis longus, *1/2;, 3/4;, 4/5;, 6R;, 6 U – radiocarpal portals.*

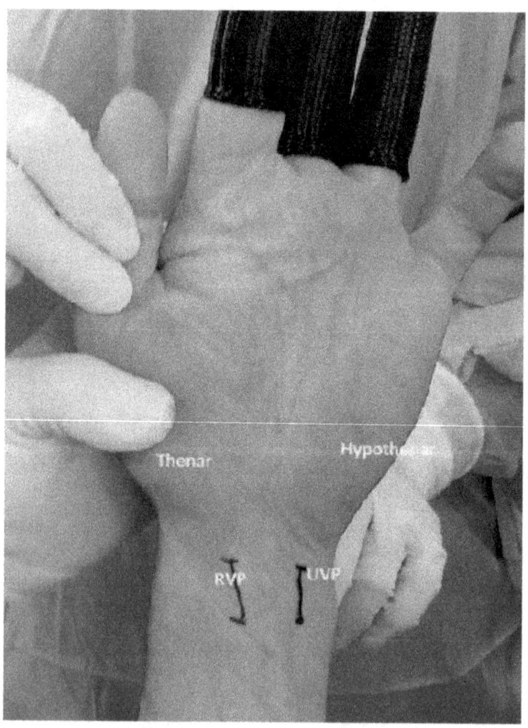

Figure 8.
Standard volar radiocarpal portals. RVP – radial volar portal, UVP – ulnar volar portal.

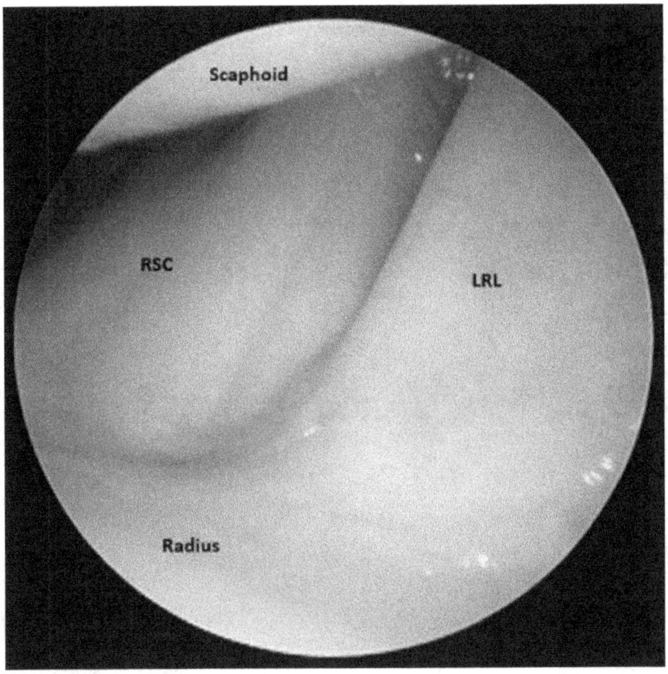

Figure 9.
Straight/radial view from 3 to 4 portal. SC – scaphoid, RSC – radioscaphocapitate ligament, LRL – long radiolunate ligament.

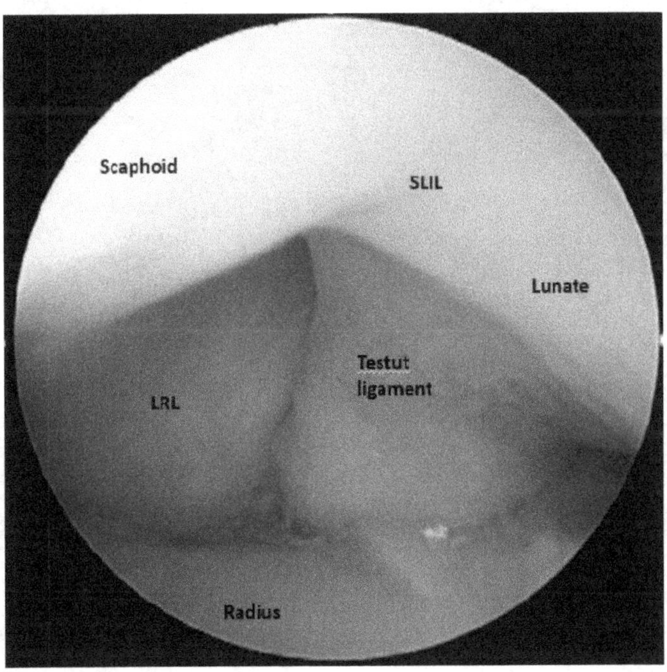

Figure 10.
Straight view from 3 to 4 portal. SC – scaphoid, RLT – radiolunotriquetral ligament, Lu – lunate, LRL – long radiolunat ligament, SLIL – scapholunate interosseous ligament.

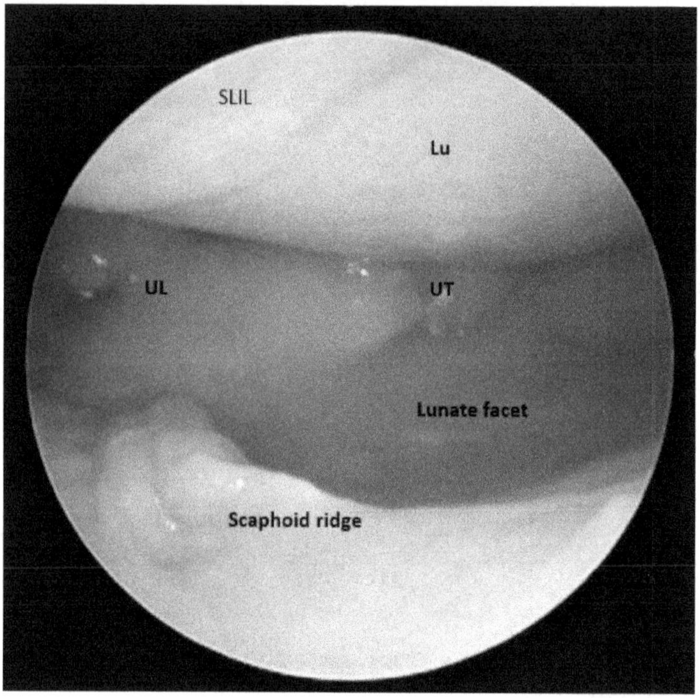

Figure 11.
Straight/ulnar view from 3 to 4 portal - Lu – lunate, SC – scaphoid, UL – ulnolunate ligament, UT – ulnotriquetral ligament, SLIL - scapholunate interosseous ligament.

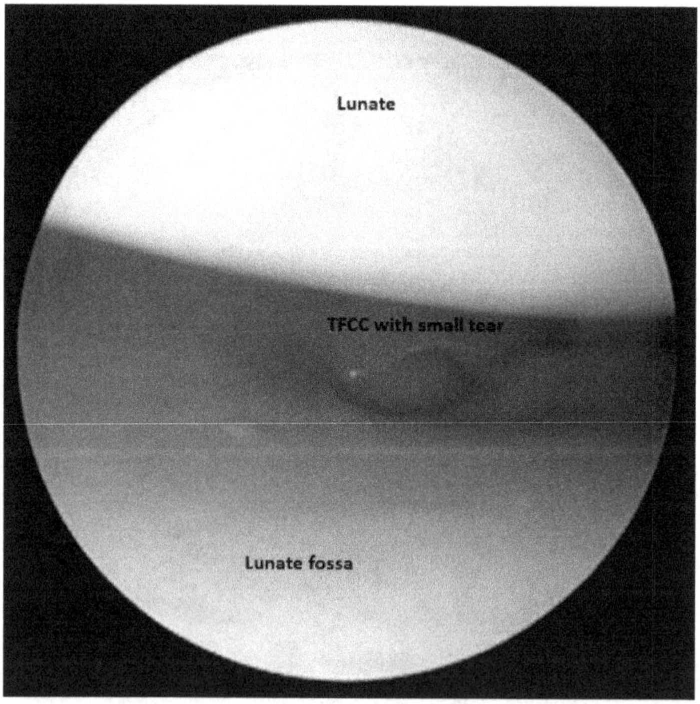

Figure 12.
Ulnar view from 3 to 4 portal over the scaphoid ridge, radial part of TFCC accessible.

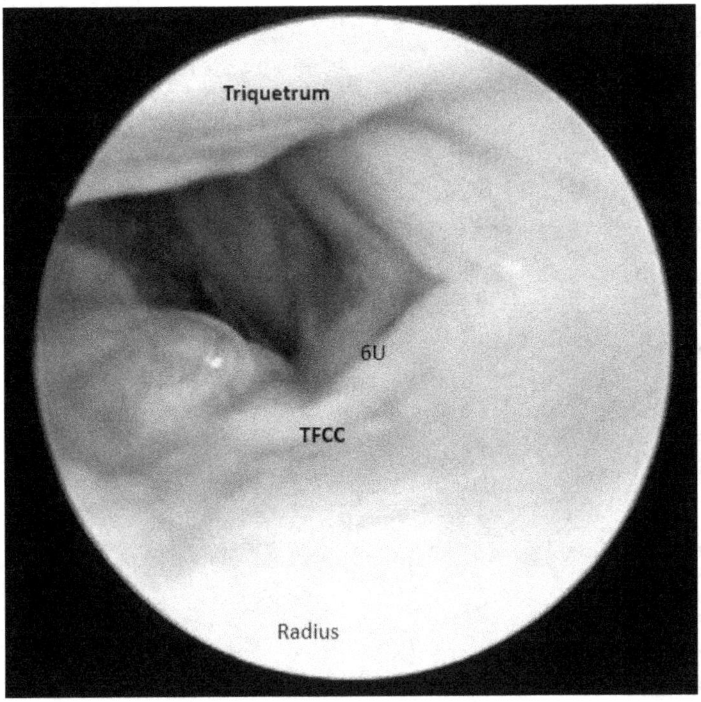

Figure 13.
Ulnar view from 3 to 4 portal – TFCC, proximal part of Triquetrum and ulnar recess. 6 U – possible location of 6 U portal.

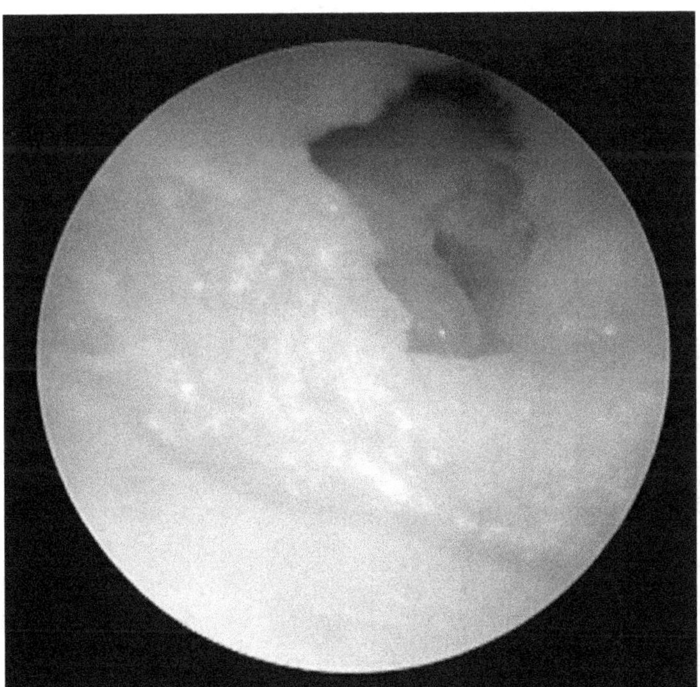

Figure 14.
Degenerative central tear of TFCC in "ulna +" variation.

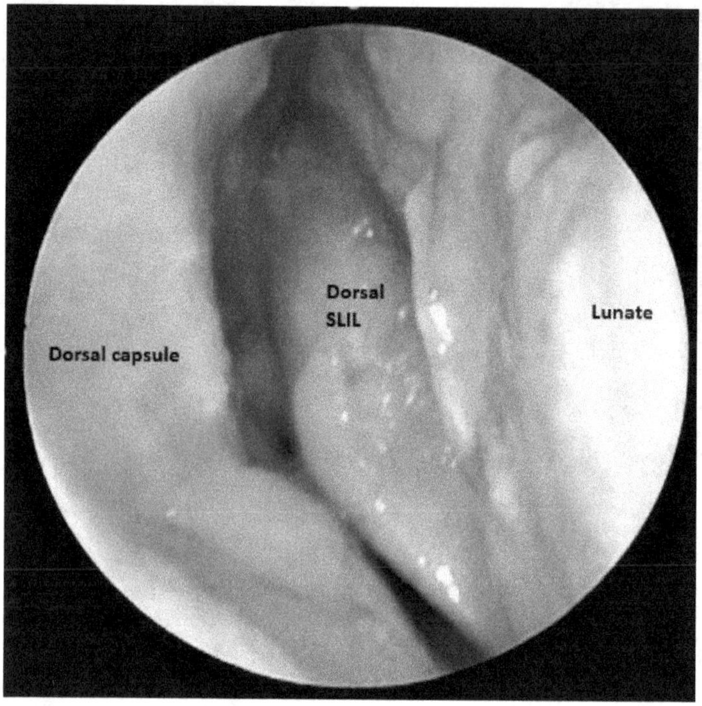

Figure 15.
Rupture of the dorsal SLIL. View from 6R portal. SLIL - scapholunate interosseous ligament.

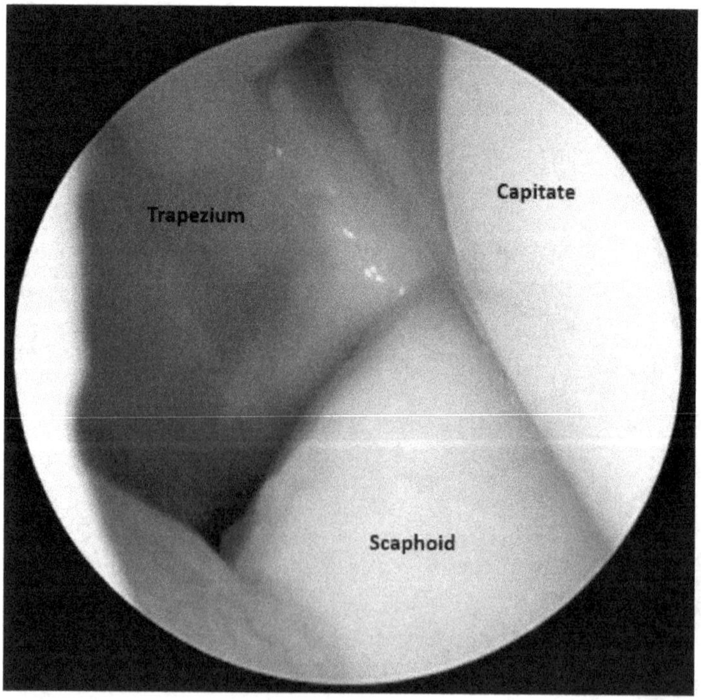

Figure 16.
View of STT joint from MCR portal. STT – Scaphotrapeziotrapezoidal joint, MCR – midcarpal radial portal.

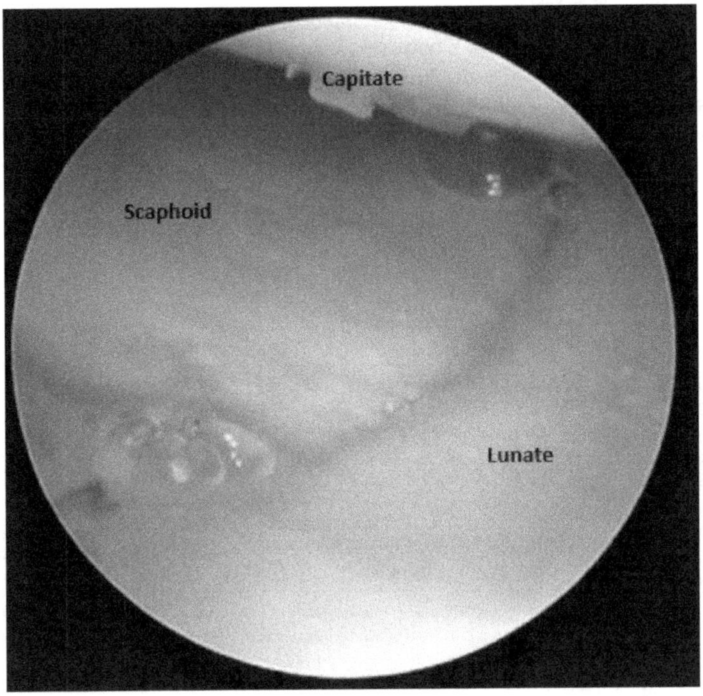

Figure 17.
View of scapholunate joint from MCR portal.

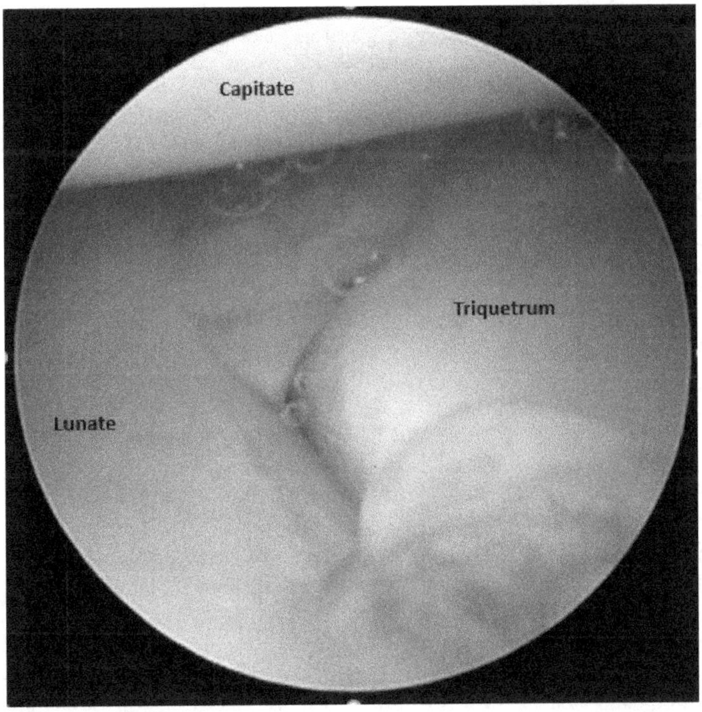

Figure 18.
View of lunotriquetral joint from MCR portal.

There are four described arthroscopy portals in the distal radio-ulnar joint. The anatomy of the DRUJ is complex because ulna articulates with both radius and proximal carpal row. Stability of the DRUJ is provided by TFCC with its volar and dorsal distal radioulnar ligaments, connecting at the fovea of the ulnar head. Even in normal wrists DRUJ is a quite narrow place for visualization and instrumentation, therefore it's suggested to use 1.9 mm scope, reduce the traction of the arm and introduce the scope in the DRUJ when the wrist is fully supinated [16–18]. Localization of the DRUJ portals, their functions and structures of the risk are described in **Table 3**.

Portals	Localization and function	Structures at risk
D-DRUJ	Localized 5-8 mm proximally from the 6R portal, between EDM and ECU tendons. Visualization of the ulnar head, undersurface of the TFCC, sigmoid notch, insertion of the volar and dorsal radioulnar ligaments in ulnar fovea	TFCC, articular cartilages of the sigmoid notch and ulnar head
P-DRUJ	Localized 1 cm proximal to the D-DRUJ portal, between EDM and ECU tendons. Visualization of the sigmoid notch, head of ulna and volar capsule,	TFCC, articular cartilages of the sigmoid notch and ulnar head
V-DRUJ	2 cm long incision parallel to ulnar margin of the flexor tendons – the same as for VU portal or can be created by pushing the blunt trocar from 6U portal towards the anterior ulnocarpal capsule between UL and UT ligaments, exiting ulnar to the flexor tendons, where small skin incision can be made. Visualization of the dorsal radioulnar ligament, possibility to proceed an arthroscopic wafer procedure when TFCC is intact	Ulnar artery, ulnar nerve and distal palmar branch of the ulnar nerve, flexor tendons
DF	Localized 1 cm proximally to the 6U portal between ECU tendon and ulnar styloid dorsally and FCU tendon volarly. Forearm must be fully supinated. Visualization of the ulnar fovea region, this portal is used as a dedicated working portal for fixation of the TFCC to the ulnar fovea in proximal TFCC lesions	Dorsal branch of the ulnar nerve, ECU and FCU tendons

ECU – m. extensor carpi ulnaris, *EDC* – m. extensor digitorum communis, *EDM* – m. extensor digiti minimi, *FCU* – m. flexor carpi ulnaris, *DF – dorsal foveal portal, D-DRUJ – dorsal distal radioulnar portal, P-DRUJ – proximal distal radioulnar portal, V-DRUJ – volar distal radioulnar portal, TFCC – triangular fibrocartilage complex, VU – volar ulnar portal.*

Table 3.
DRUJ portals.

7. Small joint arthroscopy portals

There mostly are two standard portals for STT, first carpometacarpal joint (CMC), metacarpophalangeal (MCP), proximal interphalangeal joint (PIP) and distal interphalangeal joint (DIP). Arthroscopical access to pisotriquetral (PT) [19, 20] and fourth or fifth CMC joints also are described while usefulness of these procedures is limited or not yet established [10].

First CMC portals are localized approximately 1 cm distally from STT portals on both sides of the first dorsal compartment. Accessory dorsal portal (the dorsal ulnar portal) can be used as necessary for better viewing the radial side of the joint by placing a trocar into the volar portal, across the CMC or the STT joint and out the dorsum of the hand (**Figure 19**) [21].

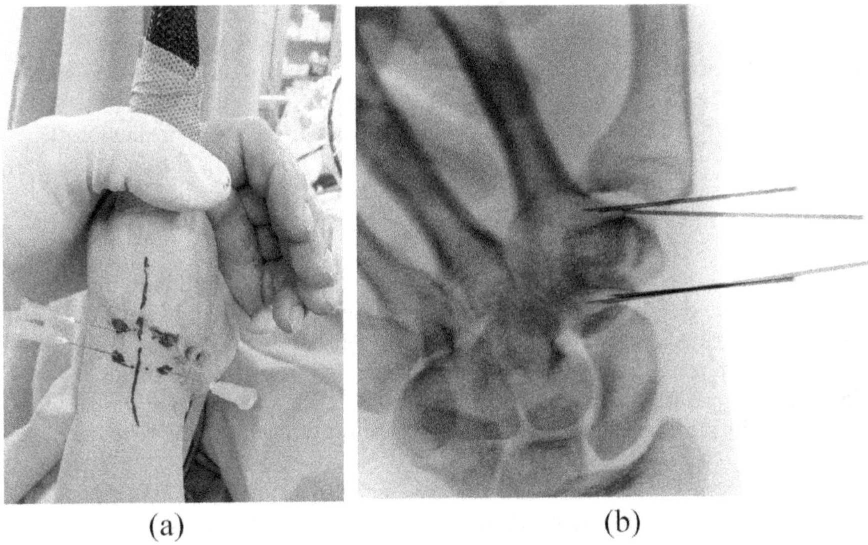

Figure 19.
CMC and STT portals. a – localization on the skin, b – verification with fluoroscope.

There are two portals – radial and ulnar for MCP, PIP and DIP joint arthroscopies, the naming of them is related to relationship with extensor tendons and they were established by Chen [2]. MCP joint arthroscopies can be successfully used in the rheumatoid conditions when synovectomy and thermal shrinkage can be performed [22–24], or in traumatic cases such as gamekeepers injury [10, 25], collateral ligament ruptures and reduction of the intraarticular metacarpal head fractures as well as in cases of complex MCP joint dislocations [26, 27]. Indications of the MCP joint arthroscopy include also chronic cases of instability, removal of the loose bodies as well as in cases of joint stiffness caused by intraarticular fibrosis or even cases of septic arthritis [18, 28].

Arthroscopy of the PIP and DIP joints has not been widely accepted because of the limited indications and technical limitations. The main indications are inflammatory or septic arthritis as well as removal of foreign bodies. Several authors suggest horizontal placement of the hand instead of using a traction tower, as it is important to be able to flex the joint freely [29, 30]. Cobb reported several cases of the DIP arthroscopic arthrodesis [10]. Since authors have no personal experience in finger joint arthroscopy, further discussion on this topic will not be continued in this chapter.

Many years the use of intra-articular fluid for wrist arthroscopy was considered essential. Francisco del Piñal *et al*. described a technique for dry arthroscopy in 2007 [5].

8. Arthroscopic treatment of ganglion cysts

Ganglion cysts are the most common benign soft-tissue tumors of the wrist. Dorsal cysts are more common than volar and surgical treatment is indicated for painful ganglions or large ones for cosmetic purposes. These ganglions usually appear in the dorsal scapholunate region which consists of three anatomical structures – the dorsal segment of scapholunate (SL) ligament, the dorsal intercarpal ligament (DICL) and the dorsal capsuloscapholunate septum (DCSS) [31]. The extra-articular part of the cyst can vary in size and location as well as in relation to dorsal ligaments. Surgical treatment of the so called "occult" ganglion cysts, who are small, intracapsular and can be very painful, is challenging by conventional methods. Arthroscopic treatment of such ganglion cysts is a method of a choice.

There are two different arthroscopical techniques for resection of the dorsal ganglia. The one is an access via radiocarpal joint and the other is through the ganglion and via the midcarpal joint [32, 33]. Some authors describe the necessity to combine radiocarpal and midcarpal portals, thus enabling a complete resection [34].

In the 2nd edition of Wrist Arthroscopy Techniques by C. Mathoulin different techniques of the dorsal ganglion artrhroscopic resections using only midcarpal portals are described and well-illustrated [35]. In our hands the midcarpal approach works perfect in most cases, except if ganglions are located very proximally (**Figure 20**). It provides also a good cosmetic result with only two almost invisible scars on the dorsal aspect of the wrist, which is important especially in younger females.

Aftertreatment – patients have to be encouraged to start early movements. In some cases, if patients have low pain malaise, short arm cast or wrist splint is recommended for first week after surgery. Recurrence rate for dorsal wrist ganglions treated arthroscopically is from 3 to 12% [34, 36–38]. Complications are rare and they are less common than in open surgeries. Most common complications reported are some stiffness (less than with open surgery), neurapraxia, extensor tenosynovitis and complex regional pain syndrom [39]. In meta-analysis presented by Head et al. in 2015, mean complication rate for arthroscopic surgical excision was 4%, and recurrence rate 6% [40]. Complication rate reported for open surgeries was 14% and recurrence rate 21%.

Volar wrist ganglions are less common than dorsal ganglions (about 20%) and they mainly occur in the radiocarpal joint, especially in the radial corner of the volar aspect. Volar ganglions in the midcarpal joint are very rare ant mostly they occur as a result of STT arthritis. The most common appearance is below FCR and FPL tendons. The technique of the arthroscopic volar ganglion resection was first described by P.C. Ho et al. in 2003 [41]. The origin and stalk of the ganglion usually locates between radioscaphocapitate (RSC) and long radiolunate (LRL) ligaments. It becomes visible

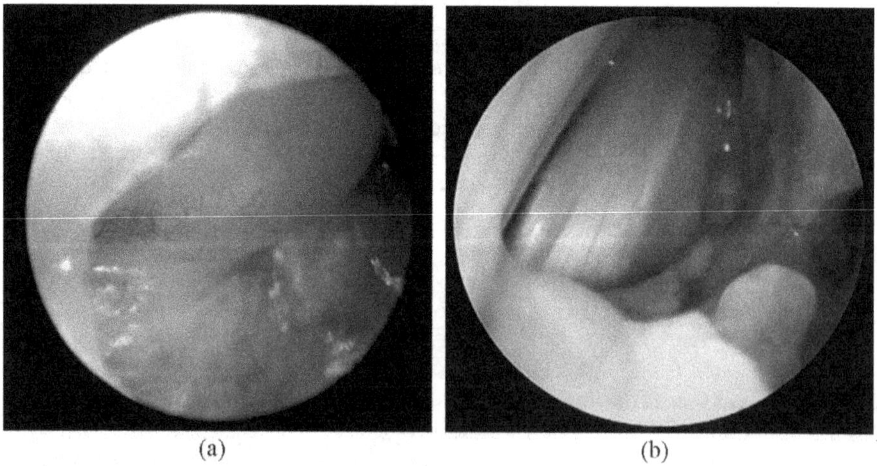

(a) (b)

Figure 20.
Dorsal ganglion, view from MCU portal, a – visualization of ganglion cyst after synovectomy, b – ganglion removed, clean extensor tendons visible.

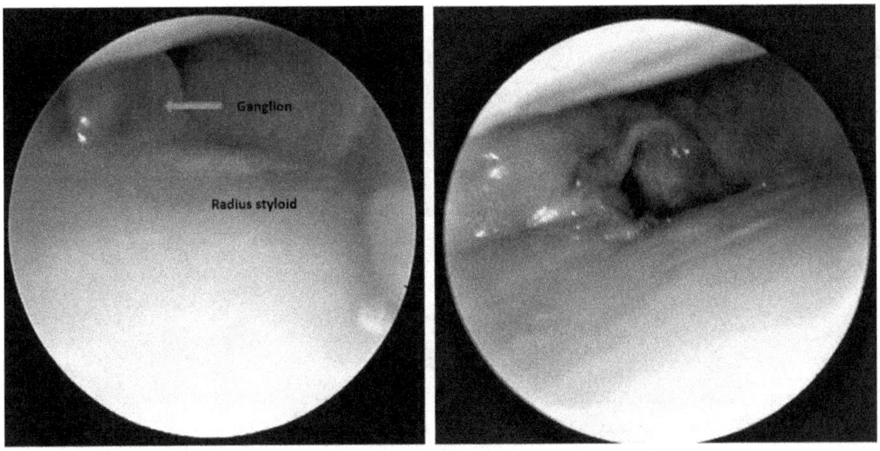

(a) (b)

Figure 21.
Volar ganglion of the wrist, a – ganglion detected in volar radial corner of the wrist, b – ganglion removed.

by gently pushing with finger on the ganglion while scope is positioned in 3-4 portal. Shaver is inserted in the 1-2 portal and ganglion has to be removed gently to avoid injuries of the neurovascular structures and flexor tendons (**Figure 21**) [39, 42].

Aftertreatment is similar to that one for dorsal ganglions. In a systemic review presented by Fernandes et al. in 2014 mean complication rate for arthroscopic volar ganglion surgeries was 6% and recurrence rate 6.9% [43]. Reported complications are increased cyst site volume during the immediate postoperative period, radial artery injuries, neuropraxia of the dorsal radial nerve, partial lesions of the median nerve [39, 43, 44].

9. Arthroscopic bone grafting of the intraosseus carpal ganglion cysts

Intraosseus ganglions (IOG) can affect all carpal bones but mostly they affect the lunate, capitate and scaphoid [45]. In patients who have dorsal wrist ganglions, the prevalence of IOGs is reported to be almost 50% [46]. Most of them are asymptomatic and can be found during the routine radiographs or CT scans because of the different complains. Surgical treatment is recommended for the symptomatic IOGs and include the curettage of the damaged bone and bone grafting.

Arthroscopically assisted treatment of the intraosseus ganglions of the lunate was first described by Ashwood and Bain in 2003 with the aim of reducing the morbidity that has been seen with open techniques [47].

Surgeries can be performed via routine radiocarpal or midcarpal portals – depending of the localization of the ganglion cyst. Usually the ganglion cyst cannot be visualized by arthroscope, because they still remain covered by the articular cartilage. The location of the drill hole has to be determined by the preoperative radiographic investigations. Once the ganglion is removed with the arthroscopic cutter and the hole is debrided with curette and shaver, it can be filled with bone grafts from the distal radius or iliac crest, which can be harvested via small incision and then delivered into the bone through a trocar under the arthroscopic visualization (**Figure 22**).

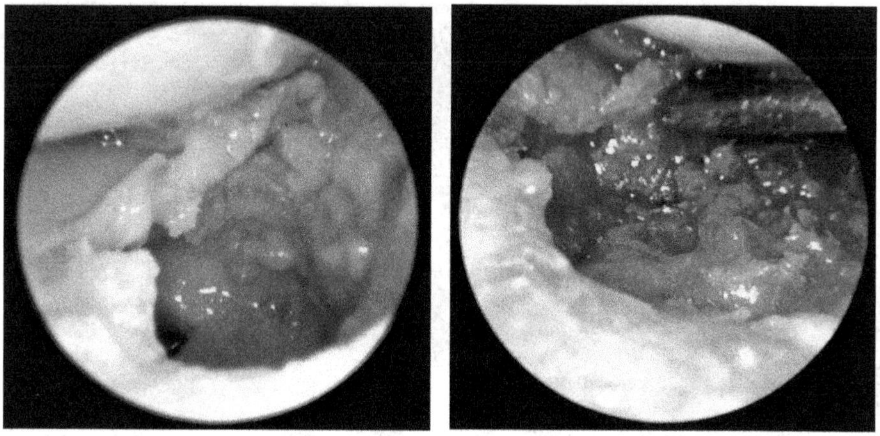

(a) (b)

Figure 22.
Arthroscopic debridement of the scaphoid cyst, a – defect of the bone after debridement, b – defect closed with autologous bone graft (ABG).

Aftetreatment includes immobilization for 10 to 14 days and patients are advised not to return to light duties until 6 weeks after the surgery, and heavy manual labor is avoided for a minimum of three months [18].

10. Arthroscopic treatment of the scapholunate ligament tears

Scapholunate interosseus ligament (SLIL) should be considered as a key stone of the intercarpal stability. It is U shaped in the sagittal plane and has three components – dorsal, volar and proximal [48]. The dorsal segment is the strongest portion with a tensile strength of 260 - 300 N and approximate thickness of 3 mm [32]. The proximal component is the weakest and avascular, The volar part has a tensile strength of 120- 150 N and approximate thickness of 1 mm. The palmar and dorsal segments work collectively to prevent rotational translation between scaphoid and lunate, whereas the intermediate segment has little role in stability [49–51].

Scapholunate stability is effectively ensured by a complex associating the dorsal and volar portions of the SLIL, the dorsal intercarpal (DIC) ligament, the dorsal radiocarpal (DRC) ligament, the radioscaphocapitate (RSC) ligament, the scaphotrapezial (ST) ligament, and the dorsal capsulo-scapholunate septum (DCSS). The integrity of these various stabilizers is taken into account while determining the arthroscopic classification of "predynamic" scapholunate instability [52].

When the SLIL is injured, the scaphoid tends to move into volarflexion, while the lunate, which is still fixed to the triquetrum, is forced, due to carpal kinematics, to follow the triquetrum into dorsal extension. The opposite happens with time when the LT interosseous ligament (LTIL) is injured. This static instability is often referred to radiologically as dorsal intercalated segment instability (DISI), following an SLIL injury and volar intercalated segment instability (VISI) following a LTIL injury [53].

The first arthroscopic classification of SLIL tears was presented in 1996 by Geissler et al. [54] using a 4-stage grading system (**Table 4**) (**Figures 23** and **24**).

In 2013 Messina et al. published the European Wrist Arthroscopy Society (EWAS) Classification of Scapholunate tears which was based on anatomical arthroscopic study and is an evolution of Geissler's classification (**Table 5**) [55].

Grade	Description
I	Attenuation or hemorrhage of interosseous ligament as seen from radiocarpal space. No incongruency of carpal alignment in mid-carpal space.
II	Attenuation or hemorrhage of interosseous ligament as seen from radiocarpal space. Incongruency or step-off of carpal space. There may be slight gap (less than width of probe) between carpal bones.
III	Incongruency or step-off of carpal alignment as seen from both radiocarpal and mid-carpal space. Probe may be passed through gap between carpal bones.
IV	Incongruency or step-off of carpal alignment as seen from both radiocarpal and mid-carpal space. There is gross instability with manipulation. 2.7-millimeter arthroscope may be passed through gap between carpal bones ("drive thru sign").

Table 4.
Geissler's arthroscopic classification of SLIL tears.

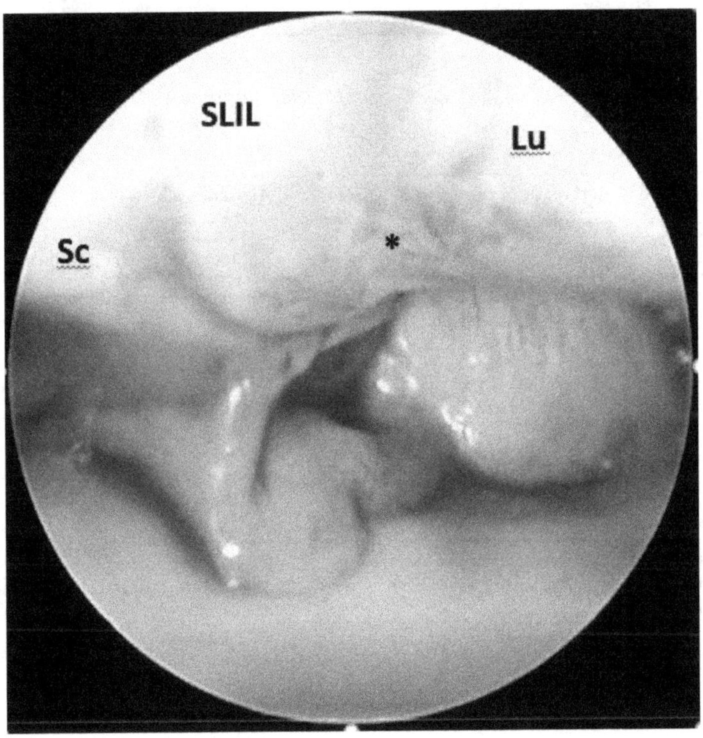

Figure 23.
Geissler grade II tear – attenuation an hemorrhage (*) of SLIL.

The existing classifications, however, describe the dynamic instability of the scapholunate joint but do not distinguish the site of ligament attenuation or tear, particularly in its volar portion.

The choice of the procedure for SLIL injuries in the absence of arthritis depends on the extent of the lesion, quality of the ligament remnants and reducibility of the joint [53].

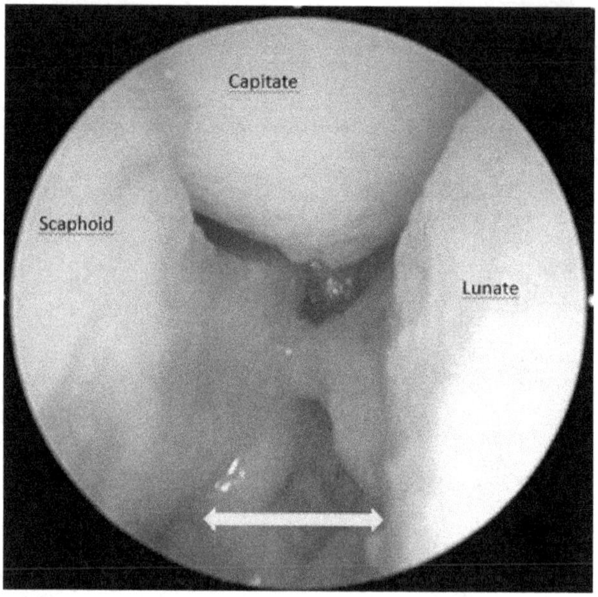

Figure 24.
Geissler grade IV tear – arrow shows gap between scaphoid and lunate. Scope easily passes between bones and slides into midcarpal joint.

Arthroscopic stage (EWAS)	Arthroscopic testing of SLIOL from MC joint	AP findings
I	No passage of the probe	Not found in cadaver specimens
II lesion of membranous SLIL	Passage of the tip of the probe in the SL space without widening (stable)	Lesion of proximal/membranous part of SLIL
III A partial lesion involving the volar SLIL	Volar widening on dynamic testing from MC joint (anterior laxity)	Lesion of anterior and proximal part of SLIL with or without lesion of RSC- LRL
III B partial lesion involving the dorsal SLIL	Dorsal SL widening on dynamic testing (posterior laxity)	Lesion of proximal and posterior part of SLIL with partial lesion of DIC
III C complete SLIL tear, joint is reducible	Complete widening of SL space on dynamic testing, reducible with removal of probe	Complete lesion of SLIL (anterior, proximal, posterior), complete lesion of one extrinsic ligament (DIC lesion or RSC/ LRL)
IV complete SLILwith SL gap	SL gap with passage of the arthroscope from MC to RC joint No radiographic abnormalities	Complete lesion of SLIL (anterior, proximal, posterior), lesion of extrinsic ligaments (DIC, and RSC/ LRL)
V	Wide SL gap with passage of the arthroscope through SL joint Frequent X Ray abnormalities such as an increased SL gap, DISI deformity	Complete lesion of SLIL, DIC, LRL, RSC, involvement of one or more other ligaments (TH, ST, DRC)

SLIL: scapholunate interosseous ligament. MC: midcarpal. RC: radiocarpal. RSC: radio-scapho-capitate. LRL: long radiolunate. DIC: dorsal intercarpal ligament. SL: scapholunate. TH: triquetro-hamate. ST: scaphotrapezial. DRC: dorso radiocarpal. DISI: dorsal intercalated segmental instability.

Table 5.
Arthroscopic EWAS (European Wrist Arthroscopy Society) Classification and corresponding anatomo-pathological (AP) findings in cadaver specimens.

Stage	1	2	3	4	5	6	7
Is the dorsal SL ligament intact?	YES	NO	NO	NO	NO	NO	NO
If repaired, has it good chances of healing?	YES	YES	NO	NO	NO	NO	NO
Is the radioscaphoid angle normal?	YES	YES	YES	NO	NO	NO	NO
Is the lunate uncovering index normal?	YES	YES	YES	YES	NO	NO	NO
Is the misalignment easily reducible?	YES	YES	YES	YES	YES	NO	NO
Are the joint cartilages normal all over the wrist?	YES	YES	YES	YES	YES	YES	NO

Table 6.
Six questions by Marc Garsia-Elias.

Garcia-Elias et al. [56] developed a set of 6 questions that provide a useful framework for developing stage-based treatment algorithms. By answering these questions in terms of yes or no, each case can be placed into one of seven categories (**Table 6**). As expected, the increasing number of negative answers indicates a progression of the dysfunction from minimal (Stage 1) to maximal (Stage 7). In general, all instabilities from the same stage will be treated similarly.

Detailed description of indications and treatment methods depending on the time after injury, the stage of SLIL disruption and stability or instability of the carpus is presented in the report of the IFSSH Committee On Carpal Instability in 2016 (part 2: Management of scapho-lunate dissociation [57].

Since this book is oriented to the arthroscopic methods of treatment further discussion on open surgical procedures will not be proceeded.

In acute injuries, arthroscopy can be used to determine the extent of scapholunate interosseous ligament injury. Partial tears may be treated by percutaneous pinning of the scaphoid and lunate, thus allowing for the possibility of primary healing or fibrosis.

Predynamic or occult SL injury results from an incomplete tear of the SL ligament. In selected cases with reducible scapholunate instability (Garcia-Elias stages 2, 3 and 4) where the ligament is partially (**Figure 25**) or completely ruptured, and where the scaphoid is well aligned or can be reduced, Mathoulin et al. proposed the arthroscopic dorsal capsuloplasty, which may be combined with K-wire fixation of the scapholunate and the scaphocapitate joints [58, 59].

This technique can be performed only in cases when ligament stumps remain attached to the scaphoid and lunate. This technique includes synovectomy of midcarpal and radiocarpal joints. Then the scope is introduced into the 6R portal to inspect the gap between the lunate and the dorsal capsule (**Figure 26**).

An absorbable monofilament suture is passed through a needle. This needle is inserted through the skin via the 3–4 portal, then shifted slightly distally so as to cross the joint capsule (**Figure 27**).

The needle is located inside the joint through the scope and then pushed through the SLIL stump on the scaphoid side. The needle is oriented dorsal to volar and angled proximal to distal, allowing it to enter the midcarpal joint (**Figure 28**). A second needle and suture are then inserted parallel to the first into the SLIL stump attached to the lunate. The scope is returned to the MCU portal. The two needles are located inside the midcarpal joint, after they have passed between the scaphoid and lunate. Both sutures are externalized via MCR portal with hemostat and the knot is tied outside the joint. Then the knot is pulled back into the midcarpal joint (**Figure 29**).

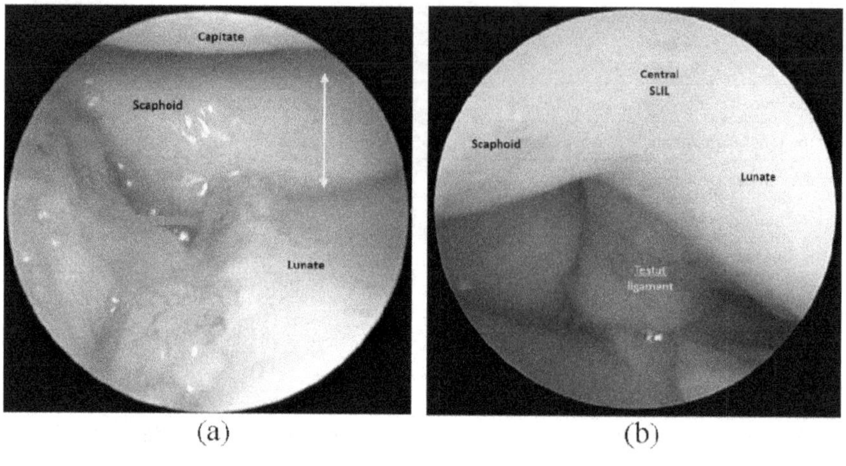

Figure 25.
Partial, reparable rupture of SLIL, a- view from MCU portal, yellow arrow shows the step off between articular surfaces od scaphoid and lunate, red arrow points detachment of SLIL from lunate, b- The same patient – normal SLIL in RC joint, view from 3 to 4 portal.

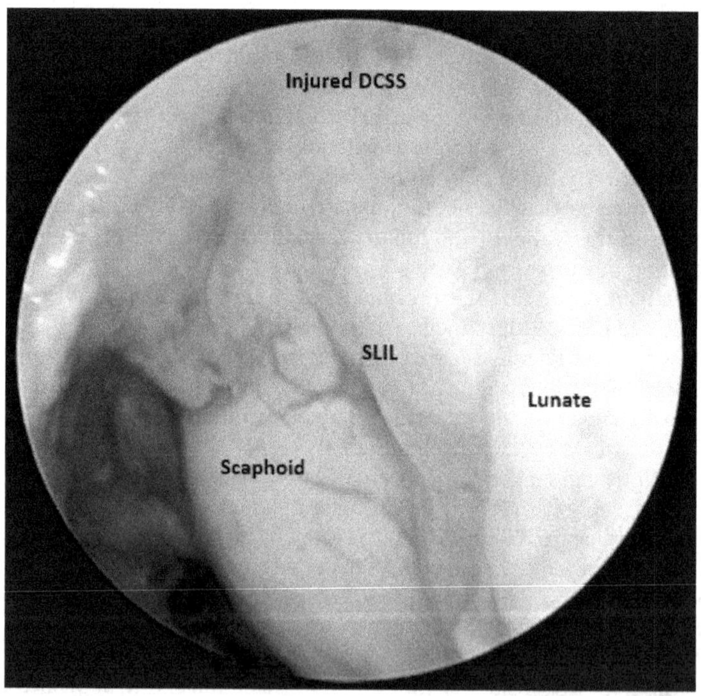

Figure 26.
View from 6R portal with detached dorsal capsule and injured dorsal capsuloligamentous scapholunate septum (DCSS).

At this point the traction of the wrist is released to reduce the gap between scaphoid and lunate. Transfixation of the scapholunate and scaphocapitate joints with K-wires can be performed if reduction is insufficient. The final knot is tied after the wrist is released from traction and positioned in slight extension [52].

DOI: http://dx.doi.org/10.5772/intechopen.99191

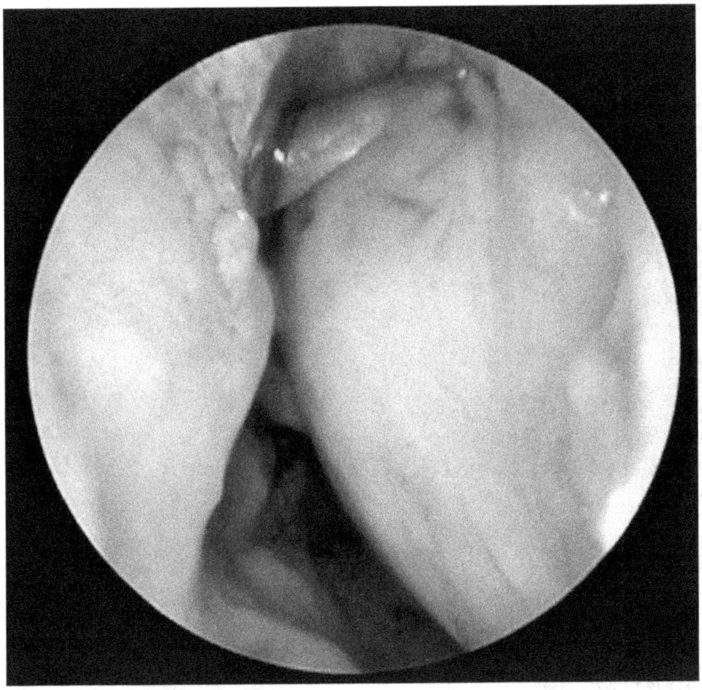

Figure 27.
Needle inserted via 3-4 portal and shifted distally to enter the midcarpal joint.

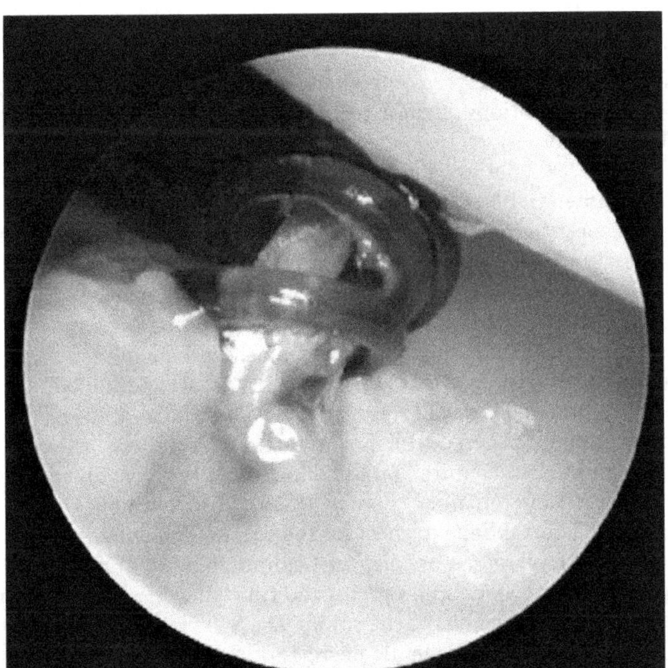

Figure 28.
View from the UMP - needle in the midcarpal joint and suture is knotted by twisting of the needle.

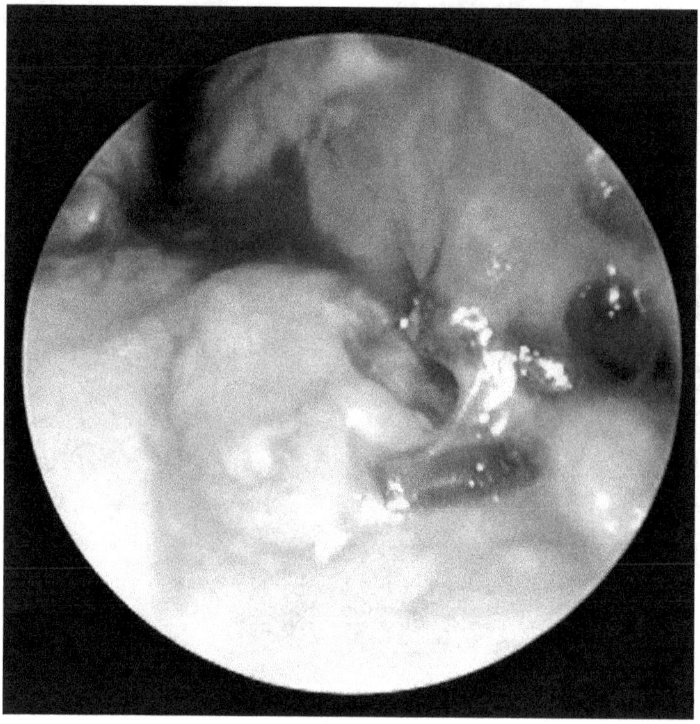

Figure 29.
The inner knot of both sutures at the level of SL joint.

After treatment includes 8 weeks of immobilization and an adequate rehabilitation.

There are several other, more complicated arthroscopic SLIL repair procedures described, but the indications of these techniques are limited to predynamic and dynamic SL instability.

P.C.Ho et al. in 2002 designed an arthroscopic assisted box reconstruction of scapholunate ligament with palmaris longus (PL) tendon graft [60]. It enables simultaneous reconstruction of the dorsal and palmar SL ligaments anatomically with the use tendon graft in a boxlike structure. With the assistance of arthroscopy and intraoperative imaging as a guide, a combined limited dorsal and volar incision exposed the dorsal and palmar SL interval without violating the wrist joint capsule. Bone tunnels of 2.4 mm are made on the proximal scaphoid and lunate. A palmaris longus tendon graft is delivered through the wrist capsule and the bone tunnels (**Figure 30**) to reduce and connect the two bones in a boxlike fashion.

Once the joint diastasis is reduced and any DISI malrotation corrected, the tendon graft is knotted and sutured on the dorsal surface of the SL joint extra-capsularly in a shoe-lacing manner (**Figure 31a,** and **b**). Additional suture anchors can be placed at the dorsal bone tunnels for the scaphoid and lunate for additional graft fixation. The RL pin is removed at the beginning of the third week. The cast is then changed to a thumb spica splint for an additional 2 weeks, at which time gentle wrist mobilization is allowed out of the splint. The SC pins are removed after 8 weeks. The potential risk of ischemic necrosis of the carpal bone is minimized by preservation of the scaphoid blood supply [52, 60].

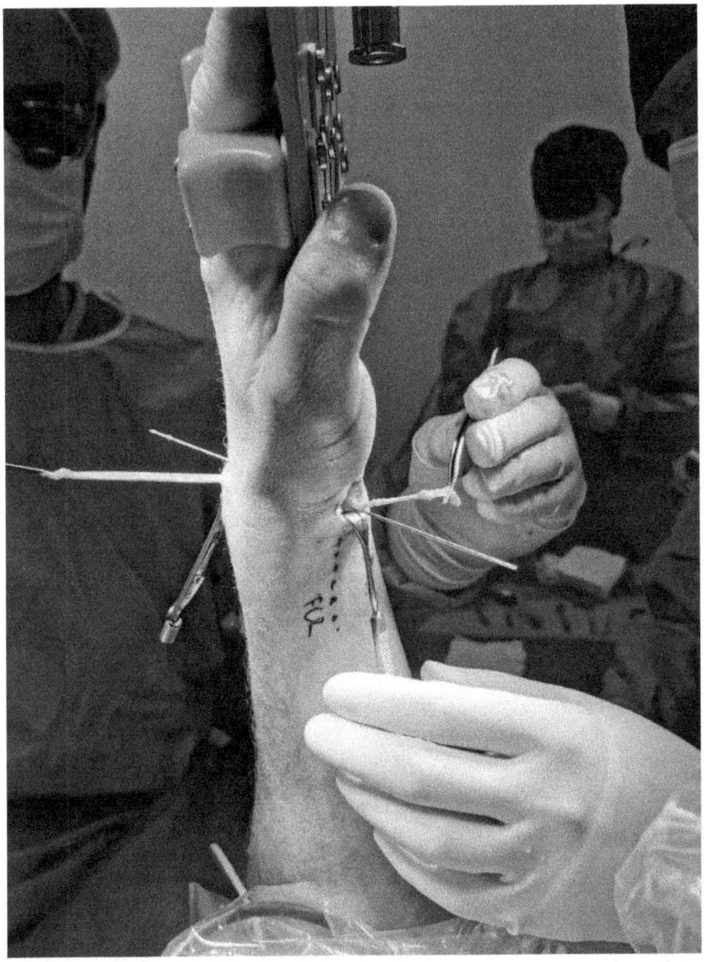

Figure 30.
A palmaris longus tendon graft deliverd through the lunate and both capsules.

Corella et al. in 2011 published a novel all arthroscopic technique for scapholunate instability [61]. They developed the BTT ligamentoplasty - Bone (base of second metacarpal bone), Tendon (flexor carpi radialis graft), Tenodesis (in the scaphoid and lunate). This technique aims to reproduce the tripple tenodesis technique proposed by Garcia-Elias et al. in 2006 [56], but with an arthroscopic approach reducing soft tissue trauma. It reconstructs both the dorsal and volar portion of the SL ligament with a 3-mm graft of the FCR tendon, which is fixed to the scaphoid and lunate tunnels with interference screws. Graft resistance and strength can be increased with the use of a 1.3 mm SutureTape. The SutureTape is passed and fixed with the screws along with the tendon graft. After the graft is fixed to the scaphoid bone with the anchor, the volar portion of the SutureTape that exits from the lunate tunnel is sutured to the portion that exits from the scaphoid tunnel. It's recommended to start early postoperative wrist mobilization with this technique – dart-throwing motion from the 3rd week and flexion/extension movements from the 5th week after surgery [62].

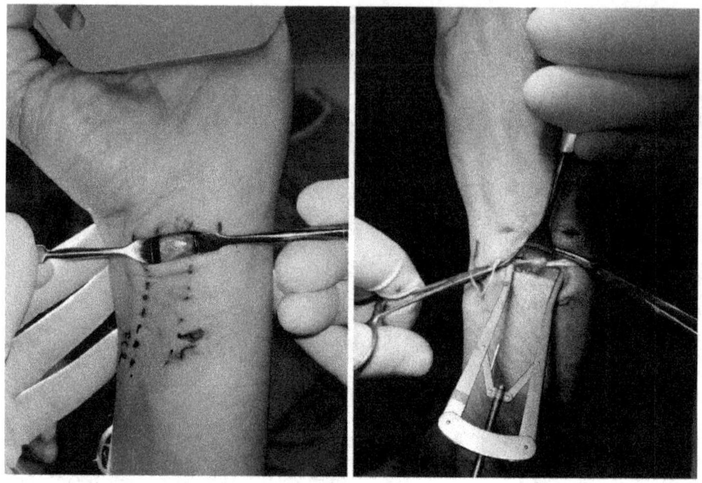

(a) (b)

Figure 31.
Tightened tendon graft, view from volar (a) and dorsla (b) side.

11. Arthroscopy in the treatment of articular distal radius fractures (DRF)

Hand surgeons began applying wrist arthroscopy to the surgical treatment of the DRF in the late 90's of the last century. Arthroscopic reduction of intraarticular fragments, as opposed to conventional methods, may improve outcomes regardless of the method of fixation, volar locking plates or external fixator and K-wires [63–69]. Failure to reduce intra-articular fractures of the distal radius predisposes to pain, restricted movement and degenerative arthritis. The functional results of treatment for articular DRF's are determined by alignment of fragments of extraarticular fracture, by restoring bone shape, length and fold, anatomical reposition of joint surface, prevention of additional damage to soft tissue, as well as potential post-operative complications [70–74]. Fluoroscopy alone provides an image that has poorer resolution than that of the magnified camera used for direct arthroscopic visualization, whereas even a small degree of displacement is obvious arthroscopically [75]. It is obvious that optical visualization of the articular space gives an opportunity to detect a greater number of soft tissue lesions more often, than only fluoroscopic and clinical evaluation or surgeon's mistrust about the possibilities of such injuries [76]. Wrist arthroscopy is currently recommended for the treatment of any articular distal radius fracture (**Figure 32a,** and **b**), but some possible contraindications have been identified. As one of these are elderly and low-active patients, open fractures and polytrauma patients, particularly at the early stage of treatment, since this procedure can significantly increase the duration of surgery. As another major objection to the use of arthroscopic treatment, is a lack of technical equipment and surgeon's experience [64, 77, 78].

There are two controversial fracture fixation techniques. In cases of volar plating, standard flexor carpi radialis approach can be used. Once the fracture is preliminarily fixed with the volar locking plate (VLP) (**Figure 33**), the wrist joint is assessed arthroscopically using the 3-4 and 4-5, 6R, 6 U or 1-2 portals to remove blood clots, small articular fragments or to make an additional reposition and

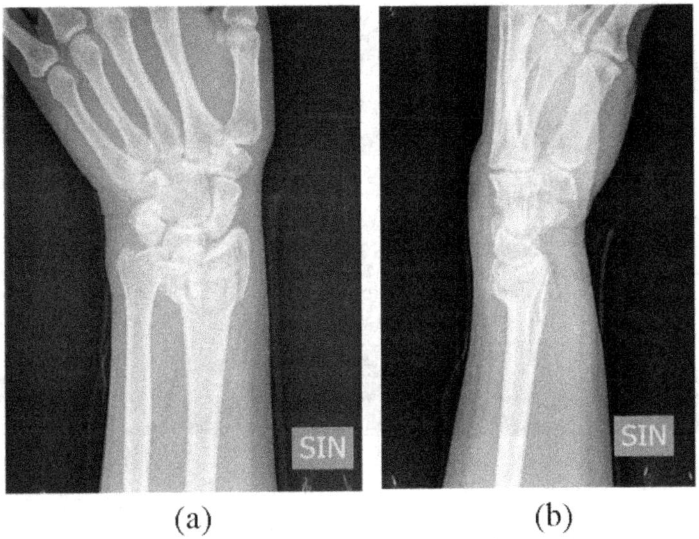

Figure 32.
Dorsally displaced articular fracture of the distal radius.

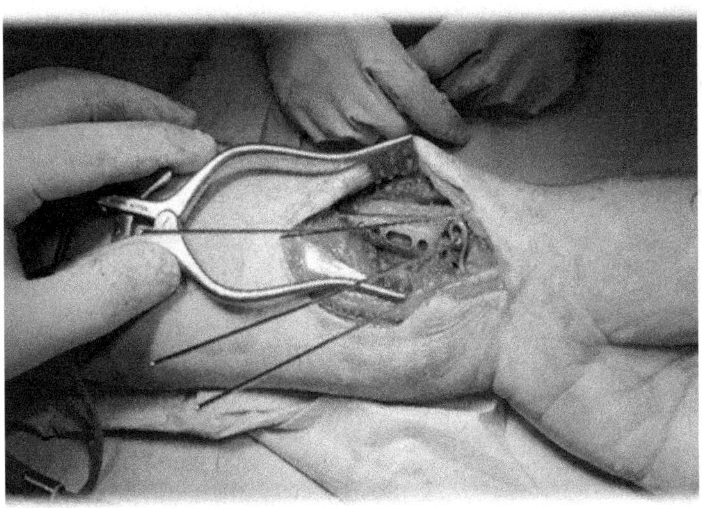

Figure 33.
Preliminary fixation of the volar plate before arthroscopic part of the surgery.

fixation with K-wires. Distal screws can be inserted only after arthroscopic inspection of the radiocarpal joint and a fluoroscopic confirmation of the correct position for the screws (**Figures 34a, b** and **35a, b**).

After treatment includes 2 weeks in short plaster cast and early mobilization can be allowed as volar locking plate provides rigid fixation.

In cases of comminuted fractures when fixation with VLP is impossible, arthroscopically assisted fracture reposition and fixation with K-wires and external fixator is recommended (**Figures 36a–c** and **37a, b**). This surgery is commenced with a primary closed reduction and fixation with several K-wires, under

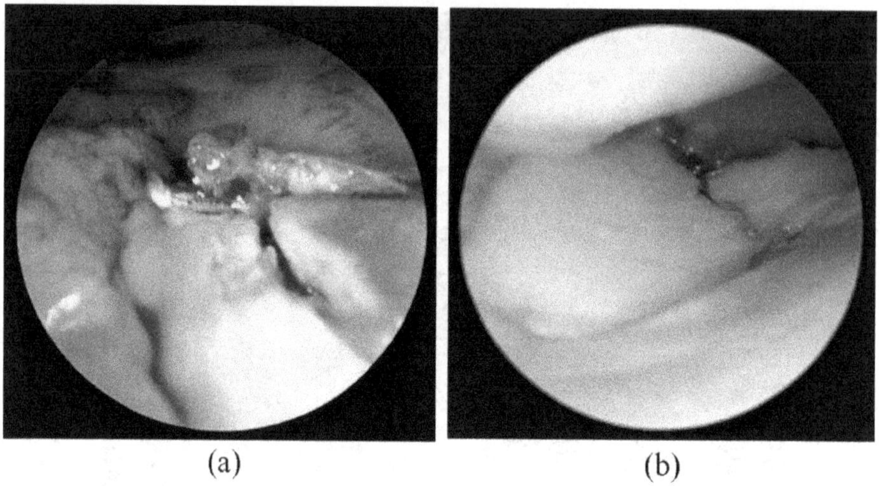

Figure 34.
Additional fragment reposition and fixation.

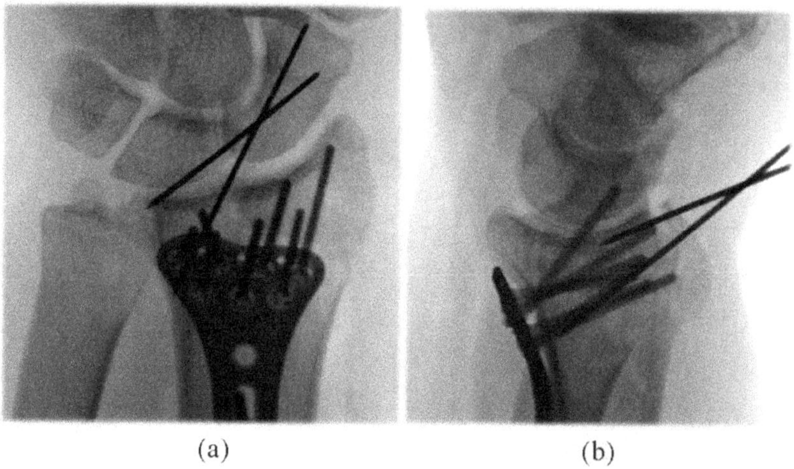

Figure 35.
Final fluoroscopic image of the surgery.

fluoroscopic guidance. Following fixation in a traction tower, the articular surfaces are assessed using the standard arthroscopic technique. Further fragment reductions are performed, if required, using a probe or K-wires as joysticks through elongated 3-4, 4-5, 1-2 and in some cases, volar portals. Additional K-wire fixation is used as required. Once satisfactory reposition is achieved, the bridging external fixator can be applied. The external fixator is removed 4 weeks after surgery. K-wires are usually removed between 4 and 6 weeks after surgery.

The associated soft tissue lesions can be found from 30 to 66% of DRFs, but not all of them require surgical treatment [79–81]. In cases of associated soft tissue injuries like SLIL and LTIL acute ruptures or TFCC lesions, arthroscopically guided, debridement of the injured ligaments or TFCC is advised, as well as trans-articular

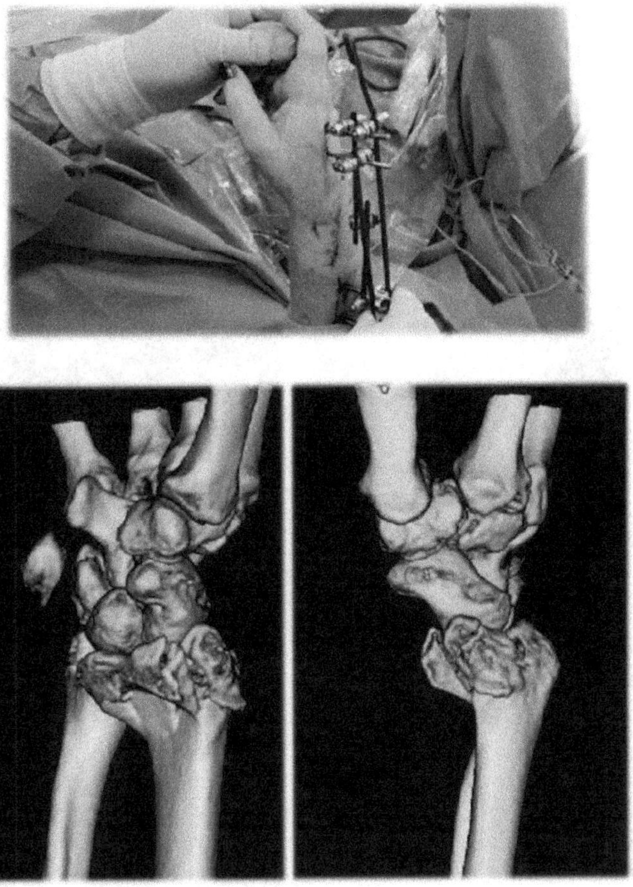

(a) (b)

Figure 36.
Position of the monolateral external fixator over the wrist joint. a and b - Comminuted volar, distal, articular fracture of the radius.

fixation of the scapholunate and/or lunotriquetral joints with K-wires, or application of peripheral sutures for TFCC tears.

Authors have never experienced severe complications as tendon ruptures or infection but we have found that the more extensive use of K-wires in reduction and/or fixation during external fixation and K-wire fixation is more likely to result in nerve damage. Furthermore, the complication of subsequent loss of position of fragments also occurred in patients treated with K-wires and external fixator [81].

In last two decades several minimally invasive plate osteosynthesis (MIPO) techniques using volar locking plates on DRF are presented [82–84]. In cases of comminuted articular DRF's this technique can be supplemented with an arthroscopic visualization. After all, two major lines of MIPO techniques evolved and got new promoters: single longitudinal incision and double transverse incision, leading to the creation of new special volar plates setups adapted to each technique's pitfalls and benefits [85, 86]. Unfortunately authors do not have any personal experience with MIPO technique.

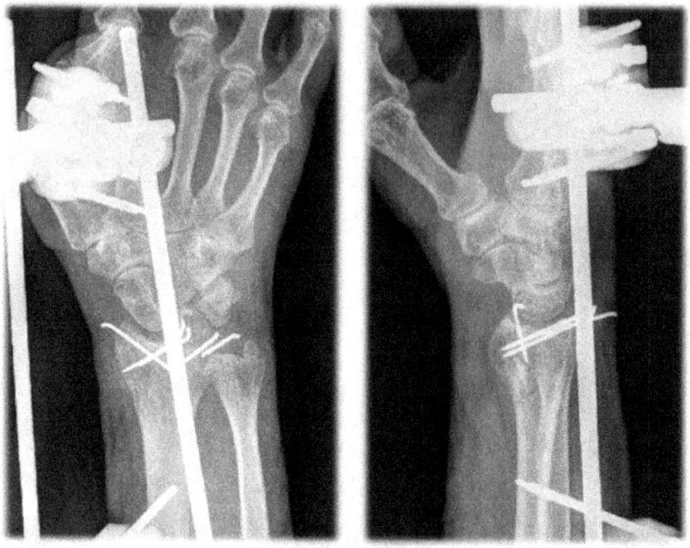

(a) (b)

Figure 37.
Final x-ray after the application of external fixation and K-wires.

12. Arthroscopic arthrolysis

Arthroscopic wrist arthrolysis is indicated in situations of posttraumatic wrist rigidity. It can be performed in radiocarpal joint, midcarpal joint and even in DRUJ. The most frequent clinical pathological conditions are adhesive capsulitis and arthrofibrosis of the wrist. Capsulitis is due to ligament and/or capsule contractures, and wrist arthrofibrosis is usually due to osseous band fibrosis of the radius and/or first row carpal bone(s) from a radius articular fracture. These two conditions can be associated in the same case [87]. The technique of the arthroscopic arthrolysis of the wrist was presented by R. Luchetti et al. in 2006. In radiocarpal joint almost all possible portals, including volar portals must be used during this surgery. It could be difficult to orient in the joint and to triangulate instruments because of the fibrotic adhesions inside the joint. Once they are removed (**Figure 38a,** and **b**), but

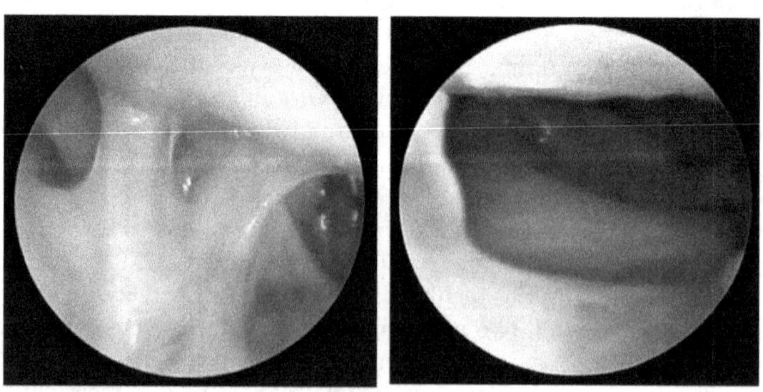

(a) (b)

Figure 38.
Intraarticular adhesions (a) after removal (b).

the range of motion (ROM) is still insufficient, resection of the volar and dorsal radiocarpal ligaments is recommended. This can be done with miniblade, laser or radiofrequency cutter. It's also recommended to leave dorsal and volar ulnar ligaments intact. The midcarpal joint also has to be inspected in the same manner but ligament resection is not recommended. Wrist stiffness is much more rarely attributable to the midcarpal joint, and any fibrosis in this joint is rarely significant [88]. Arthroscopic arthrolysis of the DRUJ is technically very challenging, because visualization of this joint is already problematic in the normal conditions and requires good arthroscopic skills of the surgeon. But once it can be done, patients achieve an improvement of prono/supination movements. If the arthroscopic arthrolysis of the DRUJ cannot be performed because of the technical difficulties it can be conversed to open surgery. Rehabilitation is started immediately after the surgery.

Complications – in cases when osteochondral lesions of various severity are present during the procedure of the arthrolysis, it is quite common for fibrotic bridges to reform in a few months and provoke partial or complete radiocarpal ankylosis. The use of articular instruments and motorized instruments can cause unwanted osteoarticular lesions (chondral scuffing, ligament injuries etc.) that can manifest themselves postoperatively in the form of pain or wrist instability [87, 89].

13. Arthroscopic treatment of scaphoid fractures

The incidence of acute scaphoid fractures is about 70% of all carpal fractures and 11% of all wrist fractures. Young men in the 2nd and 3rd decade of life are the main target population of this injury. Two-thirds of all scaphoid fractures occur in the waist area and 60 – 85% are non-dislocated fractures. Distal third is affected in 25% of cases, but proximal third in 5-10% of fractures [90]. Two morphological bone types are identified: type I or full scaphoids and type II or slender scaphoids. Type I possess more robust internal vascular network than type II scaphoids which may prove to be related to development of nonunion, avascular necrosis or Preiser disease [91]. Indications for surgical treatment are: displacement greater than 1 mm, commination, open fracture, scaphoid fracture with perilunate dislocation, associated carpal instability – scapholunate angle greater than 60°, radiolunate angle greater than 15°, as well as angulation of the scaphoid – intrascaphoid angle greater than 35° and height to length ratio greater than 0.65 [92].

In cases when volar approach with retrograde screw insertion is chosen, arthroscopic treatment of scaphoid fracture has to be started with a small, anterior volar incision through which a 1-mm K-wire is inserted into the scaphoid under fluoroscopy control. This step can be the most difficult one of the entire procedure. If a rolled-up drape is placed under the wrist to extend it to 60°, the K-wire will be about 45° to horizontal. The K-wire is angled from the distal tubercle toward the middle of the carpus. The second stage includes an arthroscopic evaluation when the wrist is placed in vertical traction. Usually midcarpal portals (MCU) are used to visualize the fracture site. If the additional reposition is required, the K-wire can be removed from the proximal pole and manual maneuvers as well as hook probe can be used to achieve the correct position. Then cannulated headless compression screw can be inserted when wrist is released from traction. After the compression of the fracture fragments it's recommended to make a final arthroscopic evaluation of the midcarpal and radiocarpal joints, to verify the compression and length of the screw [93, 94]. The alternative is a dorsal approach. It provides direct unobstructed access to the proximal scaphoid pole permitting the placement of a central axis guide-wire for antegrade screw implantation [95, 96].

Active wrist motion exercises are initiated immediately or within 10 days after surgery. Strengthening exercises were delayed until healing was well established on X-rays of the scaphoid, usually 3 to 4 months after surgery [93, 97].

14. Arthroscopic management of scaphoid nonunion

Acute scaphoid fractures are often missed and patients return with pain when delayed union or nonunion manifests (**Figure 39a**).

The natural history of untreated scaphoid nonunions is progression to carpal collapse resulting in wrist arthritis and chronic painful disability [98, 99]. Osteoarthritis at the scaphoid-radial styloid joint is significantly associated with dorsiflexed intercalated segment instability (DISI) deformity. An overall incidence of DISI deformity of the wrist is about 56%, and the frequency of DISI pattern increased with longer duration of non-union [100]. Arthroscopic management of scaphoid nonunions without severe deformities or arthritis is effective [101]. This simplifies postoperative recovery, reduces complications, and preserves the wrist's capsule-ligament complex—and, thus, the scaphoid's precarious vascularization [102]. Arthroscopic management of scaphoid nonunion is based on the following ideas: that scaphoid vascularity can be preserved because of the minimally invasive nature of arthroscopic surgeries; and that direct visualization with magnification can facilitate accurate debridement of the nonunion site, identify fibrous union and punctate bleeding from fracture site and aid perfect reduction [103].

Principles of the arthroscopic treatment of the scaphoid nonunions are the same as with other surgical techniques: excision of pseudrthrosis, correction of humpback deformity, restoration of the length of the bone, bone grafting and a stable fixation.

Surgical technique includes inspection of the radiocarpal joint via standard portals, synovectomy and arthroscopically guided styloidectomy, if necessary.

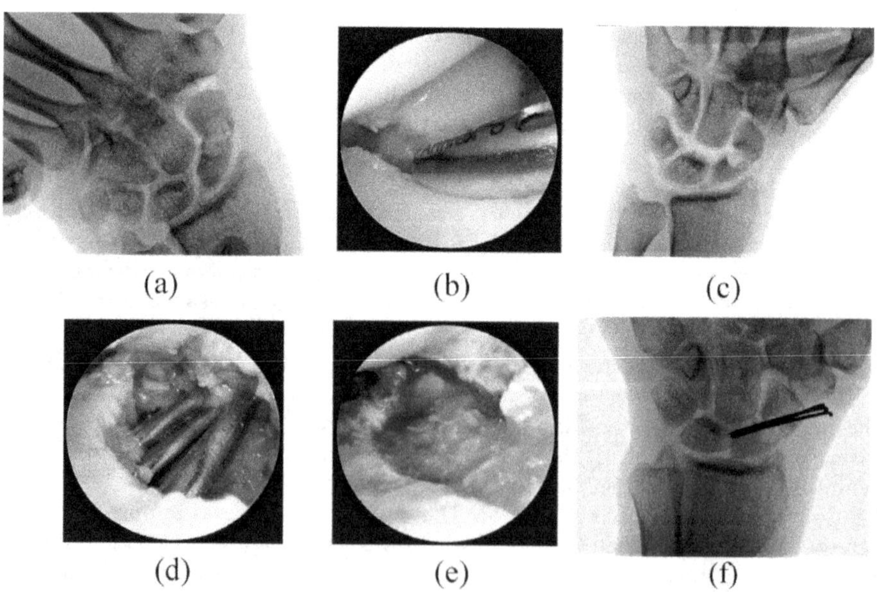

Figure 39.
(a) X-ray of scaphoid nonunion, (b) shaver in the nonunion site, (c) defect of the scaphoid after removal of debris, (d) fixation of the scaphoid with K-wires, (e) defect filled with bone graft, (f) final x-ray after the surgery.

Arthroscopic treatment of the nonunion is performed via midcarpal portals. The scope is inserted in MCU portal and instruments in MCR, accessory portal (close to the nonunion) or STT portal. If a frank bony defect is encountered, it is curetted with a fine-angled curette or motorized shaver (**Figure 39b**), until all fibrotic tissue and sclerotic bone are removed.

If the tourniquet is used, at this point it has to be released, to assess the vascularity of the bones. Any humpback and DISI deformity should be identified and corrected. Once the deformity of the scaphoid is corrected, fragments have to be transfixed with K-wires from the tubercle of the scaphoid to the proximal pole for provisional scaphoid fixation (**Figure 39c** and **d**).

This process is controlled under arthroscopic and fluoroscopic guidance. The bone graft is taken from the ipsilateral distal radius or iliac crest depending on the amount needed for filling the defect. The bone graft is inserted into a trocar and then the end of the trocar is placed at the nonunion site. The graft is pushed into the trocar with a blunt guide wire until the nonunion site is filled (**Figure 39e** and **f**).

Some surgeons recommend to add fibrin glue to protect the graft but others claim that once the scaphoid is fixed and the traction released, the capitate's native anatomical position will provide sufficient graft stabilization [102, 104]. The fragments are stabilized with screw(s) and/or K-wires. Recorded union rate with this procedure is 86 – 100% [105–107]. Arthroscopically treated patients achieve faster healing despite shorter time to surgery in the percutaneous group. Local bone grafting is considered as the main reason for this outcome [108].

15. Arthroscopic treatment of thumb carpometacarpal (CMC) osteoarthritis

Thumb CMC joint pain, instability and progressive arthritis is a common problem affecting many patients, especially middle-aged women. Once present, the symptoms of thumb CMC osteoarthritis are typically progressive and may lead to significant functional disability. There are two classifications for thumb CMC osteoarthritis: Eaton – Litter classification which is based on radiological changes [109] (**Table 7**) and arthroscopic classification developed by [110] (**Table 8**). He also presented an algorithm for management of the CMC osteoarthritis incorporating arthroscopical stages into radiological classification and subsequent treatment decision-making. Treatment methods depend on the stage of the radiologic and arthroscopic findings and can contain detriment, thermal shrinkage, correctional osteotomy of the 1st metacarpal base as well as arthroscopic resection with different interposition arthroplasties or suspensionplasties.

Class	Description
I	Synovitis phase. Subtle carpometacarpal joint space widening
II	Slight carpometacarpal joint space narrowing, sclerosis, and cystic changes with osteophytes or loose bodies < 2 mm
III	Advanced carpometacarpal joint space narrowing, sclerosis, and cystic changes with osteophytes or loose bodies > 2 mm
IV	Arthritic changes in the carpometacarpal joint as in Stage III with scaphotrapezial arthritis

Table 7.
Eaton-Litter radiological classification of 1st CMC arthritis.

Stage	Arthroscopic changes
I	Intact articular cartilage Disruption of the dorsoradial ligament and diffuse synovial hypertrophy. Inconsistent attenuation of the anterior oblique ligament (AOL)
II	Frank eburnation of the articular cartilage on the ulnar third of the base of first metacarpal and central third of the distal surface of the trapezium. Disruption of the dorsoradial ligament + more intense synovial hypertrophy. Constant attenuation of the AOL
III	Widespread, full-thickness cartilage loss with or without a peripheral rim on both articular surfaces. Less severe synovitis. Frayed volar ligaments with laxity

Table 8.
A. Badia *arthroscopic classification of 1st CMC arthritis.*

With recent advances in arthroscopic techniques, partial trapezectomy with or without different soft tissue or implant interposition has been reported with good results [111–114]. Theoretical advantages over open procedures include a decreased risk of neurovascular injuries, smaller incisions decreased postoperative pain and shorter overall recovery time. On the other side, this technique has several disadvantages, including increased setup and operative procedure time,

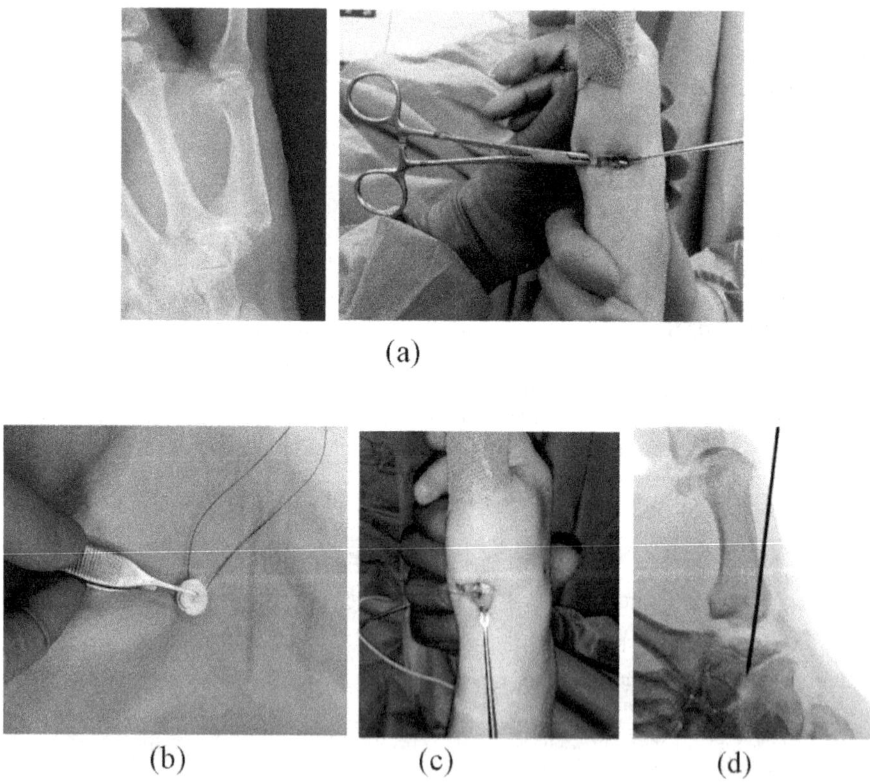

Figure 40.
(a) preopertive x-ray of 1st CMC arthritis, (b) CMC portals connected with skin incison, (c) Regjoint Scaffold sutured before insertion via elongated CMC portal, (d) Implant pulled in and positioned in the site, (e) transfixation of the bones and implant with K-wire.

increased surgical training, increased equipment cost and additional x-ray fluoroscopy time [115].

There is growing evidence that techniques involving use of no interposition result in a high rate of satisfactory outcomes [116, 117]. Cobb et al. in 2015 compared outcomes of patients treated with or without tendon interposition and found no difference in outcomes.

Another promising technique is an arthroscopic hemitrapeziectomy and suture button suspensionplasty [118, 119].

Authors have their own small experience (6 patients) with arthroscopic hemitrapezectomy and interposition arthroplasty with RegJoint™ implant (**Figure 40a–e**). The follow up is 12 to 36 months without any severe complications. Marcuzzi et al. in 2020 published long-term results with open technique [120]. They found dissapointing radiological results with an almost complete collapse of the metacarpal base on the distal pole of scaphoid in more than 80% of patients. However the results did not correspond with clinical outcomes that were very satisfactory. We hope that arthroscopical technique preserving the dorsal capsule will improve the outcomes, but further investigations are necessary.

Complication rate with arthroscopic CMC arthroplasties is about 4% and include as follows: CRPS, ulnar or radial sensory nerve neuropathy, transitory numbness near the portal, prolonged hematoma, FPL tendon rupture and superficial skin necrosis [121].

16. Arthroscopic evaluation and treatment of the triangular fibrocatilage complex (TFCC) injuries

The development of our understanding and management of TFCC tears has been developed with important contributions including Palmer's classification of TFCC tears (**Table 9**), G. Poehling's inside-out suture technique, F. Del Piñal's all inside suture technique [122], A. Atzei's and R. Luchetti's TFCC tear classification (**Figure 41**), T. Nakamura's anatomical and clinical studies [123] and J.R. Haugstvedt's

Class or subclass	Description
Class 1	**Traumatic**
1A	Central slit
1B	Ulnar avulsion with or without distal ulnar fracture
1C	Distal avulsion(carpal attachement)
1D	Radial avulsion with or without sigmoid notch fracture
Class 2	**Degenerative**
2A	TFCC wear
2B	TFCC wear, lunate or ulnar chondromalacia
2C	TFCC perforation, lunate or ulnar chondromalacia
2D	TFCC perforation, lunate or ulnar chondromalacia, lunotriquetral ligament tear
2E	TFCC perforation, lunate or ulnar chondromalacia, lunotriquetral ligament tear, ulnocarpal osteoarthritis

Table 9.
Palmer's classification of TFCC tears.

		DRUJ instability (ballotement test)	Quality of distal TFCC (appearance on RC arthroscopy)	Quality of proximal TFCC (appearance on DRUJ arthroscopy/ hook test)	Reparability of TFCC tear's margins (healing potential)	Quality of DRUJ cartilage (DRUJ arthroscopy)	Suggested treatment
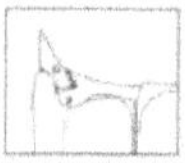	**Class 1 Repairable distal tear**	None/slight	Rupture	Intact	Good	Good	Repair: Ligament-to-capsule suture
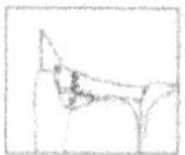	**Class 2 Repairable complete tear**	Mild/severe	Rupture	Rupture	Good	Good	Repair: Foveal refixation
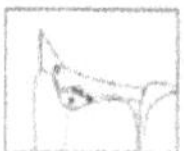	**Class 3 Repairable proximal tear**	Mild/severe	Intact	Rupture	Good	Good	Repair: Foveal refixation
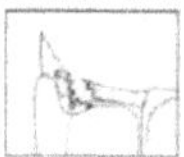	**Class 4 Non-repairable tear**	Severe	Rupture	Rupture	Poor	Good	Reconstruction: Tendon graft
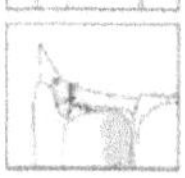	**Class 5 Arthritic DRUJ**	Mild/severe	Variable	Variable	Variable	Poor	Salvage: Arthroplasty or joint replacement

DRUJ: distal radio-ulnar joint; RC: radio-carpal; TFCC: triangular fibrocartilage complex.

Figure 41.
A. Atzei's and R. Luchetti's classification of TFCC tears (reprinted by permission).

developed techniques for the TFCC tears and lunotriquetral tears as well as studies about DRUJ functional anatomy and pathomechanics [1, 124].

TFCC – is one of the instrinsic ligaments of the wrist, with load bearing function between the lunate, triquetrum and ulnar head. TFCC acts as stabilizer for the ulnar aspect of the wrist joint [125].

TFCC consists of five parts: fibrocartilaginous disc and the meniscal homolog, volar ulnocarpal ligaments (ulnolunate and ulno-triquetral), dorsal and volar radioulnar ligaments (each with a superficial and deep part), ulnar collateral ligament as well as the floor of the fibrous 5th and 6th extensor compartments [125, 126].

Palmer had a two-dimensional view of the TFCC [127]. Nakamura described it as a three dimensional structure, and separated TFCC in three components: the distal component which acted like a hammock to suspend the carpus, the triangular ligament as the proximal component which stabilized the radius to the ulna, and the UCL as the ulnar component which stabilized the carpus to the ulna [128, 129]. Atzei and Luchetti updated previous "hammock" concept to the novel "iceberg" concept [130]. In analogy with the iceberg, during arthroscopy of the radiocarpal joint (RCJ) the TFCC shows its "emerging" tip. The tip of the iceberg represents that part of the TFCC that functions as a shock absorber. This part is much more smaller than "submerged" part which can be seen only in case of the DRUJ arthroscopy. The submerged TFCC represents the foveal insertions of the TFCC and functions as the stabilizer of the DRUJ and of the ulnar carpus. The larger size of the submerged portion of the iceberg corresponds to its greater functional importance.

TFCC biomechanics:

- TFCC stabilizes DRUJ and ulnocarpal joint
- TFCC allows the transmission and distribution of forces from wrist onto ulna and provides a gliding surface for the carpus during complex movements of the wrist.

- The central disc works as the distribution mechanism for the mechanical stress onto proximal triquetrum and the lunate

Clinical assessment of TFCC tears:

- The ulnar fovea sign is the most reliable clinical sign [131], where the patient has the point of tenderness over the ulnar capsule in the area between extensor carpi ulnaris (ECU) and flexor carpi ulnaris (FCU) tendons.

- The ballotment test evaluates DRUJ stability. This is a simple and reliable to determine DRUJ laxity [132].

Imaging assessment of TFCC tears:

- Radiographs – of limited value for TFCC injury diagnostics, but very important for acute and chronic wrist pain. The presence of ulnar styloid fracture alone or with distal radius fracture is of some importance for the diagnosis of the TFCC tear [133]. The Galeazzi fracture-subluxation is a particular condition that is associated with a TFCC tear [134].

- MRI and MRI arthrogram. MRI is more useful to exclude associated pathologies of the ulnar compartment. Comparing specificity and sensitivity of MRI, MRI arthrography and artroscopy for diagnosis of the TFCC tear, confirm the arthroscopy as the gold standard for diagnosis [135, 136].

Arthroscopic examination of TFCC. Three arthroscopic tests are used to check the type of TFCC injury:

- The "trampoline sign" – the loss of elasticity of the TFCC – seen in complete avulsion injuries of the proximal and distal portions of the TFCC

- The "hook sign"– positive in complete tears of the TFCC and negative in other cases. The hook test is more accurate than the trampoline test to detect foveal tears of the TFCC of the wrist [137]

- The "ghost sign" – reverse ""trampoline sign". This indicates an avulsion of the deep fibers of the TFCC. The sign is negative in distal lesions and positive in isolated proximal lesions.

Atzei's/Luchetti's classification also shows the stability/instability of the DRUJ joint and possible surgical treatment to corresponding TFCC tear.

An algorithm of treatment according to Atzei's/Luchetti's classification:

CLASS 0 – isolated styloid fracture without TFCC tear. Frequently associated with distal radial fractures. DRUJ is stable. If isolated treatment is wrist splinting for 3 weeks.

CLASS 1 – periferal tear of the TFCC distal component, the DRUJ may be slightly lax. Hook test negative. Small tear requires 4 weeks of wrist immobilization followed by two weeks splinting. A larger tears requires arthroscopic TFCC suture.

CLASS 3 – periferal tear of the TFCC proximal component. Mild to severe laxity of the DRUJ joint. Hook test is positive. TFCC foveal reattachment is required by transosseus sutures or a suture anchor.

CLASS 4 – nonrepairable peripheral TFCC tear due to the massive defect or poor healing potential. This condition requires reconstruction with tendon graft.

CLASS 5 – DRUJ arthritis following peripheral TFCC tear. Arthroscopy shows significant degenerative or traumatic cartilage defect. Suggested treatment – arthroplasty or prosthetic replacement.

In cases of peripheral repairable TFCC tears, authors use debridement and synovectomy to detect and refresh the site of the rupture. Usually 6R portal is used for shaver and 3-4 portal for visualization. Occasionally 6 U portal can be used if tears are localized more volarly. Once the size of tear is recognized, portal can be elongated to vizualise extensor tendons by transillumination of the capsule. Needle with suture loop is passed a little bit proximally from the margin to the TFCC to capture capsule together with the TFCC. Once recognized in the joint, suture is captured with mosquito forceps and one part of it passed via the portal or, in cases if several sutures necessary, via extra holes in the capsule. Location of the extensor tendons is evaluated to avoid capture of them in the suture and knots are tightened extra-articulary (**Figure 42a–c**). The reattachment can be performed with an inside-out, outside-in, or all-inside technique, providing good to excellent results, which tend to persist over time, in 60–90% of cases [138].

In cases of proximal reparable TFCC foveal detachment, we prefer to use the transosseus refixation of the TFCC described by T. Nakamura [139]. We use the original Arthrex target device through 6R portal and an approximately 1 cm longitudinal incision on the ulnar side of the ulnar cortex, 10–15 mm proximal from the tip of the ulnar styloid. Then target device is set on the TFCC and two parallel channels with original 1.6 mm K-wires are made from the ulnar cortex through the head of ulna and TFCC. Then follows a manipulation with needles, suture loops and main suture, where different techniques of the suture insertion are possible (**Figure 43a–c**).

After the main suture is passed through the bone channels to make outside-in pullout suture of the TFCC to the fovea and tensed with knot over the cortex. Another option is to hide the knot inside the ulna and tense with a push-lock anchor.

After treament includes 2-3 weeks in long arm plaster cast, following 3 weeks in short cast with following rehabilitation after the cast is removed.

In cases of unrepearable TFCC injuries or degenerative tears, an anatomic reconstruction with free tendon graft is recommended. The arthroscopic reconstruction is a mini invasive option of the Adams-Berger procedure [140], but it requires an experience in arthroscopic surgery. Nowadays tendon grafts can be fixed in the bone channel with interference screw, instead of the original procedure where tendons were wrapped around the bone and sutured together. Nevertheless,

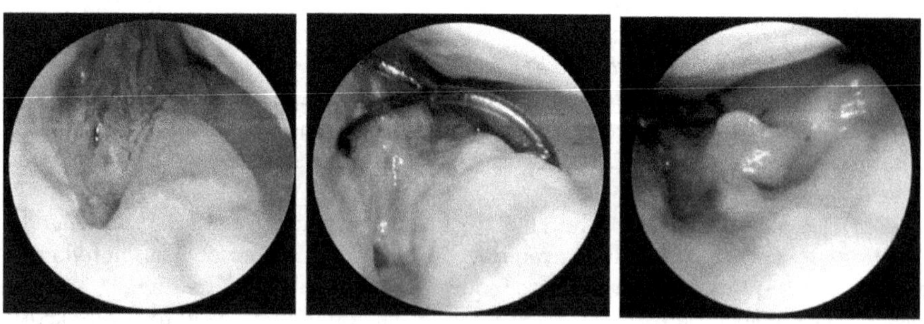

(a) (b) (c)

Figure 42.
Periferal, reconstructable TFCC tear. (a) tear after the debridement, (b) sutures passed the TFCC and capsule, (c) sutures tightened extra-articulary via 6R portal.

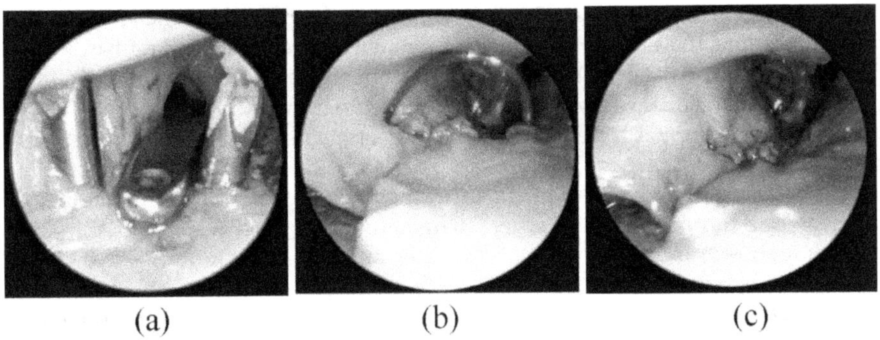

Figure 43.
Proximal reparable detachement of TFCC. (a) Arthrex targeting device over the foveal area, view from 4-5 portal, (b) sutures passed through the TFCC and head of ulna, (c) sutures tightened and TFCC reattached to foveal region.

when well done, this technique provides good stabilization of the DRUJ, while maintaining good mobility of the wrist in all directions [141].

A systemic review by Liu et al. about the surgical repair of TFCC tears confirms that arthroscopic techniques achieve overall better outcomes compared with open repair technique. For foveal tears, transosseous sutures achieve overall better functional outcomes compared with suture anchors. Current evidence demonstrates that TFCC repair achieves good clinical outcomes, with low complication rates [142].

17. Discussion

During the last 4 decades wrist arthroscopy has turned from the diagnostic tool of some enthusiasts to the widely used therapeutical complex for treatment of different wrist pathologies. Evolution of the wrist arthroscopy equipment as well as skills of the surgeons has allowed us to improve our knowledge of the wrist anatomy and biomechanics. Wrist arthroscopy is especially valuable for evaluation of intra-articular soft tissue pathologies. Furthermore - arthroscopic classification systems have been described for TFCC, SLIL and LTIL lesions, Kienböck disease, 1st CMC joint, etc.

Wrist arthroscopy techniques have proved superiority over the open techniques with lower complication rates and recurrence rates. For example in wrist ganglion surgery open surgical excision had a mean recurrence of 21%, compared with a recurrence rate of 59% for aspiration. The lowest rate was observed with arthroscopic excision, with a recurrence of 6% across all studies [40].

Arthroscopic scapho-lunate ligamentous repair is now considered the less damaging and denervating than open repair [143]. Although several arthroscopic SLIL reconstruction methods as well as arthroscopic reconstruction technique for LTIL tears have been described, these surgeries are challenging, therefore different modalities and variations of open procedures are still actual and used. Some arthroscopic techniques require a long learning curve and years of practice.

A systematic review about arthroscopic vs. open TFCC surgeries shows comparable results between open and arthroscopic procedures, in terms of DRUJ re-instability and functional outcome scores. There is insufficient evidence to recommend one technique over the other in clinical practice [144]. However arthroscopic procedures are less aggressive and may allow quicker recovery, especially in athletes [145]. In combination with a TFCC procedure, the ulnar variance can readily be assessed. Ulnar abutment or impingement can be directly visualized through dynamic assessment. Whilst ulnar shortening is an extra-articular procedure, the arthroscopic wafer procedure allows for intra-articular treatment without the need for hardware. This overcomes the issues of hardware prominence and circumvents non-union rates of about 10%, while also allowing for a quicker return to work [145, 146].

Wrist arthroscopy is beneficial also in the treatment of distal radius articular fractures, because it helps to visualize articular gaps and step-offs unrecognized with the fluoroscope alone. Although arthroscopically assisted DRF surgeries have superior long-term outcomes in several parameters [76], the advantage of this procedure, however, is the recognition of associated soft tissue lesions which can be prevented if recognized.

The next aspect is professional training and experience of the surgeon. Leclercq et al. in the multicenter study organized by EWAS found that surgeons who perform less than 25 wrist arthroscopies per year have a complication rate of 12.06%, whereas among the surgeons who perform more than 75 wrist arthroscopies per year, the complication rate is 3.95%. Surgeon with less than 5 years of practice in wrist arthroscopy have complication rate 13.6%, whereas surgeons who had 15 or more years of practice complication rate is only 2.3%. Surgeons with longer practice and greater amount of wrist artrhroscopies performed per year, more often are doing therapeutical arthroscopies. This ratio is up to 87% of procedures comparing to less experienced colleagues who perform therapeutical procedures in about 60.5% of cases [147].

18. Conclusions

Arthroscopy has assumed an important place in wrist surgery. It requires specific operative skills, training, technical equipment and patience, because these surgeries sometimes take more time than expected, even if you think, you are trained enough (my personal experience). Minimally invasive surgery is a trend of our century and arthroscopic treatment of wrist pathologies has already demonstrated promising outcomes and it's superiority over open surgical procedures.

Author details

Uldis Krustins* and Jānis Krustins
Microsurgery Centre of Latvia, Riga, Latvia

*Address all correspondence to: uldis.krustins@mcl.lv

References

[1] Baker A WT, Poehling GG, Bain GI. 2020;1(1):44-64. History of wrist arthroscopy. J Arthrosc Surg Sport Med 2020;1(1):44-64.

[2] Chen YC. Arthroscopy of the wrist and finger joints. Orthop Clin North Am. 1979;10(3):723-733.

[3] Whipple TL, Marotta JJ, Powell JH, 3rd. Techniques of wrist arthroscopy. Arthroscopy. 1986;2(4):244-252.

[4] Ong MT, Ho PC, Wong CW, Cheng SH, Tse WL. Wrist Arthroscopy under Portal Site Local Anesthesia (PSLA) without Tourniquet. J Wrist Surg. 2012;1(2):149-152.

[5] del Pinal F, Garcia-Bernal FJ, Pisani D, Regalado J, Ayala H, Studer A. Dry arthroscopy of the wrist: surgical technique. J Hand Surg Am. 2007;32(1): 119-123.

[6] Badur N. LR, Atzei A. Arthroscopy has assumed an important place. Arthroscopic Wrist Anatomy and Setup. In: W. G, editor. Wrist and Elbow Arthroscopy: A Practical Surgical Guide to Techniques. New York, NY.: Springer; 2015.

[7] Mathoulin C. Materials and Set-Up. In: Mathoulin C, editor. Wrist Arthroscopy Techniques. 2nd Edition ed.: Thieme Medical Publishers, Inc.; 2019.

[8] Ekman EF PG. Principles of arthroscopy and wrist arthroscopy equipment. Hand Clin. 1994 Nov:;10(4): 557-66.

[9] Abrams RA, Petersen M, Botte MJ. Arthroscopic portals of the wrist: an anatomic study. J Hand Surg Am. 1994; 19(6):940-944.

[10] Cobb TK, Berner SH, Badia A. New frontiers in hand arthroscopy. Hand Clin. 2011;27(3):383-394.

[11] Bettinger PC, Cooney WP, 3rd, Berger RA. Arthroscopic anatomy of the wrist. Orthop Clin North Am. 1995;26 (4):707-719.

[12] Abe Y, Doi K, Hattori Y, Ikeda K, Dhawan V. A benefit of the volar approach for wrist arthroscopy. Arthroscopy. 2003;19(4):440-445.

[13] Slutsky DJ. Wrist arthroscopy through a volar radial portal. Arthroscopy. 2002;18(6):624-630.

[14] Slutsky DJ. The use of a volar ulnar portal in wrist arthroscopy. Arthroscopy. 2004;20(2):158-163.

[15] Slutsky DJ. Clinical applications of volar portals in wrist arthroscopy. Tech Hand Up Extrem Surg. 2004;8(4): 229-238.

[16] Mathoulin C. Wrist Arthroscopy Techniques. 2nd ed.: Thieme; 2019.

[17] Atzei A, Rizzo A, Luchetti R, Fairplay T. Arthroscopic foveal repair of triangular fibrocartilage complex peripheral lesion with distal radioulnar joint instability. Tech Hand Up Extrem Surg. 2008;12(4):226-235.

[18] Slutsky D, Nagle D. Techniques in wrist and hand arthroscopy. Philadelphia: Churchill Livingstone; 2007.

[19] Katolik LI. Arthroscopic resection of pisotriquetral joint loose body: a case report. J Hand Surg Am. 2008;33(2): 206-209.

[20] John C. Arthroscopic Management of Piso-Triquetral Conditions. Piñal Fd, editor: Springer, Berlin, Heidelberg; 2012.

[21] Cobb T, Sterbank P, Lemke J. Arthroscopic resection arthroplasty for

treatment of combined carpometacarpal and scaphotrapeziotrapezoid (pantrapezial) arthritis. J Hand Surg Am. 2011;36(3):413-419.

[22] Badia A. Arthroscopy of the trapeziometacarpal and metacarpophalangeal joints. J Hand Surg Am. 2007;32(5):707-724.

[23] Sekiya I, Kobayashi M, Taneda Y, Matsui N. Arthroscopy of the proximal interphalangeal and metacarpophalangeal joints in rheumatoid hands. Arthroscopy. 2002; 18(3):292-297.

[24] Wei N, Delauter SK, Erlichman MS, Rozmaryn LM, Beard SJ, Henry DL. Arthroscopic synovectomy of the metacarpophalangeal joint in refractory rheumatoid arthritis: a technique. Arthroscopy. 1999;15(3):265-268.

[25] Xie X, Xie X, Qin H, Shen L, Zhang C. Comparison of internal and external fixation of distal radius fractures. Acta Orthop. 2013;84(3): 286-291.

[26] Choi AK, Chow EC, Ho PC, Chow YY. Metacarpophalangeal joint arthroscopy: indications revisited. Hand Clin. 2011;27(3):369-382.

[27] Abernathie BL, Lovy AJ, Koehler SM, Hausman MR. Arthroscopic Repair of Collateral Ligaments in Metacarpophalangeal Joints. Arthrosc Tech. 2015;4(2):e97-e100.

[28] Borisch N. [Arthroscopy of the proximal interphalangeal joint]. Oper Orthop Traumatol. 2017;29(4):353-359.

[29] Sekiya I, Kobayashi M, Okamoto H, Otsuka T. Progress and Role of Finger Joint Arthroscopy. Hand Clin. 2017;33 (4):819-829.

[30] Thomsen NO, Nielsen NS, Jorgensen U, Bojsen-Moller F. Arthroscopy of the proximal interphalangeal joints of the finger. J Hand Surg Br. 2002;27(3):253-255.

[31] Overstraeten LV, Camus EJ, Wahegaonkar A, Messina J, Tandara AA, Binder AC, et al. Anatomical Description of the Dorsal Capsulo-Scapholunate Septum (DCSS)-Arthroscopic Staging of Scapholunate Instability after DCSS Sectioning. J Wrist Surg. 2013;2(2): 149-154.

[32] Rizzo M, Berger RA, Steinmann SP, Bishop AT. Arthroscopic resection in the management of dorsal wrist ganglions: results with a minimum 2-year follow-up period. J Hand Surg Am. 2004;29(1): 59-62.

[33] Chen AC, Lee WC, Hsu KY, Chan YS, Yuan LJ, Chang CH. Arthroscopic ganglionectomy through an intrafocal cystic portal for wrist ganglia. Arthroscopy. 2010;26(5): 617-622.

[34] Gallego S, Mathoulin C. Arthroscopic resection of dorsal wrist ganglia: 114 cases with minimum follow-up of 2 years. Arthroscopy. 2010; 26(12):1675-1682.

[35] Mathoulin. C. Arthroscopic Treatment of Dorsal Wrist Ganglia. In: Mathoulin C, editor. Wrist Arthroscopy Techniques. 2nd Edition ed.: Thieme; 2019.

[36] Fernandes CH, Meirelles LM, Raduan Neto J, Fernandes M, Dos Santos JBG, Faloppa F. Arthroscopic Resection of Dorsal Wrist Ganglion: Results and Rate of Recurrence Over a Minimum Follow-up of 4 Years. Hand (N Y). 2019;14(2):236-241.

[37] Ahsan ZS, Yao J. Arthroscopic dorsal wrist ganglion excision with color-aided visualization of the stalk: minimum 1-year follow-up. Hand (N Y). 2014;9(2): 205-208.

[38] Borisch N. [Arthroscopic resection of dorsal wrist ganglion cysts]. Oper Orthop Traumatol. 2016;28(4): 270-278.

[39] Mathoulin C, Gras M. Arthroscopic Management of Dorsal and Volar Wrist Ganglion. Hand Clin. 2017;33(4): 769-777.

[40] Head L, Gencarelli JR, Allen M, Boyd KU. Wrist ganglion treatment: systematic review and meta-analysis. J Hand Surg Am. 2015;40(3):546-553 e8.

[41] Ho PC, Lo WN, Hung LK. Arthroscopic resection of volar ganglion of the wrist: A new technique. Arthroscopy. 2003;19(2):218-221.

[42] Rocchi L, Canal A, Fanfani F, Catalano F. Articular ganglia of the volar aspect of the wrist: arthroscopic resection compared with open excision. A prospective randomized study. Scand J Plast Reconstr Surg Hand Surg. 2008; 42(5):253-259.

[43] Fernandes CH, Miranda CD, Dos Santos JB, Faloppa F. A systematic review of complications and recurrence rate of arthroscopic resection of volar wrist ganglion. Hand Surg. 2014;19(3): 475-480.

[44] Oliveira RK, Brunelli JPF, Bayer LR, Aita M, Mantovani G, Delgado PJ. Artrhoscopic Resection of Volar Wrist Ganglion: Surgical Technique and Case Series. Rev. Bras Ortop (Sao Paulo). 2019;54(6):721-30.

[45] Schrank C, Meirer R, Stabler A, Nerlich A, Reiser M, Putz R. Morphology and topography of intraosseous ganglion cysts in the carpus: an anatomic, histopathologic, and magnetic resonance imaging correlation study. J Hand Surg Am. 2003;28(1):52-61.

[46] Van den Dungen S, Marchesi S, Ezzedine R, Bindou D, Lorea P. Relationship between dorsal ganglion cysts of the wrist and intraosseous ganglion cysts of the carpal bones. Acta Orthop Belg. 2005;71(5):535-539.

[47] Ashwood N, Bain GI. Arthroscopically assisted treatment of intraosseous ganglions of the lunate: a new technique. J Hand Surg Am. 2003; 28(1):62-68.

[48] Berger RA. The gross and histologic anatomy of the scapholunate interosseous ligament. J Hand Surg Am. 1996;21(2):170-178.

[49] Geissler WB. Arthroscopic management of scapholunate instability. J Wrist Surg. 2013;2(2):129-135.

[50] Sammer DM, Shin AY. Wrist surgery: management of chronic scapholunate and lunotriquetral ligament injuries. Plast Reconstr Surg. 2012;130(1):138e-56e.

[51] Wahed K, Deore S, Bhan K, Vinay S, Jayasinghe G, Dutta A, et al. Management of chronic scapholunate ligament injury. J Clin Orthop Trauma. 2020;11(4):529-536.

[52] Mathoulin C. wrist artrhroscopy techniques. 2nd ed.: thieme; 2019.

[53] Andersson JK. Treatment of scapholunate ligament injury: Current concepts. EFORT Open Rev. 2017;2(9): 382-393.

[54] Geissler WB, Freeland AE, Savoie FH, McIntyre LW, Whipple TL. Intracarpal soft-tissue lesions associated with an intra-articular fracture of the distal end of the radius. J Bone Joint Surg Am. 1996;78(3):357-365.

[55] Messina JC, Van Overstraeten L, Luchetti R, Fairplay T, Mathoulin CL. The EWAS Classification of Scapholunate Tears: An Anatomical Arthroscopic Study. J Wrist Surg. 2013;2 (2):105-109.

[56] Garcia-Elias M, Lluch AL, Stanley JK. Three-ligament tenodesis for the treatment of scapholunate dissociation: indications and surgical technique. J Hand Surg Am. 2006;31(1): 125-134.

[57] Instability ISCoC. Part 2: Management of scapho-lunate dissociation. IFSSH Scientific Committee on Carpal Instability; 2016.

[58] Mathoulin CL, Dauphin N, Wahegaonkar AL. Arthroscopic dorsal capsuloligamentous repair in chronic scapholunate ligament tears. Hand Clin. 2011;27(4):563-572, xi.

[59] Wahegaonkar AL, Mathoulin CL. Arthroscopic dorsal capsulo-ligamentous repair in the treatment of chronic scapho-lunate ligament tears. J Wrist Surg. 2013;2(2):141-148.

[60] Ho PC, Wong CW, Tse WL. Arthroscopic-Assisted Combined Dorsal and Volar Scapholunate Ligament Reconstruction with Tendon Graft for Chronic SL Instability. J Wrist Surg. 2015;4(4):252-263.

[61] Corella F, Del Cerro M, Larrainzar-Garijo R, Vazquez T. Arthroscopic ligamentoplasty (bone-tendon-tenodesis). A new surgical technique for scapholunate instability: preliminary cadaver study. J Hand Surg Eur Vol. 2011;36(8):682-689.

[62] Corella F, Del Cerro M, Ocampos M, Simon de Blas C, Larrainzar-Garijo R. Arthroscopic Scapholunate Ligament Reconstruction, Volar and Dorsal Reconstruction. Hand Clin. 2017;33(4): 687-707.

[63] Doi K, Hattori Y, Otsuka K, Abe Y, Yamamoto H. Intra-articular fractures of the distal aspect of the radius: arthroscopically assisted reduction compared with open reduction and internal fixation. J Bone Joint Surg Am. 1999;81(8):1093-1110.

[64] Abe Y. Plate presetting and arthroscopic reduction technique (PART) for treatment of distal radius fractures. Handchir Mikrochir Plast Chir. 2014;46(5):278-285.

[65] Freeland AE, Geissler WB. The arthroscopic management of intra-articular distal radius fractures. Hand Surg. 2000;5(2):93-102.

[66] Ruch DS, Vallee J, Poehling GG, Smith BP, Kuzma GR. Arthroscopic reduction versus fluoroscopic reduction in the management of intra-articular distal radius fractures. Arthroscopy. 2004;20(3):225-230.

[67] Varitimidis SE, Basdekis GK, Dailiana ZH, Hantes ME, Bargiotas K, Malizos K. Treatment of intra-articular fractures of the distal radius: fluoroscopic or arthroscopic reduction? J Bone Joint Surg Br. 2008;90(6): 778-785.

[68] Ono H, Furuta K, Fujitani R, Katayama T, Akahane M. Distal radius fracture arthroscopic intraarticular displacement measurement after open reduction and internal fixation from a volar approach. J Orthop Sci. 2010;15 (4):502-508.

[69] Ono H, Katayama T, Furuta K, Suzuki D, Fujitani R, Akahane M. Distal radial fracture arthroscopic intraarticular gap and step-off measurement after open reduction and internal fixation with a volar locked plate. J Orthop Sci. 2012;17(4): 443-449.

[70] Geissler WB. Arthroscopically assisted reduction of intra-articular fractures of the distal radius. Hand Clin. 1995;11(1):19-29.

[71] Mehta JA, Bain GI, Heptinstall RJ. Anatomical reduction of intra-articular fractures of the distal radius. An arthroscopically-assisted approach. J Bone Joint Surg Br. 2000;82(1):79-86.

[72] Catalano LW, 3rd, Barron OA, Glickel SZ. Assessment of articular displacement of distal radius fractures. Clin Orthop Relat Res. 2004(423):79-84.

[73] Wadsten MA, Buttazzoni GG, Sjoden GO, Kadum B, Sayed-Noor AS. Influence of Cortical Comminution and Intra-articular Involvement in Distal Radius Fractures on Clinical Outcome: A Prospective Multicenter Study. J Wrist Surg. 2017;6(4):285-293.

[74] Ardouin L, Durand A, Gay A, Leroy M. Why do we use arthroscopy for distal radius fractures? Eur J Orthop Surg Traumatol. 2018;28(8):1505-1514.

[75] Lutsky K, Boyer MI, Steffen JA, Goldfarb CA. Arthroscopic assessment of intra-articular distal radius fractures after open reduction and internal fixation from a volar approach. J Hand Surg Am. 2008;33(4):476-484.

[76] Krustiņš U NV, Bringina D, Jaudzema A, Jumtiņš A. Comparison of Fluoroscopically and Arthroscopically Assisted Volar Plating of Articular Distal Radius Fractures Proceedings of the Latvian Academy of Sciences Section B Natural, Exact, and Applied Sciences 2021;75(2021)(1 (February 2021)):58-64.

[77] Del Pinal F. Technical tips for (dry) arthroscopic reduction and internal fixation of distal radius fractures. J Hand Surg Am. 2011;36(10):1694-1705.

[78] Kastenberger T, Kaiser P, Schmidle G, Schwendinger P, Gabl M, Arora R. Arthroscopic assisted treatment of distal radius fractures and concomitant injuries. Arch Orthop Trauma Surg. 2020.

[79] Lindau T. Arthroscopic Evaluation of Associated Soft Tissue Injuries in Distal Radius Fractures. Hand Clin. 2017;33(4):651-658.

[80] del Piñal F. 9 Mini Approaches. Distal Radius Fractures and Carpal Instabilities: FESSH IFSSH 2019 Instructional Book. 2019.

[81] Krustins U, Krustins J, Bringina D, Laurane K, Jumtins A. Comparison of volar locking plates with external fixation and K-wires in arthroscopically assisted intra-articular distal radial fracture fixation. J Hand Surg Eur Vol. 2020;45(4):333-338.

[82] Imatani J, Noda T, Morito Y, Sato T, Hashizume H, Inoue H. Minimally invasive plate osteosynthesis for comminuted fractures of the metaphysis of the radius. J Hand Surg Br. 2005;30 (2):220-225.

[83] Sen MK, Strauss N, Harvey EJ. Minimally invasive plate osteosynthesis of distal radius fractures using a pronator sparing approach. Tech Hand Up Extrem Surg. 2008;12(1):2-6.

[84] Igeta Y, Vernet P, Facca S, Naroura I, Hidalgo Diaz JJ, Diaz JJH, et al. The minimally invasive flexor carpi radialis approach: a new perspective for distal radius fractures. Eur J Orthop Surg Traumatol. 2018;28 (8):1515-1522.

[85] Ruggiero GM. 9 Mini Approaches. In: del Piñal F, editor. Distal Radius Fractures and Carpal Instabilities: FESSH IFSSH 2019 Instructional Book. 1st Edition ed.: Thieme Medical Publishers, Inc.; 2019.

[86] Abe Y, Tsubone T, Tominaga Y. Plate presetting arthroscopic reduction technique for the distal radius fractures. Tech Hand Up Extrem Surg. 2008;12(3): 136-143.

[87] Luchetti R, Atzei A, Fairplay T. Arthroscopic wrist arthrolysis after wrist fracture. Arthroscopy. 2007;23(3): 255-260.

[88] Mathoulin C. Arthroscopic Arthrolysis of the Wrist. In: Mathoulin C, editor. Wrist Arthroscopy

Techniques. 2nd Edition ed.: Thieme Medical Publishers, Inc.; 2019.

[89] Luchetti R, Atzei A, Papini Zorli I. [Arthroscopic wrist arthrolysis]. Chir Main. 2006;25 Suppl 1:S244-53.

[90] Clementson M, Bjorkman A, Thomsen NOB. Acute scaphoid fractures: guidelines for diagnosis and treatment. EFORT Open Rev. 2020;5(2): 96-103.

[91] Morsy M, Sabbagh MD, van Alphen NA, Laungani AT, Kadar A, Moran SL. The Vascular Anatomy of the Scaphoid: New Discoveries Using Micro-Computed Tomography Imaging. J Hand Surg Am. 2019;44(11):928-938.

[92] VD. K. Scaphoid fractures and nonunions. In: Trumble TE BJ, Cornwall R., editor. Hand, Elbow, & Shoulder: Core Knowledge in Orthopedics. Philadelphia, PA:: Mosby Elsevier; 2006. p. 116-31.

[93] Mathoulin C. Arthroscopic-Assisted Scaphoid Fracture Fixation. In: Mathoulin C, editor. Wrist Arthroscopy Techniques. 2nd Edition ed.: Thieme Medical Publishers, Inc.; 2019.

[94] Martinache X, Mathoulin C. [Percutaneous fixation of scaphoid fractures with arthroscopic assistance.]. Chir Main. 2006;25S1:S171-S7.

[95] Slutsky DJ, Trevare J. Use of arthroscopy for the treatment of scaphoid fractures. Hand Clin. 2014;30 (1):91-103.

[96] Slade JF, 3rd, Gillon T. Retrospective review of 234 scaphoid fractures and nonunions treated with arthroscopy for union and complications. Scand J Surg. 2008;97(4):280-289.

[97] Slade JF, Lozano-Calderon S, Merrell G, Ring D. Arthroscopic-assisted percutaneous reduction and screw fixation of displaced scaphoid fractures. J Hand Surg Eur Vol. 2008;33 (3):350-354.

[98] Gehrmann S, Roeger T, Kaufmann R, Schaedle A, Logters T, Windolf J. Wrist motion analysis in scaphoid nonunion. Eur J Trauma Emerg Surg. 2016;42(1):11-14.

[99] Ruby LK, Leslie BM. Wrist arthritis associated with scaphoid nonunion. Hand Clin. 1987;3(4):529-539.

[100] Inoue G, Sakuma M. The natural history of scaphoid non-union. Radiographical and clinical analysis in 102 cases. Arch Orthop Trauma Surg. 1996;115(1):1-4.

[101] Kang HJ, Chun YM, Koh IH, Park JH, Choi YR. Is Arthroscopic Bone Graft and Fixation for Scaphoid Nonunions Effective? Clin Orthop Relat Res. 2016;474(1):204-212.

[102] Mathoulin C. Arthroscopic Bone Grafting for Scaphoid Nonunion. In: Mathoulin C, editor. Wrist Arthroscopy Techniques. 2nd Edition ed.: Thieme Medical Publishers, Inc.; 2019.

[103] Mathoulin CL, Arianni M. Treatment of the scaphoid humpback deformity - is correction of the dorsal intercalated segment instability deformity critical? J Hand Surg Eur Vol. 2018;43(1):13-23.

[104] Wong WC, Ho PC. Arthroscopic Management of Scaphoid Nonunion. Hand Clin. 2019;35(3):295-313.

[105] Delgado PJ. Arthroscopic Reconstruction of Chronic Unstable Scaphoid Nonunion. J Wrist Surg 2015; 04 - A002.

[106] Jeff E. Nonunion of the Scaphoid with Flexion ("Humpback") Deformity Comparison of Arthroscopic Bone Graft (ABG) and Vascularised Medial Femoral Bone Graft (VMFBG). J Wrist Surg. 2015;2015; 04 - A018.

[107] Kim JP, Seo JB, Yoo JY, Lee JY. Arthroscopic management of chronic unstable scaphoid nonunions: effects on restoration of carpal alignment and recovery of wrist function. Arthroscopy. 2015;31(3):460-469.

[108] Gvozdenovic R, Joergensen RW, Joerring S, Jensen CH. Arthroscopically Assisted Bone Grafting Reduces Union Time of Scaphoid Nonunions Compared to Percutaneous Screw Fixation Alone. J Wrist Surg. 2020;9(1):13-18.

[109] Eaton R G LJW. Ligament reconstruction for the painful thumb carpometacarpal joint. J Bone Joint Surg Am.1973;55(08::1655–66. .

[110] Badia A. Trapeziometacarpal arthroscopy: a classification and treatment algorithm. Hand Clin. 2006; 22(2):153-163.

[111] Ma C, Deng Q, Pu H, Cheng X, Kan Y, Yang J, et al. External fixation is more suitable for intra-articular fractures of the distal radius in elderly patients. Bone Res. 2016;4:16017.

[112] Diaconu M, Mathoulin C, Facca S, Liverneaux P. Arthroscopic interposition arthroplasty of the trapeziometacarpal joint. Chir Main. 2011;30(4):282-287.

[113] Cobb TK, Walden AL, Cao Y. Long-Term Outcome of Arthroscopic Resection Arthroplasty With or Without Interposition for Thumb Basal Joint Arthritis. J Hand Surg Am. 2015;40(9): 1844-1851.

[114] Taleb C, Berner S, Mantovani Ruggiero G. First metacarpal resurfacing with polyvinyl alcohol implant in osteoarthritis: preliminary study. Chir Main. 2014;33(3):189-195.

[115] Logli AL, Twu J, Bear BJ, Lindquist JR, Schoenfeldt TL, Korcek KJ. Arthroscopic Partial Trapeziectomy With Soft Tissue Interposition for Symptomatic Trapeziometacarpal Arthritis: 6-Month and 5-Year Minimum Follow-Up. J Hand Surg Am. 2018;43(4):384 e1- e7.

[116] Adams JE. Does arthroscopic debridement with or without interposition material address carpometacarpal arthritis? Clin Orthop Relat Res. 2014;472(4):1166-1172.

[117] Cobb TK. Arthroscopic Resection Arthroplasty of Thumb Carpometacarpal Joint. In: Mathoulin C, editor. Wrist Arthroscopy Techniques. 2nd Edition ed.: Thieme Medical Publishers, Inc.; 2019.

[118] Landes G, Gaspar MP, Goljan P, Jacoby SM, Bachoura A, Culp RW. Arthroscopic Trapeziectomy With Suture Button Suspensionplasty: A Retrospective Review of 153 Cases. Hand (N Y). 2016;11(2):232-237.

[119] Ozcelik IB, Ugurlar M, Sari A. Arthroscopic Hemitrapeziectomy and Suture Button Suspensionplasty in the Treatment of First Carpometacarpal Joint Eaton-Littler Stage 2-3 Arthrosis. J Wrist Surg. 2019;8(2):132-138.

[120] Marcuzzi A, Colzani G, Acciaro AL, Rosa ND, Landi A. Retrospective Review of Long-term Outcomes of Patients Undergoing CMC Arthroplasty With Interposition Scaffold. Hand (N Y). 2020: 1558944720918366.

[121] Wilkens SC, Bargon CA, Mohamadi A, Chen NC, Coert JH. A systematic review and meta-analysis of arthroscopic assisted techniques for thumb carpometacarpal joint osteoarthritis. J Hand Surg Eur Vol. 2018;43(10):1098-1105.

[122] del Pinal F, Garcia-Bernal FJ, Cagigal L, Studer A, Regalado J, Thams C. A technique for arthroscopic all-inside suturing in the wrist. J Hand Surg Eur Vol. 2010;35(6):475-479.

[123] Nakamura TN, S. Gakai, Z. 1995 168-80.PMID: 7782655 Japanese. Triangular fibrocartilage complex: functional anatomy and histology. 1995; Apr;69(4):168-80.

[124] Haugstvedt JR, Langer MF, Berger RA. Distal radioulnar joint: functional anatomy, including pathomechanics. J Hand Surg Eur Vol. 2017;42(4):338-345.

[125] Mathoulin C. Anatomy of the TFCC: Current Concepts. In: Mathoulin C, editor. Wrist Arthroscopy Techniques. 2nd Edition ed.: Thieme Medical Publishers, Inc.; 2019.

[126] Palmer AKW, F.K. The triangular fibrocartilage complex of the wrist—Anatomy and function. J Hand Surg Am. 1981;Mar;6(2):153-62.

[127] Palmer AK. Triangular fibrocartilage complex lesions: a classification. J Hand Surg Am. 1989 Jul; 14(4):594-606.

[128] Nakamura T, Yabe Y, Horiuchi Y. Functional anatomy of the triangular fibrocartilage complex. J Hand Surg Br. 1996;21(5):581-586.

[129] Nakamura T, Yabe Y. Histological anatomy of the triangular fibrocartilage complex of the human wrist. Ann Anat. 2000;182(6):567-572.

[130] Atzei A, Luchetti R. Foveal TFCC tear classification and treatment. Hand Clin. 2011;27(3):263-272.

[131] Tay SC, Tomita K, Berger RA. The "ulnar fovea sign" for defining ulnar wrist pain: an analysis of sensitivity and specificity. J Hand Surg Am. 2007;32(4): 438-444.

[132] Moriya T, Aoki M, Iba K, Ozasa Y, Wada T, Yamashita T. Effect of triangular ligament tears on distal radioulnar joint instability and evaluation of three clinical tests: a biomechanical study. J Hand Surg Eur Vol. 2009;34(2):219-223.

[133] May MM, Lawton JN, Blazar PE. Ulnar styloid fractures associated with distal radius fractures: incidence and implications for distal radioulnar joint instability. J Hand Surg Am. 2002;27(6): 965-971.

[134] Rettig ME, Raskin KB. Galeazzi fracture-dislocation: a new treatment-oriented classification. J Hand Surg Am. 2001;26(2):228-235.

[135] Meier R, Schmitt R, Krimmer H. [Wrist lesions in MRI arthrography compared with wrist arthroscopy]. Handchir Mikrochir Plast Chir. 2005;37 (2):85-89.

[136] Pederzini LL, R.; Soragni,O.; Alfarano, M.; Montagna, G.; Cerofolini, E.; Colombini, R.; Roth, J. Evaluation of the triangular fibrocartilige complex tears by arthroscopy, arthrography and MRI. Arthroscopy. 1992(1992;8(2)): 191-7.

[137] Atzei A, Luchetti R, Carletti D, Marcovici LL, Cazzoletti L, Barbon S. The Hook Test Is More Accurate Than the Trampoline Test to Detect Foveal Tears of the Triangular Fibrocartilage Complex of the Wrist. Arthroscopy. 2021.

[138] Haugstvedt JR, Soreide E. Arthroscopic Management of Triangular Fibrocartilage Complex Peripheral Injury. Hand Clin. 2017;33(4):607-618.

[139] Nakamura T, Sato K, Okazaki M, Toyama Y, Ikegami H. Repair of foveal detachment of the triangular fibrocartilage complex: open and arthroscopic transosseous techniques. Hand Clin. 2011;27(3):281-290.

[140] Adams BD, Berger RA. An anatomic reconstruction of the distal radioulnar ligaments for posttraumatic distal radioulnar joint instability. J Hand Surg Am. 2002;27(2):243-251.

[141] Mathoulin C. Arthroscopic Reconstruction of the TFCC Using a Free Tendon Graft. In: Mathoulin C, editor. Wrist Arthroscopy Techniques. 2nd Edition ed.: Thieme Medical Publishers, Inc.; 2019.

[142] Liu EH, Suen K, Tham SK, Ek ET. Surgical Repair of Triangular Fibrocartilage Complex Tears: A Systematic Review. J Wrist Surg. 2021; 10(1):70-83.

[143] Mathoulin C, Gras M. Role of wrist arthroscopy in scapholunate dissociation. Orthop Traumatol Surg Res. 2020;106(1S):S89-S99.

[144] Andersson JK, Ahlen M, Andernord D. Open versus arthroscopic repair of the triangular fibrocartilage complex: a systematic review. J Exp Orthop. 2018;5(1):6.

[145] Franca Bisneto EN, de Paula EJL, Mattar R. Wrist Arthroscopy in Athletes. Rev. Bras Ortop (Sao Paulo). 2020;55(1):1-7.

[146] Viswanath A TS. Recent advances and future trends in wrist arthroscopy. J Arthrosc Surg Sport Med 2020;1(1): 65-72.

[147] Leclercq C, Mathoulin C, Members of E. Complications of Wrist Arthroscopy: A Multicenter Study Based on 10,107 Arthroscopies. J Wrist Surg. 2016;5(4):320-326.

Section 3

Shoulder

Chapter 7

Arthroscopic Bankart Repair Using a Lasso-Loop Stitch

Christian Konrads and Stefan Döbele

Abstract

Anterior inferior shoulder dislocation is a common injury. After primary traumatic shoulder dislocation and conservative treatment, the risk of re-dislocation is very high in patients younger than 35 years. With age, the risk of re-dislocation after traumatic shoulder dislocation and conservative treatment decreases. Surgical treatment via either open or arthroscopic stabilization minimizes the risk of re-dislocation. Today, anterior shoulder stabilization by arthroscopic refixation of the labroligamentous complex with suture anchors is a standard procedure, if there is no severe chronic bony defect at the glenoid site. Lafosse et al. described the so-called „Lasso-loop stitch". This technique allows for positioning of the knot away from the joint and at the same time it establishes a labral bump that stabilizes the humeral head against (sub)luxation. The surgical principle and aim consist of refixation of the anterior labrum-capsule-ligament complex to the glenoid with positioning of the knot at distance to the joint as well as bulging up the labrum. This stabilizes the shoulder joint and therefore avoids further dislocations and associated pathologies. The aim of this work is to give an illustrated instruction of the surgical technique of arthroscopic Bankart repair using the lasso-loop stitch.

Keywords: Shoulder instability, Dislocation, ALPSA, Perthes lesion, Hill Sachs

1. Introduction

After traumatic first-time shoulder dislocation followed by conservative treatment, the re-dislocation rate is >70% in patients <30 years. With age, the risk of re-dislocation after traumatic shoulder dislocation and conservative treatment decreases. Surgical treatment via either open or arthroscopic stabilization minimizes the risk of re-dislocation [1–4].

In cases without severe chronic bone loss at the glenoid site, anterior shoulder stabilization by arthroscopic refixation of the labroligamentous complex with suture anchors is the standard therapeutic procedure [1, 5]. The so-called „Lasso-loop stitch "was described by Lafosse et al [6–9]. This technique allows positioning of the knot away from the joint and at the same time it establishes the sought labral bump. With the "Oblique mattress lasso-loop stitch" Parnes et al. published a resembling arthroscopic technique, but without giving clinical results [10].

The goal of the surgery is refixation of the anterior labrum-capsule-ligament complex to the glenoid with positioning of the knot at distance to the joint as well as bulking up the labrum. This stabilizes the gleno-humeral joint and therefore avoids further dislocations and associated pathologies. Using lasso-loop stitches probably leads to more bulging up of the labrum than other stitching techniques as for example the single interrupted stitch or the mattress stitch. The lasso-loop stitch accentuates the physiological bumper effect of the glenoid labrum and can therefore avoid re-dislocation.

Indications for this operation are shoulder instabilities with repairable damage to the labrum: Bankart lesion, bony Bankart lesion, ALPSA, Perthes lesion, and reversed (posterior) Bankart lesions as well as injuries to the long head biceps tendon anchor (SLAP). Contraindications for this operation are arbitrary shoulder dislocations during growth period without damage to the labrum and chronic bony glenoid defects >15% of the glenoid surface [11–13]. HAGL lesions require soft-tissue refixation at the humeral site [14].

Patient consent should contain the following issues apart from the standard operation risks: cartilage damage, lesion to the axillary nerve, suture rupture, switching to open surgical procedure in case of larger bony defects, standardized postoperative treatment, restriction of motion (especially external rotation), re-dislocation, anchor dislocation, osteolysis in case of resorbable anchors, post-traumatic arthritis, pain, hospitalization for 1–2 days, day surgery possible, work leave dependent on job and arm dominance 2 days to 16 weeks.

While recording the patient history, it is critical to differentiate between traumatic and habitual cause and evaluate the main symptom, either pain or instability. It is followed by a standardized clinical examination including apprehension sign and determination of the instability direction as well as evaluating an existing hyperlaxity. X-rays of the shoulder in three planes (true a.p., y-view, axial) and MRI (**Figure 1**) are performed [15, 16]. The surgical site should be shaved, if strongly covered by hair. An examination under anesthesia is performed to record the passive glenohumeral range of motion following the neutral-zero method as well as evaluation of glenohumeral stability and translation according to the modified Hawkins classification [6] and exclusion of multidirectional instability. In case of larger glenoid defects, a CT scan is necessary [17].

With this technical modification to the classic arthroscopic Bankart repair, we reliably experienced very good clinical results and high patient satisfaction. It is the aim of this work to give an illustrated instruction of the surgical technique of arthroscopic Bankart repair using the lasso-loop stitch.

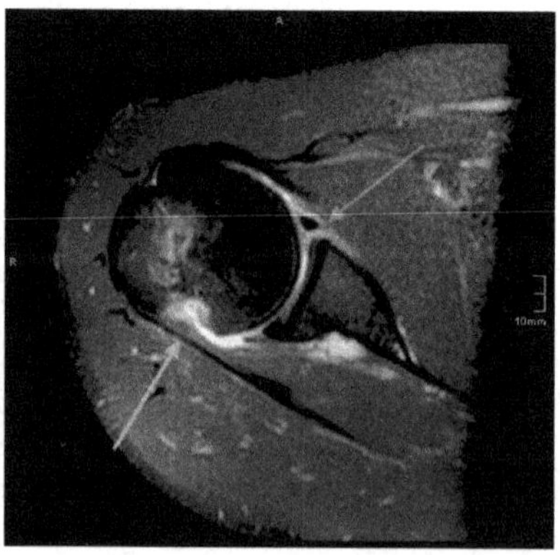

Figure 1.
MRI of the right shoulder of a 20-year-old male after primary traumatic anterior-inferior shoulder dislocation. The red arrow marks a classic Bankart lesion. The green arrow marks a concomitant hill-Sachs lesion.

2. Surgery

2.1 Setup

Surgery is performed under general anesthesia. Preoperatively, a prophylactic antibiotic single shot dose of 2 g Ampicillin and 1 g Sulbactam i. v. is administered. Dependent on preference, the operation can be done in beach chair position or lateral decubitus position with lateral tension. The latter increases the intraarticular space by putting traction on the arm. Alternatively, a special arm holder with free positioning of the arm in slight abduction and external rotation can be used. We routinely used the latter option.

After diagnostic arthroscopy, fixation of the anterior capsulo-labral complex with suture anchors in lasso-loop technique is performed. The following arthroscopy equipment and instruments are used during surgery:

- Arthroscopy tower with arthroscope (4 mm, 30°), monitor, camera, and documentation unit, cold light source, light cable, shaver, hook probe
- Working cannula 8.25 mm x 70 mm (transparent)
- Working cannula 5.5 mm x 72 mm (transparent)
- Bankart raspatory 30°
- Bankart rasp 30°
- PDS no. 0 as hold-suture
- Birdpeak
- Optional: Suture-lasso
- Drill
- Gliding all-suture anchor (Alternatively: singular armed resorbable suture anchor)

2.2 Surgical technique

For developing a posterior arthroscopy portal, a stab incision of the skin is made 2 cm caudal and 2 cm medial of the posterolateral corner of the acromion. After entering the glenohumeral joint with a switching stick, the arthroscopy sheath is introduced, the joint is filled up with water, and the arthroscope is inserted. At first, a diagnostic arthroscopic evaluation and incision for the anterior inferior working portal in outside-in technique just above the subscapular tendon is performed. In this antero-inferior working portal, a working cannula (8.25 mm) is inserted. Alternatively, a 5:30 o'clock portal can be used about 8 cm distal to the coracoid through the inferior (muscular) part of the subscapularis tendon. This facilitates placement of the first suture anchor as low as recommended.

An additional antero-superior portal is developed directly anterior to the acromio-clavicular joint (ACJ) in outside-in technique and a working cannula (5.5 mm) is introduced here. The **Figures 2–4** illustrate the surgical technique:

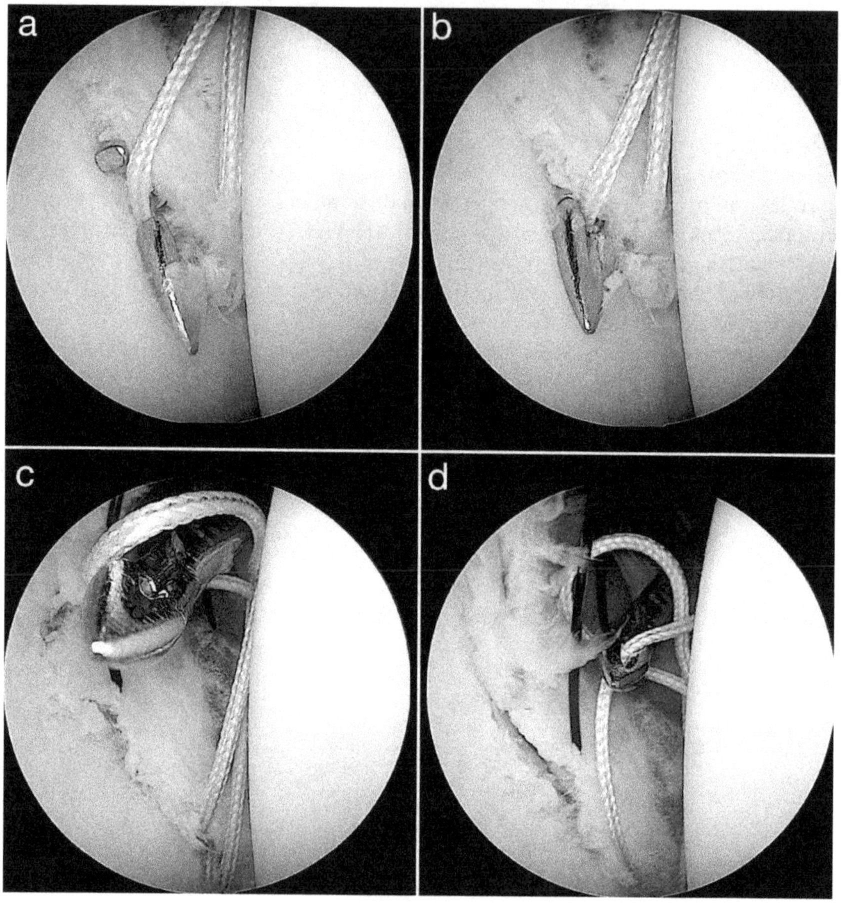

Figure 2.
The lasso-loop stitch (a-d). A Birdpeak is pushed through the capsulolabral complex from anterior (a). Then, one suture end of the anchor is grasped (b), pulled through the capsulolabral complex anteriorly, and formed into an intraarticular loop (c). The Birdpeak is pushed through the loop and the same suture end is grasped again (d). Now, the Birdpeak is kept closed and the suture end is pulled out of the shoulder joint through the working cannula. During this procedure, the other suture end outside of the shoulder joint is secured by a clamp.

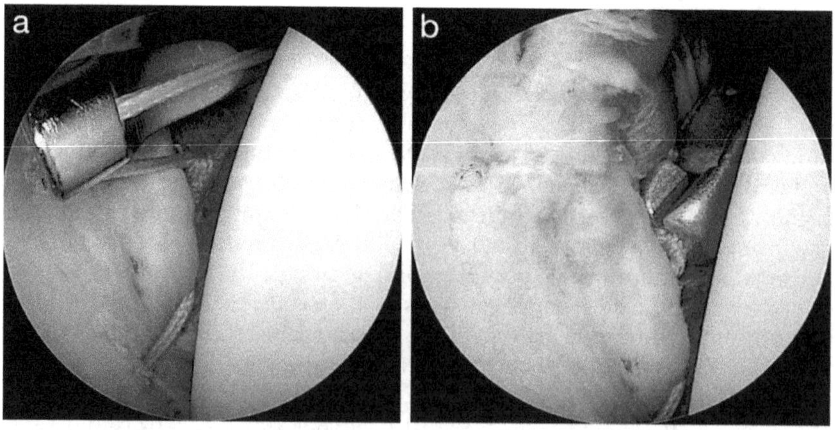

Figure 3.
Tying of the knot (a) and shortening of both FibreWire ends with arthroscopic scissors (b).

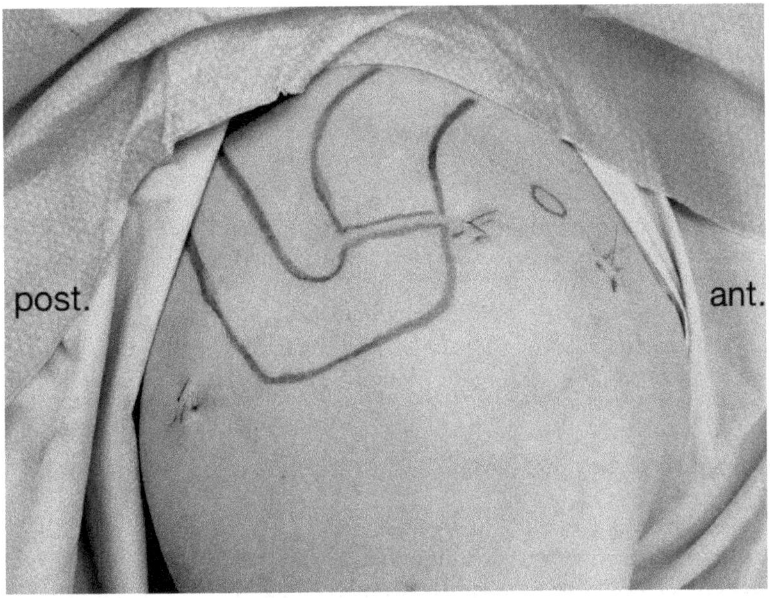

Figure 4.
Right shoulder after arthroscopic anterior stabilization.

Examination with a hook probe, mobilization of the labrum with the Bankart raspatory and debridement of the glenoid neck with the Bankart rasp.

Trial cranialisation of the capsulo-labral complex is performed via a grasper through the anterior superior portal followed by insertion of a hold-suture (PDS no. 0).

The first single-armed resorbable suture anchor is positioned through the anterior inferior portal onto the anterior glenoid rim as caudal as possible at the anterior cartilage border. The anchor is inserted ca. 135° to the glenoid plane. Not too steep and not too flat. The anchor should not be inserted too deep either; under no circumstances should the end of the anchor stick out. Because this could lead to cartilage damage and it could potentially cause anchor dislocation.

Cranialisation of the labrum is accomplished using the hold-suture. Then, refixation of the capsulo-labral complex in lasso-loop technique is performed. Also the second suture end is stitched through and behind the labrum, so the knot comes to lie away from the joint. This suture end represents the drawstring. Seven singular knots are made.

Then, the clamp is switched and with the birdpeak (or a suture lasso) the second suture end is pulled anteriorly through the labrum and outside of the joint through the antero-inferior working cannula.

Now, the hold-suture can be removed as it is no longer needed after tying of the first antero-inferior suture anchor.

Slightly further cranial, labral refixation is undertaken in the same way with the second anchor. A further hold-suture is not needed after the first anchor is sutured.

In most cases, an additional third anchor is necessary further cranial for secure labral refixation using the same technique. Enough distance has to be kept from the long head biceps tendon origin not to compromise this tendon mobility.

Final examination of labrum stability with a hook probe and careful clinical verification of joint stability.

Removal of instruments, skin disinfection, closure of the arthroscopic portals via interrupted single Donati backstitches, and sterile wound dressing as well as immobilization with a sling.

2.2.1 Tips and tricks

For improved arthroscopic evaluation of potential glenoid bone loss and subluxation of the humeral head, we recommend arthroscopic view via the anterior superior portal.

Only if the second suture end is also positioned behind the labrum, the knot will come to lie away from the joint surface.

Pulling on the one suture end without the loop reattaches the capsulo-labral ligament complex to the glenoid. Strain to the other suture end – the one creating the loop – would pull the tissue away from the glenoid. Therefore, the singular stitched suture end has to be the drawstring while tying the knot.

When using the lasso-loop technique, only one of the anchor dependent suture ends can slide through the tissue. Therefore, no arthroscopic slip knots can be made. Seven half hitches come into use. Alternating half hitches lead to a secure blocking of the knot.

2.3 Postoperative treatment

Postoperatively, physical therapy out of a sling or Gilchrist bandage for four to six weeks with external rotation limited to 20° is applicated. Clinical follow up with the surgeon at six weeks postoperatively is recommended for clinical control. Then, careful unlimited motion is allowed. No forced external rotation should be performed for further six weeks. Training of the active and dynamic stabilizers of the shoulder girdle is important. Throwing and contact sports can be taken up again at the earliest six months postoperatively, if power and coordination are fully restored [18–22].

3. Results

For one year, we followed up our operatively treated patients using the described technique after antero-inferior shoulder dislocation with damage to the glenoid labrum. We identified all 30 consecutive patients (3 females, 27 males), who had been treated for shoulder dislocation with anterior-inferior damage to the glenoid labrum by arthroscopic refixation of the anterior capsulolabral complex with suture anchors in lasso-loop technique. Patients with relevant anterior-inferior bone loss or Bankart fracture >15% of the glenoid joint surface received either bony augmentation or osteosynthesis and were not part of the patient cohort used for this analysis.

Five patients were either not available or not prepared to take part in the follow-up examination. 25 of 30 patients could be followed up. One patient had to be excluded for a recent ipsilateral elbow fracture dislocation. In this case, no shoulder re-dislocation occurred. In total, we followed up three female and 21 male patients completely. The mean age was 27.8 years (17–49 years). The average follow-up took place 30.4 months (25–36 months) postoperatively.

In 96% of all cases, there was an excellent subjective and objective outcome. The average Rowe Score was 96.3 points (80–100 points; SD = 3.9). The mean QuickDash was 2.8 points (0–14 points, SD = 3.9). The Constant Score had an average of 93.7 points (65–100 points, SD = 8.8). The average pain level on the numeric analogue pain scale (NAS 0–10) was very low with reported 0.4 points (0-3 points, SD = 1.0). The average passive and active range of motion of the operated glenohumeral joint was Ext/Flex 30/0/170°, Abd/Add 70/0/20°, and Ero/Iro 60/0/95°. There was no restriction of movement greater than 10° compared to the other side. No significant difference in passive or active range of motion in comparison to the healthy side could be seen. The rotator cuff tests were negative. The anterior apprehension sign was negative in all cases; in one case accompanied by slight pain. Apart from one traumatic re-dislocation during handball there were no further complications.

4. Discussion

An anatomic reconstruction of the capsulo-labral complex is one of the advantages of the described surgical technique. It is possible to address SLAP lesions (Superior labrum anterior to posterior) and rotator cuff tears at the same time. The subscapular muscle or its insertion are not compromised as in an open surgical procedure. Compared to other arthroscopic techniques, the procedure presented here leads to an accentuated labral bump and enables secure knot-tying with positioning of the knot away from the articular cartilage while avoiding the suture cutting through the tissue.

As shown, the arthroscopic Bankart repair using the lasso-loop stitch leads to very good results, which are comparable to other studies of arthroscopic shoulder stabilization with good clinical outcomes [16–18]. Possible disadvantages of the lasso-loop stitch compared to arthroscopic single interrupted or mattress sutures are a relatively demanding and slightly more time-consuming technique, and not being able to use slip knots. Iatrogenic cartilage damage, misplacement of anchors, or lesions to the axillary nerve can occur intraoperatively; the latter when too much tissue is taken while performing a capsular shift in the anterior inferior recessus.

Malcompliance by the patient with risk to the healing process of the anterior capsulo-labral complex with strong tensile forces during external rotation require extensive patient consent and education. In the event of re-dislocation, a detailed investigation of causes in the patient history and further diagnostics including MRI should be performed before possibly attempting revision surgery [23, 24]. Postoperative infection requires arthroscopic irrigation and systemic antibiotics, beginning with Ampicillin/Sulbactam and possibly changing to the antibiogram.

If a bony Bankart fragment is big enough to allow screw fixation, this should be undertaken either openly or arthroscopically. If the labrum remains partially unstable, a further labrum reconstruction following screw fixation may be necessary [25].

The arthroscopic refixation of the capsulo-labral complex with suture anchors using the lasso-loop stitch is slightly more elaborate due to the suturing technique than single interrupted sutures or mattress sutures. But this technique leads to a stronger bulging of the glenoid labrum and might therefore increase the physiological bumper effect of the labrum. At the same time, the knot can be positioned away from the joint to avoid irritation without cutting through the tissue like it is possible with mattress sutures for glenoid labrum refixation [26]. For further clarification of possible advantages and disadvantages of this technical modification, prospective studies comparing the described procedure with other stitching techniques are recommended.

5. Conclusions

The lasso-loop stitch in arthroscopic Bankart repair is useful and safe. It leads to an accentuated labral bump and enables secure knot-tying with positioning of the knot away from the articular cartilage while avoiding the suture cutting through the tissue.

Conflict of interest

The authors declare that they have no Conflict of Interest.

Abbreviations and definitions

ACJ	Acromio-clavicular joint
ALPSA	Anterior Labroligamentous Periosteal Sleeve Avulsion
Bankart	A Bankart lesion is a tear of the labrum-capsule-ligament complex from the glenoid
GLAD	Glenoid-Labral Articular Disruption
HAGL	Humeral Avulsion of the Glenohumeral Ligament
MRI	Magnetic Resonance Imaging
PDS	Polydioxanone (Suture)
Perthes	The Perthes lesion is a soft-tissue decollement at the scapular neck (no tissue rupture) leading to a pouch of the joint capsule
SLAP	Superior Labrum Anterior to Posterior

Author details

Christian Konrads* and Stefan Döbele
Department of Trauma, Reconstructive Surgery, Sports Medicine and Arthroscopy, BG Klinik, University of Tübingen, Tübingen, Germany

*Address all correspondence to: christian.konrads@gmail.com

References

[1] Aboalata M, Plath JE, Seppel G, Juretzko J, Vogt S, Imhoff AB, et al. Results of arthroscopic Bankart repair of anterior-inferior shoulder instability at 13-year follow- up. Am J Sports Med. 2017;45:782-787.

[2] Martetschläger F, Imhoff AB. Shoulder dislocation in athletes: current therapy con- cepts. Orthopade. 2014;43:236-243.

[3] Minkus M, Böhm E, Moroder P, Scheibel M. Initial management of traumatic ventral shoulder dislocation. Unfallchirurg. 2018;121:100-107.

[4] Martetschläger F, Tauber M, Habermeyer P. Diagnostics and treatment concepts for anteroinferior shoulder instability: current trends. Orthopade. 2017;46(October (10)):877-892.

[5] Balke M, Shafizadeh S, Bouillon B, et al. Management of shoulder instability: the current state of treatment among German orthopaedic surgeons. Arch Orthop Trauma Surg. 2016;136: 1717-1721.

[6] Lafosse L, Van Raebroeckx A, Brzoska R. A new technique to improve tissue grip: "the lasso-loop stitch. Arthroscopy. 2006;22(1246):e1-3.

[7] Toussaint B, Schnaser E, Lafosse L, Bahurel J, Gobezie R, et al. A new approach to improving the tissue grip of the medial-row repair in the suture-bridge technique: the "modified lasso-loop stitch". Artrhoscopy. 2009;25: 691-695.

[8] Ponce BA, Hosemann CD, Raghava P, Tate JP, Eberhardt AW, Lafosse L, et al. Biomechanical evaluation of 3 arthroscopic self-cinching stitches for shoulder ar- throscopy: the lasso-loop, lasso-mattress, and double-cinch stitches. Am J Sports Med. 2011;39:188-194.

[9] Lafosse L, Meller R. Arthroskopische stabilisierung bei vorderer schulterinstabilität. In: Agneskirchner JD, Lafosse L, Lobenhoffer P, eds. Arthroskopische schulterchirurgie. Cologne: deutscher Ärzte-Verlag; 2013; 2013.

[10] Parnes N, Blevins M, Morman M, Carey P. The oblique mattress lasso-loop stitch for arthroscopic capsulolabral repair. Arthrosc Tech. 2016;5:e959-963.

[11] Mahure SA, Mollon B, Capogna BM, Zuckerman JD, Kwon YQ, Rokito AS. Risk factors for recurrent instability or revision surgery following arthroscopic Bankart repair. Bone Jt J. 2018;100-B:324-330.

[12] Porter DA, Birns M, Hobart SJ, Kowalsky M, Galano GJ. Arthroscopic treatment of osseous instability of the shoulder. HSS J. 2017;13:292-301.

[13] Cartucho A, Moura N, Sarmento M. Evaluation and management of failed shoulder instability surgery. Open Orthop J. 2017;11:897-908.

[14] Fritz EM, Pogorzelski J, Hussain ZB, Godin JA, Millett PJ. Arthroscopic repair of humeral avulsion oft he glenohumeral ligament lesion. Arthrosc Tech. 2017;6:e1195-1200.

[15] Hawkins RJ, Bokor DJ. Clinical evaluation of shoulder problems. In: Rockwood CA, JrMatsen FA, IIIeds. The shoulder. Philadelphia: Saunders; 1998.

[16] Ng DZ, Kumar VP. Arthroscopic bankart repair using knot-tying versus knotless suture anchors: is there a difference? Arthroscopy. 2014;30: 422-427.

[17] Ockert B, Biermann N, Nebelung W, Wiedemann E. Arthroscopic soft tissue stabili- zation of posttraumatic anterior shoulder instability: techniques,

limitations and long-term results. Unfallchirurg. 2018;121:108-116.

[18] Boughebri O, Maqdes A, Moraiti C, Dib C, Leclère FM, Valenti P. Results of 45 arthroscopic bankart procedures: does the ISIS remain a reliable prognostic assessment after 5 years? Eur J Orthop Surg Traumatol. 2015;25: 709-716.

[19] Ma R, Brimmo OA, Li X, Colbert L. Current concepts in rehabilitation for traumatic anterior shoulder instability. Curr Rev Musculoskelet Med. 2017;10:499-506.

[20] DeFroda SF, Mehta N, Owens BD. Physical therapy protocols for arthroscopic Bankart repair. Sports Health. 2018;10:250-258.

[21] Kim K, Saper MG. Postoperative management following arthroscopic Bankart repair in adolescents and young adults: a systematic review. Arthrosc Sports Med Rehabil. 2020;2:e839-e845.

[22] Wilson KW, Popchak A, Li RT, Kane G, Lin A. Return to sport testing at 6 months after arthroscopic shoulder stabilization reveals residual strength and functional deficits. J Shoulder Elbow Surg. 2020;29:S107-S114.

[23] Lacheta L, Siebenlist S, Imhoff AB, Willinger L. Recurrent instability and instability arthropathy. Unfallchirurg. 2018;121:142-151.

[24] Waterman BR, Leroux T, Frank RM, Romeo AA. The evaluation and management of the failed primary arthroscopic Bankart repair. J Am Acad Orthop Surg. 2020;28:607-616.

[25] Nolte PC, Elrick BP, Bernholt DL, Lacheta L, Millett PJ. The bony Bankart: clinical and technical considerations. Sports Med Arthrosc Rev. 2020;28: 146-152.

[26] Konrads C, Jovic S, Rueckl K, Fenwick A, Barthel T, Rudert M, Plumhoff P. Surgical technique and clinical outcome of arthroscopic shoulder stabilization via suture anchors using the lasso-loop stitch. 2018;15:553-557.

CPSIA information can be obtained
at www.ICGtesting.com
Printed in the USA
LVHW060127060422
715457LV00007B/275